Schizophrenia and Psychoses in Later Life

New Perspectives on Treatment, Research, and Policy

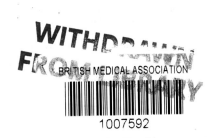

"Professors Cohen and Meesters have provided a timely, comprehensive, and scholarly review of the state of the science in late life psychotic disorders. This volume bridges epidemiology, diagnostic, treatment, health systems, and health policy issues. It accords special emphasis to the voices of those living with these disorders. The roster of contributors to this volume—scientists, clinicians, health services researchers, policy experts, and consumers—is greatly to be admired. It doesn't get any better than this."

Charles F. Reynolds III MD
Distinguished Professor of Psychiatry and UPMC Endowed Professor in Geriatric Psychiatry emeritus, University of Pittsburgh School of Medicine
Editor-in-Chief, American Journal of Geriatric Psychiatry

Despite the recent focus on schizophrenia that has nearly exclusively targeted the prodrome and early psychosis and despite the unfortunate fact people with schizophrenia have extensively shortened life expectancies, there are lots of older people with schizophrenia and this number will only keep rising. This book does it all: it covers all aspects of functioning, treatment, medical concerns, and policy. It is the definitive current reference on schizophrenia and aging and is required reading for anyone interested in schizophrenia, aging, or both.

Philip D. Harvey, PhD Leonard M. Miller Professor of Psychiatry and Behavioral Sciences

Within Schizophrenia and Psychoses in Later Life, an international panel of distinguished authors comprehensively review the scientific literature, current best practice recommendations and outstanding research questions. Through concise and well-written chapters, features of the most important diagnoses are described, together with interventions and strategies for management. Many of the authors express justified optimism that successful aging for older adults with schizophrenia is possible and the evidence-based ingredients for achieving this are detailed. This brilliant book stands as a definitive and practical state of the art resource for clinicians, researchers and those who plan and commission services for this patient population.

Robert Howard, Professor of Old Age Psychiatry, University College London.

The number of older people living with psychotic illnesses is increasing and it is straining available resources. This outstanding volume provides both a sobering and an optimistic view of the challenges in assisting these individuals. On the one hand, this is a diverse population with a broad range of medical and psychiatric problems; on the other hand, new paradigms are available for meeting the needs of these patients and improving health and functioning. Many older age people with schizophrenia view themselves as having opportunities for enhancing the quality of their lives. Contributions by leading authorities span epidemiology, social needs, pharmacologic and psychosocial treatment. It is essential reading for clinicians and researchers with an interest in this population, especially psychiatrists, psychologists, nurses, and therapists.

Stephen R Marder, M.D.
Daniel X. Freedman Professor of Psychiatry

As attention increasingly shifts to early intervention and prevention in both research and treatment of psychosis, this volume provides welcome attention to those at the other end of the spectrum. Cohen and Meesters have marshalled researchers, practitioners and those with lived experience to address the full range of issues that confront us in these patients. The international perspective that animates many of the contributions insures that the volume will be of value to a wide range of readers, including policy makers who can influence provision of services and the future well-being of this underserved population.

Nina R. Schooler, PhD.
Professor of Psychiatry & Behavioral Sciences
SUNY Downstate Medical Center
Brooklyn NY USA

"This book is an important achievement in the field of geriatric psychiatry, integrating new insights from both aging perspectives and recent schizophrenia research in later life. The composition of the chapters have been particularly well chosen with clear sections covering all relevant topics for both clinicians and other disciplines working with geriatric and psychiatric patients in different care settings. For this book the editors, from the USA and Europe, have succeeded in engaging a long list of specialists within the field of psychosis in later life offering the reader a well balanced view on new approaches of this topic e.g. a more dynamic view on outcome in late life psychosis and applying the recovery approach when treating these patients. This book offers a comprehensive view on all topics important for researchers and health workers in the field."

Max Stek, professor in old age psychiatry, UMC Amsterdam/GGZinGeest.

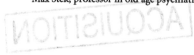

Schizophrenia and Psychoses in Later Life

New Perspectives on Treatment, Research, and Policy

Edited by

Carl I. Cohen
SUNY Downstate Medical Center

Paul D. Meesters
Friesland Mental Health Services

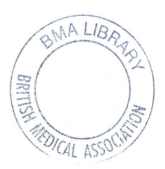

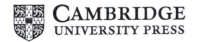

CAMBRIDGE
UNIVERSITY PRESS

CAMBRIDGE
UNIVERSITY PRESS

University Printing House, Cambridge CB2 8BS, United Kingdom

One Liberty Plaza, 20th Floor, New York, NY 10006, USA

477 Williamstown Road, Port Melbourne, VIC 3207, Australia

314–321, 3rd Floor, Plot 3, Splendor Forum, Jasola District Centre, New Delhi – 110025, India

79 Anson Road, #06-04/06, Singapore 079906

Cambridge University Press is part of the University of Cambridge.

It furthers the University's mission by disseminating knowledge in the pursuit of education, learning, and research at the highest international levels of excellence.

www.cambridge.org
Information on this title: www.cambridge.org/9781108727778
DOI: 10.1017/9781108539593

First published 2019

Printed and bound in Great Britain by Clays Ltd, Elcograf S.p.A.

A catalogue record for this publication is available from the British Library.

ISBN 978-1-108-72777-8 Paperback

Contents

Contributors

Hila Avieli, Ph.D.
Ariel University
Ariel, Israel

Tova Band-Winterstein, Ph.D.
University of Haifa,
Haifa, Israel

Stephen J. Bartels, M.D., M.S.
Department of Psychiatry, Geisel
School of Medicine at Dartmouth,
The Dartmouth Institute for Health Policy
and Clinical Practice, and Dartmouth
Centers for Health and Aging, NH, USA

Michael B. Centorino, M.D.
James A. Haley Veterans Hospital
Mental Health and Behavioral Science and
University of South Florida, Tampa, FL,
USA

Carl I. Cohen, M.D.
Division of Geriatric Psychiatry, SUNY
Downstate Medical Center, NY, USA

Alisa Coleman, M.D.
St John's Episcopal Hospital,
NY, USA

Frank Copeli
Harvard South Shore,
Brockton, MA, USA

Peter R. DiMilia, M.P.H.
The Dartmouth Institute for Health
Policy and Clinical Practice and
Dartmouth Centers for Health and
Aging, NH, USA

Graham Eglit, Ph.D.
Department of Psychiatry and Sam
and Rose Stein Institute for Research
on Aging, University of California, CA,
USA

Michael B. Friedman, M.S.W.
School of Social Work, Columbia
University and Geriatric Mental Health
Alliance, NY, USA

Lisa Furst, M.S.W., M.P.H.
Vibrant Emotional Health and Geriatric
Mental Health Alliance, NY, USA

Brian R. Ghezelaiagh, M.D.
Department of Psychiatry,
SUNY at Stony Brook, USA

Dina Ghoneim, M.D.
SUNY Downstate Medical Center
Brooklyn, NY, USA

Deborah Gustafson, Ph.D.
Department of Neurology, SUNY
Downstate Medical Center, NY, USA

Dilip V. Jeste, M.D.
Department of Psychiatry, Sam
and Rose Stein Institute for Research
on Aging, and Department of Neurosciences,
University of California, CA, USA

Rujvi Kamat, Ph.D.
Department of Psychiatry, University
of California, San Diego, CA, USA

John Kasckow, M.D., Ph.D.
Deputy Director of Psychiatry
Perry Point VA Medical Center
Maryland VA Health Care System
Perry Point, MD 21902
and
University of Pittsburgh Physicians
3471 Fifth Ave
Pittsburgh, PA 15213

Harriet P. Lefley, Ph.D.
University of Miami,
Miami, FL, USA

Heather Leutwyler, R.N., Ph.D., N.P.
Department of Physiological Nursing,
University of California, San Francisco,
CA, USA

Subramoniam Madhusoodanan, M.D.
St John's Episcopal Hospital
and S.U.N.Y. Health Science Center at
Brooklyn, NY, USA

Donna McAlpine, Ph.D.
Division of Health Policy and
Management, School of Public Health,
University of Minnesota, MN, USA

Ellen McCreedy, Ph.D.
Center for Gerontology and Healthcare
Research, Brown University, School of
Public Health, RI, USA

Paul D. Meesters, M.D.
Department of Research and Education,
Friesland Mental Health Services,
Leeuwarden, the Netherlands

Shifra Mincer
SUNY Downstate Medical Center
Brooklyn, NY, USA

Samir T. Mukherjee, M.D.
Center for Occupational and
Environmental Health, University of
California, Irvine, CA, USA

Tessa Murante, D.O.
Weill Cornell Medicine/New York
Presbyterian Westchester Division
White Plains, NY, USA

Peli Mushkin, M.S.W.
University of Haifa,
Haifa, Israel

Eric Nelson
SUNY Downstate Medical Center
Brooklyn, NY, USA

Paul S. Nestadt, M.D.
Department of Psychiatry and Behavioral
Sciences, Johns Hopkins School of Medicine,
Department of Mental Health Johns Hopkins
Bloomberg School of Public Health, USA

Barton W. Palmer, Ph.D.
Department of Psychiatry, Sam and Rose
Stein Institute for Research on Aging,
University of California, and Veterans Affairs
San Diego Healthcare System, CA, USA

Tarek K. Rajji, M.D., F.R.C.P.C.
Geriatric and Adult Neurodevelopmental
Psychiatry Division, Centre for Addiction
and Mental Health, and Department of
Psychiatry, University of Toronto, Canada

Michael Reinhardt, M.D.
Geriatric Psychiatry Fellowship Program
and the Center of Excellence for
Alzheimer's Disease at SUNY Downstate
Medical Center, Brooklyn, NY, USA

Lina Rodriguez, M.S.W.
Legal Advocates for Children and Youth:
A Program of The Law Foundation of
Silicon Valley, USA

Susan K. Schultz, M.D.
James A. Haley Veterans Hospital
Mental Health and Behavioral Science and
University of South Florida, Tampa, FL,
USA

Robert Sigström, M.D., Ph.D.
Department of Psychiatry and
Neurochemistry, Institute of Neuroscience
and Physiology, University of Gothenburg,
Sweden

Paulina Vargas
SUNY Downstate Medical Center
Brooklyn, NY, USA

Aninditha Vengassery, M.D.
SUNY Downstate Medical Center
Brooklyn, NY, USA

Kimberly A. Williams, M.S.W.
Vibrant Emotional Health,
Geriatric Mental Health Alliance, and
National Coalition on Mental Health and
Aging, NY, USA

Preface

There is a looming crisis in the care of older adults with schizophrenia. During the first quarter of the twenty-first century, the number of older adults (defined as age 55 and over) with schizophrenia is expected to double in the United States and Europe. By 2025, in the United States, older adults will comprise one-fourth of the population with schizophrenia. Worldwide, the number of people aged 60 years and older with schizophrenia will double by 2050 and will reach about 10 million people. This growth will place enormous strains on a care system that has been structured to treat younger people. This prediction is especially ominous in developing countries because of the pronounced changes occurring in traditional social structures in the wake of increased urbanization and industrialization, and the resultant isolation or even abandonment faced by elderly persons.

There have been no recent books that have addressed the gaps in research, policy, and treatment with this population. A seminal publication by Nancy Miller and Gene Cohen, *Schizophrenia and Aging*, appeared in 1987. In 2003, one of the editors of this volume (Carl Cohen) published *Schizophrenia into Later Life* that largely updated the findings of the 1987 book and included more information on clinical care and policy. Two subsequent books, *Schizophrenia in Late Life: Aging Effects on Symptoms and Course of Illness* by Phillip Harvey, published in 2004, and *Psychoses in the Elderly* by Anne M. Hassett, David Ames, and Edmond Chiu, published in 2005, covered many of the same topics as the Cohen book. Thus, it has been more than a decade since the last book on this topic was published.

There has been an increase in new research about older adults with schizophrenia

Notably, over the past decade there has been an appreciable expansion in the quantity and quality of research papers on the course, associated risk factors, and treatment of older adults with schizophrenia. For example, there have been a range of studies in the United States and Europe on remission, recovery, depression, negative symptoms, quality of life, community integration, successful aging, cognitive functioning, adaptive functioning, coping strategies, and physical health. Novel treatment strategies have been fashioned, such as cognitive remediation therapy, social skills training, cognitive behavioral treatment, and self-management techniques along with various model programs such as collaborative care and case management strategies. Moreover, in recent years, longitudinal data have emerged that provide important insights into the course of symptoms and long-term outcomes. Importantly, the longitudinal data have challenged prevailing beliefs about late adulthood being a "state of quiescence" for individuals with schizophrenia.

There is a growing interest in other psychoses occurring among older adults

There is increased interest in the diagnosis and management of other psychotic illnesses in older adults. Psychosis is one of the most common experiences in later life, with a lifetime risk of 23%. Among persons aged 55 and over, the prevalence rate of psychoses is 3%, and this rate rises considerably with age. Psychoses can be either primary (caused by a psychiatric disorder) or secondary (due to a medical or neurological disorder). About three-fifths of psychotic disorders in later life are secondary conditions. Elderly patients with late-life-onset psychosis require careful evaluation. There are no reliable pathognomonic signs to distinguish primary from secondary psychosis. Moreover, symptoms thought to indicate a primary disorder may reveal themselves over time to be due to a secondary disorder. Although this book focuses primarily on schizophrenia, we have added material on psychoses in later life in recognition of the need to pay greater attention to its diagnosis and treatment.

A new paradigm of schizophrenia in later life is emerging

Much of the work in this volume will incorporate results of studies conducted with community-dwelling middle-aged and older adults with schizophrenia by research groups in North America and Europe. These studies have provided important data about symptom outcomes (e.g., positive symptoms, cognition) as well as global outcomes (e.g., remission, recovery). As they have generally included age-matched community comparison groups, readers are able to assess the relative performance of the older adult with schizophrenia. Notably, investigators have found a wide range of favorable outcomes. Moreover, many of the individual and global outcome measures are associated with a variety of potentially ameliorable social and clinical variables.

Taken together, recent studies support the emergence of a new paradigm that conceptualizes the outcome of schizophrenia in later life as a more dynamic process comprising diverse, predominantly non-overlapping indicators. *This paradigmatic shift has implications with respect to how we conceptualize research, policy, and clinical care for this aging population.* The scaffolding for this book will be this new paradigm that is emerging with respect to schizophrenia in later life. The paradigm includes several elements that will be elaborated in this volume:

1. A more nuanced approach to outcome has emerged based on symptoms (e.g., positive and negative symptoms, depression, cognitive functioning) and global parameters (e.g., remission, recovery, community integration, successful aging) that are only weakly associated with each other.
2. Diagnostic assessment is much more complex in later life and sharp demarcations of disorders may not be obtained.
3. In general, outcomes for most measures are more favorable than had been believed during much of the twentieth century, although long-term remission appears to be more modest and there are many possible trajectories.
4. Schizophrenia in later life is not a state of quiescence with little change in symptoms or outcome.
5. Course and outcome of schizophrenia in later life can well be viewed within the psychiatry recovery model and the life course perspective of gerontology.
6. Treatment requires a combination of comprehensive pharmacological and innovative psychosocial approaches that address the various outcome dimensions. Given the variety of outcomes, an individualized approach to care is essential.

The book will provide guidelines for clinical care, research, and policy that are consistent with these emerging paradigmatic changes occurring with respect to schizophrenia in later life. A particular strength of this volume has been to merge various perspectives about aging and schizophrenia. Many authors have backgrounds in aging as well as other disciplines, e.g., biological psychiatry, social psychiatry, sociology, anthropology, social work, psychology, neuropsychology. Clinicians, researchers, service providers, and policy makers are among the target audiences for this book that provides in-depth information on demographic and clinical characteristics of older persons with schizophrenia, treatment approaches, research strategies, and economic and health policy issues.

Finally, the book should also be of value to patients and their relatives. In this respect, we quote Mary V. Seeman, psychiatrist and Professor Emerita at the University of Toronto. In 2005, at age 70, in a paper titled *Parallels Between Aging and Schizophrenia* she offered some highly personal insight: "As I grow old and struggle to cope with the infirmities of age, I marvel at the resilience of my patients who grapple with and overcome the indignities of schizophrenia. Schizophrenia research is mainly about the deficits, about the many difficulties patients face. It rarely celebrates the accomplishments of patients, their ability, on the whole, to accommodate and adapt to the constraints of their illness." Clearly, patients do not have a choice on whether or not to deal with their schizophrenia, but clinicians and society as a whole certainly do. Clinicians should overcome their prejudices about older schizophrenia patients, who still too often are merely seen as "lost cases." Society may actively seek ways to counteract the double stigma that is attached to being old and having a severe mental illness. Doing so will benefit not only patients, but society itself.

Acknowledgments

We express heartfelt thanks to the late Richard Marley who persisted in encouraging us to develop this book. He was unwaveringly kind and supportive. He will be missed. We also thank the rest of the Cambridge staff who helped guide this book through production: Catherine Barnes, who picked up Richard's baton, Noah Tate, Jessica Papworth, Susan Skakel, and Jo Tyszka. Carl Cohen thanks SUNY Downstate Medical Center and his Chair in the Department of Psychiatry, Dr. Ayman Fanous, for providing resources and assistance, Barbara Singh for administrative assistance, and the National Institute of Health that provided funding over his career for studies of mental illness in later life. Most importantly, thanks to his family – his wife Kate, his children Sara and Zack, and grandchildren Melanie, Libby, and Max – for just being there. Paul David Meesters thanks his colleagues Willeke van der Plas, Paul Mutsaers, Lex Wunderink, Ton Dhondt, and Adriaan Jansen at GGZ Friesland (Leeuwarden, the Netherlands), for facilitating his studies of schizophrenia in later life. Last, but not least, thanks to his wife Maaike, his sons Michaël and Simon, and their partners Katharina and Kristien for their unconditional love and encouragement.

Finally, we thank those who generously participated in our research studies and the patients who taught us so much.

Acknowledgments

Chapter

1

Epidemiology of Psychotic Disorders: Methodological Issues and Empirical Findings

Robert Sigström, M.D. Ph.D. and
Deborah Gustafson, Ph.D.

Introduction

This chapter will begin with a discussion of several general topics regarding the study of psychiatric symptoms and disorders in older adults that are relevant to the research findings presented throughout this volume. This discussion will be followed by a review of the empirical findings on the epidemiology of psychotic disorders in older adults.

Epidemiology

The field of epidemiology includes studies of disease burden (as measured by prevalence and incidence), as well as studies of risk factors for diseases, their course and their consequences. Apart from being a way of understanding the etiology of disease, epidemiology is also of use in service planning and guidance of clinicians (for example in raising awareness of a disease that is common in a particular segment of the population). Since global and regional variations in living conditions influence exposures during the life-span, epidemiological studies of a particular disease may yield different results across societies over space and time. Thus, epidemiological studies must be conducted in different types of societies and conducted repeatedly to discover secular trends in the prevalence and incidence of diseases, their risk factors and their prognosis [1]. Epidemiological studies may utilize different data sources and different methods in this pursuit. Most epidemiological studies are observational, i.e., studied at the population or group level rather than the individual level, and without intervention. The observational epidemiology study designs commonly used in psychiatry are:

- *Longitudinal "cohort" studies*: one or more samples or "cohorts" are followed prospectively over time with respect to an outcome and associated risk factors.
- *"Case–control" studies*: retrospective examinations that compare patients or "cases" that have a disease or outcome of interest with patients who do not have the disease or outcome (controls) on various risk factors.
- *Cross-sectional studies*: examine data at one point in time. Cross-sectional studies can be distinguished from case–control studies in that they provide data on the entire population under study, whereas case–control studies usually focus on only people with a specific disease or disorder and compare them with those without the disease or disorder.

Case–control studies are more often used in psychiatric epidemiology because they are less expensive and time-consuming than prospective studies. For example, one frequently employed approach is to select a sample of the population in a catchment area and to define cases of a disorder on the basis of information gathered by interviews with participants or self-report questionnaires. Another approach is to utilize health care registers and/or hospital records to identify cases of a disorder within a catchment area; remaining inhabitants of the catchment area are assumed not to have the disorder. The strengths and weaknesses of these different designs will be reviewed with respect to the study of late-life psychosis.

General considerations when evaluating the observational epidemiological literature on psychoses

It is important to consider several general issues in evaluating the observational epidemiologic literature prior to a more specific discussion of psychotic disorders:

1. It is essential to define clinical outcome. As described in the next section, this is not a straightforward task with respect to psychosis. Consistently operationalized methods for defining symptoms and functioning, and making diagnoses across studies, are lacking in epidemiologic studies of psychosis. Comparison and replication of studies are, as a result, limited. However, when similar associations are observed despite differences in diagnostic criteria and/or operationalizing these criteria, this may denote a more robust association.

2. Overlap of psychiatric symptoms among disorders is known. For example, underlying dementia neuropathologies may induce psychotic symptoms, thereby confusing the diagnosis.

3. Socioethnodemographic characteristics of global populations at risk are important. Adequate descriptions of study samples are imperative for proper interpretation of the data, planning follow-up measures and ancillary studies, and identifying areas of intervention and ultimately prevention.

4. Age of exposure and age at which outcomes occur are critical in psychiatric epidemiology. Psychiatric outcomes have early-, mid- and later-life onsets and characteristics. Risk associations may differ depending on when an exposure is measured and when the outcome is manifest.

5. The timing of association between exposure and outcome is critical due to the influence of underlying neuropathological changes on physiological "exposures," as well as manifestation of intermediate and clinical phenotypes. For example, in the epidemiology of dementia, when measured in mid-life, body weight, blood pressure and blood cholesterol levels have been associated with increased late-onset dementia risk; however, when measured in late-life, they may not be risk factors, and are sometimes protective.

6. Duration of exposures may convey information regarding "load." Individual differences in susceptibility and length of exposure to stressors are linked to behavioral responses to environmental challenges that are coupled to physiologic and pathophysiologic responses.

7. Survival time of the population being studied is important in evaluating the population at risk for later-life psychiatric outcomes. Psychiatric outcomes in older ages are observed among survivors, i.e., those who have lived to old age.

8. Birth cohort is a primary consideration regarding the role of exposures, as well as outcome characteristics, not only based on neurodevelopmental hypotheses, but secular trends in exposures, such as diet and air pollution. In addition, birth cohort reflects rapid technological changes, as well as advancement of pharmacologic interventions for psychiatric disorders and comorbid conditions.

9. It is imperative to take note of the study design and the analysis strategy used to arrive at the conclusions of any research study. Longitudinal studies with comprehensive follow-up, adequate assessment of exposures and definitive outcomes data, including mortality, are the only ones whereby "true" risk can be calculated. Other study designs, e.g., case–control studies, provide provisional data on estimation of risks and correlations.

10. Competing risks are and will continue increasing in their importance with aging of the global population. Competing risk generally refers to the presence of multimorbidities, which increase with age, making it more difficult to identify the etiologic exposure or indicator.

11. The increasing availability of genetic or other biomarkers such as those provided by neuroimaging or fluid-based biomarkers will allow for novel approaches to risk stratification as well as refinement of both exposures and outcomes.

These points are summarized in Table 1.1.

Defining psychosis in epidemiological studies

It is fair to say that the epidemiology of late-life psychosis has been considerably less extensively studied than that of, for example, late-life depression. This may partly be explained by a long-prevailing lack of consensus on nomenclature and research diagnostic criteria for late-life psychosis [2]. Another explanation is that the study of psychosis is considered to present greater methodological challenges than the study of depression.

Measurement versus evaluation

Psychiatry is a "hybrid science" aiming at both explanation and interpretation. These aims have been in dialectic tension throughout its history [3,4]. Explanatory, quantitative

Table 1.1 General considerations when evaluating the observational epidemiological literature on psychoses

- Outcome definitions and measurements
- Overlapping symptoms across various psychiatric outcomes
- Age of exposure or onset of outcome
- Timing of exposure in relation to outcome, e.g., mid-life versus late-life exposure
- Exposure level ("load")
- Duration and persistence of exposure
- Survival factors
- Birth cohort
- Study design and analysis strategy
- Competing risks
- Biomarkers

research strives for objectivity by using methods of the natural sciences. However, psychiatric research is always dependent on interpretation of subjective experience, because psychiatric symptoms and signs are not objects ("things") that can be measured in the sense that, for example, blood levels of glucose are measured [5]. From this should follow that all data collection, whether it be via interviews or questionnaires, in routine health care or research contexts, includes evaluation or some kind of judgment, on the part of both the study participant and the interviewer [6–8].

Gathering information on psychotic symptoms

The problem of objectifying and quantifying subjective experiences is a problem of validity, i.e., whether a scientific method captures something that is relevant to the matter in question and is in concordance with reality [9]. A review of methods used in epidemiological studies of late-life psychosis suggests that assumptions about valid methods in the study of psychosis differ from the assumptions behind epidemiological studies of, for example, mood and anxiety disorders. Most of the epidemiological studies of psychosis rely on information gathered and/or reviewed by clinical experts. Thus, detection and evaluation of psychotic symptoms is considered to require the clinical skill to evaluate a person's beliefs and perceptions. This assumption does not seem to be made in most epidemiological studies of late-life depression, which often utilize structured interviews conducted by trained laypersons or even self-report symptom scales.

The basis of this methodological assumption may be as follows. Loss of contact with reality, or "lack of insight," is considered to be one important quality of psychosis. Thus, contrary to most individuals with depression or anxiety, most individuals with psychosis do not evaluate their beliefs and experiences as psychiatric symptoms per se. A question about whether they "have delusions or hallucinations" will obviously lead to "false negative" cases[1] [10]. To acquire valid information, questions about psychotic symptoms must be indirect, and there must be room for clarifying questions. This reduces the face validity of questions regarding psychotic symptoms, meaning that their intention should not be understood by study participants. However, beliefs and experiences similar to psychotic symptoms (such as beliefs in telepathic communication) are not uncommon in the population [11,12]. A poor conception of what kind of experiences are sought, either by the interviewer or by the interviewed, results in a rate of "false positive" cases that outnumbers the "true positives" [10,13–15]. Such psychosis-like experiences may be on a continuum with clinical psychotic disorders, so that research into the former may help to explain the latter [11,16–18]. However, if there are important qualitative differences between these phenomena, the psychosis-like experiences may blur the picture instead [19,20].

For other reasons, qualitative aspects of psychotic symptoms are of special importance in studies of older adults. In this age group, psychotic symptoms may often appear in the context of dementia, delirium, medication usage and/or physical disorders [21]. In fact, such conditions have been found to be the final diagnosis in a significant proportion of older patients presenting with new-onset psychotic symptoms, even in psychiatric settings [22–24]. Hallucinations and delusions due to, for example, medication or physical disorders are not by definition different from hallucinations and delusions due to a psychiatric disorder. An expert judgment of the quality (e.g., modality of hallucinations,

---

[1] These expressions are put between quotation marks since they are made with reference to a non-existent "gold standard" for when the symptoms actually are present. However, the expression is useful for the purposes of this discussion.

delusional content) and context of psychotic symptoms is crucial for studies aiming to report on psychotic symptoms that are primarily due to psychiatric disorders ("primary" psychotic disorders) and to study correlates of such symptoms. It is important to recognize that older persons may have two coexisting causes for psychotic symptoms that may affect their form and content, e.g., physical or neurological disease and schizophrenia.

Individuals with psychotic symptoms may be reluctant to reveal them because of previous negative experiences from doing so [26]. This may be of greater importance for a case finding of delusional disorder and isolated psychotic symptoms than for schizophrenia, since schizophrenia may be more likely to reveal itself by behavioral disturbances or signs of global functional impairment [27]. Thus, cases of psychosis may be missed if studies rely only on interviews with participants. Other important information sources are key informant interviews and medical records [28].

Apart from these problems with the detection of psychosis, individuals with psychosis may be more reluctant than others to participate in epidemiological studies [29]. Since the phenomenon studied is fairly rare, a selection bias involving a small number of individual non-participants can have a high relative impact on, for example, prevalence estimates [30].

Studies based on health care registers

Drawing information from health care registers and/or hospital records avoids the problem of non-participation. Many studies utilizing health care data use registered diagnostic codes to define a case of a disorder, while others add information by reviewing medical records of patients recorded to have a certain diagnosis. Since register studies require limited human resources to establish whether someone fulfills the diagnostic criteria for psychotic disorders or not, it is possible to obtain very large study samples, sometimes including the population of a whole country, which is a major advantage of this design. However, although researchers can expect an expert judgment to be involved in detection and diagnosis of psychosis in routine health care, and that the diagnosis is based on observations collected over an extended time period, they do not have control over the diagnostic process and have to rely on disorders being diagnosed adequately by clinicians within the health care system. Expert review of medical records avoids this problem, but requires more human resources and may limit the size of the catchment area. Another problem is that register studies only capture cases that have been identified by health care services. The magnitude of this bias is unknown, but may be significant, even for schizophrenia. A longitudinal study following a birth cohort with repeated examinations up to age 38 years identified a 2% cumulative incidence of schizophrenia that could be confirmed by pharmacological treatment or hospital records [31]. An additional 1.7% of this cohort formally met the diagnostic criteria for schizophrenia, but had not (yet) been diagnosed by health care services. Cases not (currently) identified by health care services may be less severe, but their identification is of importance for estimating the true disease burden and for studying the true risk factors and consequences of late-life psychosis [32].

Epidemiology of late-life psychosis

Prevalence

The prevalence of psychotic symptoms in older adults has been estimated to be between 1% and 13.4% [28,33–44]. The median prevalence in the included studies is 3%. One review study from Western Europe found increasing prevalence of psychotic symptoms with advancing age, so that rates were under 2% in persons aged 65–74, but 4% and 7% in those aged 85–94 and 95–104, respectively [36].

The prevalence of non-affective psychotic disorders in older adults is reported to be between 0.1% and 4.7%. References are displayed in Table 1.2. The median prevalence of the reviewed studies is 1.2%. The majority of studies find schizophrenia to be the most common disorder. One study reported the prevalence of schizophrenia by age of onset, giving a prevalence of 0.35% for early-onset schizophrenia, 0.14% for late-onset schizophrenia (between the ages of 40 and 59 years) and 0.05% for very-late-onset schizophrenia-like psychosis (VLOSLP, onset at age 60 or older) [45]. Two studies reporting the current prevalence of delusional disorder in older adults found it to be very rare, 0.04% [26] and 0.03% [45]. Others found a life-time prevalence of 0.46% [46] and one study found it to be more common than schizophrenia (2.0%) [47]. The very low prevalence of delusional disorder reported by some studies may be due to underestimations related to methodological factors mentioned above.

Since psychotic disorders most often have an onset before age 40 and the mortality rate in the most common psychotic disorder, schizophrenia, is two to three times higher than in the general population [48], it might be expected that the point prevalence of psychotic disorders declines with age. Only one of the reviewed prevalence studies examined this and suggested schizophrenia to be slightly less common with increasing age among older adults [45]. Because of its rarity, age trends in the prevalence of delusional disorder are difficult to examine.

Incidence

The incidence of psychotic symptoms in older adults has been reported by few studies. The cumulative incidence has been found to be 6% with a follow-up duration of 3.6 years [33], 8% with a follow-up duration of 7 years [49], and 4.8% among 70 year olds followed until death or age 90 [50].

A meta-analysis of studies of the incidence of very-late-onset psychotic disorder (after 65 years) has been published [51]. It identified a total of 41 relevant studies between 1960 and 2016, of which 25 could be used to calculate a pooled incidence. Given this large time-span, the included studies were heterogeneous in important aspects such as diagnostic criteria, case definition and data sources. The study reported a pooled incidence of schizophrenia of 7.5 cases per 100 000 person-years. Of note, the incidence of affective psychosis was considerably higher (30.9 cases per 100 000 person-years), although this was based on a smaller number of studies.

Risk factors

The life-time risk for the most common psychotic disorder, schizophrenia, is higher in men than in women [52,53], but no significant gender differences were found in the prevalence of psychotic disorders in old age (Table 1.2). Women have been reported to have a later age at onset for schizophrenia [54]. One study [45] found the prevalence of schizophrenia in older adults to be two times higher in women than in men. This may partly reflect a higher likelihood of survival to old age in women with early-onset schizophrenia, but older women also seem to have higher incidence rates of psychosis than older men [51].

Table 1.2 Studies reporting prevalence estimates of psychotic disorders according to DSM criteria in old age

Study [Reference]	Year	Diagnostic instrument	Diagnostic criteria	Age	N	Prevalence (%)		
						Women	Men	Total
Gothenburg H85 [47]	1986	CPRS/expert judgment	DSM-III-R schizophrenia, delusional disorder, psychotic NOS	85	484	4.6	4.9	4.7
MRC ALPHA [26]	1986	GMS/expert judgment	DSM-III-R schizophrenia, delusional disorder, psychotic NOS	≥65	5222	N.R	N.R	0.2
NCS-R [13]	2002	CIDI screen, SCID	DSM-IV non-affective psychosis	≥60	≥60	≥60	≥60	0.2
PIF Study[a] [46]	2002	CIDI screen, SCID, medical records, expert judgment	DSM-IV non-affective psychosis	≥65	N.R.	2.67	1.71	2.32
ESPRIT [68][b]	2000	MINI, expert judgment	DSM-IV affective and non-affective psychosis	≥65	1873	1.5	1.9	1.7
Amsterdam Study[c] [45]	2008	MINI-plus, expert judgment	DSM-IV schizophrenia spectrum	≥60	185/26351[d]	0.90	0.44	0.71

DSM: Diagnostic and Statistical Manual of Mental Disorders. CPRS: Comprehensive Psychopathological Rating Scale. NOS: Not otherwise specified. GMS: Geriatric Mental State. CIDI: Composite International Diagnostic Interview. SCID: Structured Clinical Interview for DSM-IV-Axis-1 Disorders. MINI: Mini International Neuropsychiatric Interview. All prevalence estimates are current to one year except *a*, which is life-time prevalence estimate. Dementia was an exclusion criterion for psychotic disorder in all studies except *b*. Prevalence figures include whole population including individuals with dementia except *c* which excluded individuals with moderate–severe dementia from the study sample. Year denotes year in which study was initiated. *d* Case-register study of patients (numerator) in a catchment area population (denominator).

Based on clinical experience, cross-sectional population studies and case–control studies, it is generally believed that sensory impairment (visual or hearing), social isolation and premorbid paranoid personality traits are risk factors for psychotic symptoms in old age [28,39,55]. Furthermore, there are reported associations between psychotic symptoms and structural brain pathology [55], for example basal ganglia calcification [56].

One systematic review of risk factors for late-onset psychosis has been published [57]. It included 11 studies, all with a longitudinal design. Temporal antecedence is one of the prerequisites for a causal relationship between a possible risk factor and a disease [58]. However, the review included studies that were very heterogeneous with respect to important factors such as study design, case definition, baseline age of the samples and length of follow-up. In this review, visual impairment, a history of psychotic symptoms, cognitive dysfunction, poor physical health and negative life events emerged as risk factors. Increasing age and female gender were not found to be risk factors for late-onset psychosis and results on social isolation were ambiguous.

Prognosis and consequences

Mortality

Psychotic disorder [59–63] and psychotic symptoms [28,33] have been associated with mortality in older adults. Thus, the well-known health gap between individuals with psychotic disorders and the general population persists into old age. However, the difference in mortality between individuals with and without schizophrenia may be smaller in older adults compared to younger age groups [62]. Excess mortality is higher among men than among women [59,61]. Physical disease dominates as cause of death in individuals with late-life psychosis, with circulatory diseases being the most common cause of death (as in the general population) [62]. Individuals with VLOSLP seem to have a higher mortality rate than age- and gender-matched individuals with early-onset schizophrenia [61], but disease duration seems to have little or no effect on mortality after adjustment for other variables [59,61]. Findings of higher mortality may, to an unknown extent, be explained by cases erroneously diagnosed as VLOSLP that may instead represent cases of dementia, which is strongly associated with mortality [61].

Association with dementia

Schizophrenia [64], as well as late-onset schizophrenia [65], has been associated with an increased risk for dementia. This association is likely to be multifactorial. Possible causes include higher rates of cerebrovascular disease and substance abuse compared to the general population [65]. An important etiological question is to what extent new-onset psychotic symptoms in later life represent prodromal symptoms of dementia. Several population studies, with a follow-up of between three and ten years, have reported an elevated relative risk for incident dementia among older individuals with prevalent [28,44,49] or first-onset [50] psychotic symptoms, late-onset delusional disorder [66] and VLOSLP [65]. In the studies of individuals with psychotic symptoms, the proportion who were later diagnosed with dementia varies widely (between 15% and 60%). To some extent, these findings corroborate an early clinical study of late-life psychosis which found that only a minority of these patients developed dementia within two years [67].

Conclusions

- Epidemiological studies of late-life psychosis pose several methodological challenges and there are relatively few high-quality studies regarding the risk factors and prognosis of late-life psychosis.
- Reports on the prevalence of late-life psychosis are highly variable, ranging from 1–13.4% for psychotic symptoms and 0.2–4.7% for non-affective psychotic disorders.
- Risk factors that have been found to be associated with late-life psychosis include sensory impairment, social isolation, paranoid personality, structural brain abnormalities, cognitive dysfunction, poor physical health and negative life events.
- Individuals with late-life psychosis have a markedly higher mortality rate than the general population and an increased risk for developing dementia.
- New-onset psychotic symptoms in older adults without dementia confer a greater risk for the subsequent development of dementia, but the proportion of persons at risk varies considerably between studies. Future investigations need to be undertaken to clarify those that are at greater risk for developing dementia.
- Some of the methodological goals for future research include: greater standardization of outcome definitions; increased inclusion of genetic and other biomarkers; improved understanding of critical exposures, their accumulation and duration over the life course; acknowledgment of multimorbidities accompanying aging and psychiatric disease; attention to the polypharmaceutical milieu and effects on psychiatric outcomes.

References

1. Skoog I. Dementia: dementia incidence – the times, they are a-changing. *Nature Reviews Neurology.* 2016;**12**(6):316–18.

2. Howard R, Rabins PV, Seeman MV, Jeste DV; The International Late-Onset Schizophrenia Group. Late-onset schizophrenia and very-late-onset schizophrenia-like psychosis: an international consensus. *American Journal of Psychiatry.* 2000;**157**(2):172–8.

3. Kendler KS, Muñoz RA, Murphy G. The development of the Feighner criteria: a historical perspective. *American Journal of Psychiatry.* 2010;**167**:134–42.

4. Kandel ER. A new intellectual framework for psychiatry. *American Journal of Psychiatry.* 1998;**155**:457–69.

5. Marková IS, Berrios GE. Epistemology of psychiatry. *Psychopathology.* 2012;**45**(4):220–7.

6. Berrios GE, Marková IS. Is the concept of "dimension" applicable to psychiatric objects? *World Psychiatry.* 2013;**12**(1):76–8.

7. Stanghellini G. The puzzle of the psychiatric interview. *Journal of Phenomenological Psychology.* 2004;**35**(2):173–95.

8. Brugha TS, Bebbington PE, Jenkins R. A difference that matters: comparisons of structured and semi-structured psychiatric diagnostic interviews in the general population. *Psychological Medicine.* 1999;**29**(5):1013–20.

9. Kendell R, Jablensky A. Distinguishing between the validity and utility of psychiatric diagnoses. *American Journal of Psychiatry.* 2003;**160**(1):4–12.

10. Spitzer RL. Psychiatric diagnosis: are clinicians still necessary? *Comprehensive Psychiatry.* 1983;**24**(5):399–411.

11. van Os J, Hanssen M, Bijl RV, Ravelli A. Strauss (1969) revisited: a psychosis continuum in the general population? *Schizophrenia Research.* 2000;**45**(1–2):11–20.

12. Johns LC, Cannon M, Singleton N, et al. Prevalence and correlates of self-reported

psychotic symptoms in the British population. *British Journal of Psychiatry.* 2004;**185**:298–305.

13. Kessler RC, Birnbaum H, Demler O, et al. The prevalence and correlates of nonaffective psychosis in the National Comorbidity Survey Replication (NCS-R). *Biological Psychiatry.* 2005;**58**(8):668–76.

14. Schultze-Lutter F, Renner F, Paruch J, et al. Self-reported psychotic-like experiences are a poor estimate of clinician-rated attenuated and frank delusions and hallucinations. *Psychopathology.* 2014;**47**(3):194–201.

15. Ochoa S, Haro JM, Torres JV, et al. What is the relative importance of self reported psychotic symptoms in epidemiological studies? Results from the ESEMeD–Catalonia Study. *Schizophrenia Research.* 2008;**102**(1):261–9.

16. McGrath JJ, Saha S, Al-Hamzawi A, et al. Psychotic experiences in the general population: a cross-national analysis based on 31261 respondents from 18 countries. *Journal of the American Medical Association Psychiatry.* 2015;**72**(7):697–705.

17. Nuevo R, Chatterji S, Verdes E, et al. The continuum of psychotic symptoms in the general population: a cross-national study. *Schizophrenia Bulletin.* 2012;**38**(3):475–85.

18. Bebbington PE, McBride O, Steel C, et al. The structure of paranoia in the general population. *British Journal of Psychiatry.* 2013;**202**:419–27.

19. David A. Why we need more debate on whether psychotic symptoms lie on a continuum with normality. *Psychological Medicine.* 2010;**40**(12):1935–42.

20. Stanghellini G, Langer ÁI, Andra Ambrosini A, Cangas AJ. Quality of hallucinatory experiences: differences between a clinical and a non-clinical sample. *World Psychiatry.* 2012;**11**(2):110–13.

21. Reinhardt MM, Cohen CI. Late-life psychosis: diagnosis and treatment. *Current Psychiatry Reports.* 2015;**17**(2):1–13.

22. Webster J, Grossberg GT. Late-life onset of psychotic symptoms. *American Journal of Geriatric Psychiatry.* 1998;**6**(3):196–202.

23. Javadpour A, Sehatpour M, Mani A, Sahraian A. Assessing diagnosis and symptoms profiles of late-life psychosis. *GeroPsych.* 2013;**26**(4):205.

24. Louhija UM, Saarela T, Juva K, Appelberg B. Brain atrophy is a frequent finding in elderly patients with first episode psychosis. *International Psychogeriatrics.* 2017;**29**(11):1925–9.

25. Knäuper B, Wittchen H-U. Diagnosing major depression in the elderly: evidence for response bias in standardized diagnostic interviews? *Journal of Psychiatric Research.* 1994;**28**(2):147–64.

26. Copeland JR, Dewey ME, Scott A, et al. Schizophrenia and delusional disorder in older age: community prevalence, incidence, comorbidity, and outcome. *Schizophrenia Bulletin.* 1998;**24**(1):153–61.

27. American Psychiatric Association. *Diagnostic and Statistical Manual of Mental Disorders,* 5th edn. Arlington, VA: American Psychiatric Association; 2013.

28. Östling S, Skoog I. Psychotic symptoms and paranoid ideation in a nondemented population-based sample of the very old. *Archives of General Psychiatry.* 2002;**59**(1):53–9.

29. Allgulander C. Psychoactive drug use in a general population sample, Sweden: correlates with perceived health, psychiatric diagnoses, and mortality in an automated record-linkage study. *American Journal of Public Health.* 1989;**79**(8):1006–10.

30. Kessler RC, Little RJ, Groves RM. Advances in strategies for minimizing and adjusting for survey nonresponse. *Epidemiologic Reviews.* 1995;**17**(1):192–204.

31. Fisher HL, Caspi A, Poulton R, et al. Specificity of childhood psychotic symptoms for predicting schizophrenia by 38 years of age: a birth cohort study. *Psychological Medicine.* 2013;**43**(10):2077–86.

32. Cohen P, Cohen J. The clinician's illusion. *Archives of General Psychiatry*. 1984;**41**(12):1178–82.

33. Henderson AS, Korten AE, Levings C, et al. Psychotic symptoms in the elderly: a prospective study in a population sample. *International Journal of Geriatric Psychiatry*. 1998;**13**(7):484–92.

34. Sigström R, Skoog I, Sacuiu S, et al. The prevalence of psychotic symptoms and paranoid ideation in non-demented population samples aged 70–82 years. *International Journal of Geriatric Psychiatry*. 2009;**24**(12):1413–19.

35. Östling S, Börjesson-Hanson A, Skoog I. Psychotic symptoms and paranoid ideation in a population-based sample of 95-year-olds. *American Journal of Geriatric Psychiatry*. 2007;**15**(12):999–1004.

36. Östling S, Bäckman K, Waern M, et al. Paranoid symptoms and hallucinations among the older people in Western Europe. *International Journal of Geriatric Psychiatry*. 2013;**28**(6):573–9.

37. Soares WB, Ribeiz SR, Bassitt DP, De Oliveira MC, Bottino CM. Psychotic symptoms in older people without dementia from a Brazilian community-based sample. *International Journal of Geriatric Psychiatry*. 2014;**30**(5):437–45.

38. Livingston G, Kitchen G, Manela M, Katona C, Copeland J. Persecutory symptoms and perceptual disturbance in a community sample of older people: the Islington study. *International Journal of Geriatric Psychiatry*. 2001;**16**(5):462–8.

39. Forsell Y, Henderson AS. Epidemiology of paranoid symptoms in an elderly population. *British Journal of Psychiatry*. 1998;**172**:429–32.

40. Christenson R, Blazer D. Epidemiology of persecutory ideation in an elderly population in the community. *American Journal of Psychiatry*. 1984;**141**(9):1088–91.

41. Cohen CI, Magai C, Yaffe R, Walcott-Brown L. Racial differences in paranoid ideation and psychoses in an older urban population. *American Journal of Psychiatry*. 2004;**161**(5):864–71.

42. Lyketsos CG, Steinberg M, Tschanz JT, et al. Mental and behavioral disturbances in dementia: findings from the Cache County Study on Memory in Aging. *American Journal of Psychiatry*. 2000;**157**(5):708–14.

43. Subramaniam M, Abdin E, Vaingankar J, et al. Prevalence of psychotic symptoms among older adults in an Asian population. *International Psychogeriatrics*. 2016;**28**(7):1211–20.

44. Köhler S, Allardyce J, Verhey FR, et al. Cognitive decline and dementia risk in older adults with psychotic symptoms: a prospective cohort study. *American Journal of Geriatric Psychiatry*. 2013;**21**(2):119–28.

45. Meesters PD, de Haan L, Comijs HC, et al. Schizophrenia spectrum disorders in later life: prevalence and distribution of age at onset and sex in a Dutch catchment area. *American Journal of Geriatric Psychiatry*. 2012;**20**(1):18–28.

46. Perälä J, Suvisaari J, Saarni SI, et al. Lifetime prevalence of psychotic and bipolar I disorders in a general population. *Archives of General Psychiatry*. 2007;**64**(1):19–28.

47. Skoog I, Nilsson L, Landahl S, Steen B. Mental disorders and the use of psychotropic drugs in an 85-year-old urban population. *International Psychogeriatrics*. 1993;**5**(1):33–48.

48. Saha S, Chant D, McGrath J. A systematic review of mortality in schizophrenia: is the differential mortality gap worsening over time? *Archives of General Psychiatry*. 2007;**64**(10):1123–31.

49. Soares WB, Dos Santos EB, Bottino CMC, Elkis H. Psychotic symptoms in older people without dementia from a Brazilian community-based sample: a seven years' follow-up. *PLoS One*. 2017;**12**(6):e0178471.

50. Östling S, Palsson SP, Skoog I. The incidence of first-onset psychotic symptoms and paranoid ideation in a representative population sample followed from age 70-90 years. Relation to mortality and later development

of dementia. *International Journal of Geriatric Psychiatry.* 2007;**22**(6):520–8.

51. Stafford J, Howard R, Kirkbride JB. The incidence of very late-onset psychotic disorders: a systematic review and meta-analysis, 1960–2016. *Psychological Medicine.* 2017:1–12.

52. Pedersen CB, Mors O, Bertelsen A, et al. A comprehensive nationwide study of the incidence rate and lifetime risk for treated mental disorders. *Journal of the American Medical Association Psychiatry.* 2014;**71**(5):573–81.

53. McGrath J, Saha S, Welham J, El Saadi O, MacCauley C, Chant D. A systematic review of the incidence of schizophrenia: the distribution of rates and the influence of sex, urbanicity, migrant status and methodology. *British Medical Council Medicine.* 2004;**2**(1):13.

54. Castle DJ, Murray RM. The epidemiology of late-onset schizophrenia. *Schizophrenia Bulletin.* 1993;**19**(4):691–700.

55. Almeida OP, Howard RJ, Levy R, David AS. Psychotic states arising in late life (late paraphrenia): the role of risk factors. *The British Journal of Psychiatry.* 1995;**166**(2):215–28.

56. Östling S, Andreasson LA, Skoog I. Basal ganglia calcification and psychotic symptoms in the very old. *International Journal of Geriatric Psychiatry.* 2003;**18**(11):983–7.

57. Brunelle S, Cole MG, Elie M. Risk factors for the late-onset psychoses: a systematic review of cohort studies. *International Journal of Geriatric Psychiatry.* 2012;**27**(3):240–52.

58. Hill AB. The environment and disease: association or causation? *Proceedings of the Royal Society of Medicine.* 1965;**58**(5):295.

59. Meesters PD, Comijs HC, Smit JH, et al. Mortality and its determinants in late-life schizophrenia: a 5-year prospective study in a Dutch catchment area. *American Journal of Geriatric Psychiatry.* 2016;**24**(4):272–7.

60. Talaslahti T, Alanen HM, Hakko H, et al. Mortality and causes of death in older patients with schizophrenia. *International Journal of Geriatric Psychiatry.* 2012;**27**(11):1131–7.

61. Talaslahti T, Alanen HM, Hakko H, et al. Patients with very-late-onset schizoprhenia-like psychosis have higher mortality rates than elderly patients with earlier onset schizophrenia. *International Journal of Geriatric Psychiatry.* 2015;**30**(5):453–9.

62. Kredentser MS, Martens PJ, Chochinov HM, Prior HJ. Cause and rate of death in people with schizophrenia across the lifespan: a population-based study in Manitoba, Canada. *Journal of Clinical Psychiatry.* 2014;**75**(2):154–61.

63. Almeida OP, Hankey GJ, Yeap BB, et al. Mortality among people with severe mental disorders who reach old age: a longitudinal study of a community-representative sample of 37892 men. *PloS One.* 2014;**9**(10):e111882.

64. Ribe AR, Laursen TM, Charles M, et al. Long-term risk of dementia in persons with schizophrenia: a Danish population-based cohort study. *Journal of the American Medical Association Psychiatry.* 2015;**72**(11):1095–101.

65. Kørner A, Lopez AG, Lauritzen L, Andersen PK, Kessing LV. Late and very-late first-contact schizophrenia and the risk of dementia – a nationwide register based study. *International Journal of Geriatric Psychiatry.* 2009;**24**(1):61–7.

66. Kørner A, Lopez AG, Lauritzen L, Andersen PK, Kessing LV. Delusional disorder in old age and the risk of developing dementia – a nationwide register-based study. *Aging and Mental Health.* 2008;**12**(5):625–9.

67. Roth M. The natural history of mental disorder in old age. *The British Journal of Psychiatry.* 1955;**101**(423):281–301.

68. Ritchie K, Artero S, Beluche I, et al. Prevalence of DSM-IV psychiatric disorder in the French elderly population. *British Journal of Psychiatry.* 2004;**184**:147–52.

Patterns of Care for Older People with Schizophrenia

Donna McAlpine, Ph.D. and Ellen McCreedy, Ph.D.

While, on average, people with schizophrenia live shorter lives than people without schizophrenia [1], many with schizophrenia are now living well into older age. Coupled with demographic shifts that are increasing the percentage of the population that is elderly, there is growing attention to the mental health care needs of older adults, including those with schizophrenia [2–4]. For some people with schizophrenia, aging is associated with reduction in symptoms or even remission. However, across the life course, schizophrenia is considered one of the most severe mental health conditions, and is associated with profound disability, disruptions in social roles, socioeconomic disadvantage and reduced overall quality of life [2,4,5]. While estimates of the total economic burden of schizophrenia vary widely [6], there is consensus that they are substantial. The most recent estimate in the United States suggests that the total direct and indirect cost of schizophrenia in 2013 was about 156 billion, with direct medical costs accounting for about one-quarter of the total [7]. Costs of caring for people with schizophrenia increase with age and accumulation of other comorbid conditions [8].

While the weight of research attention has focused on younger people with schizophrenia, the problems faced by older people are likely to be different and warrant dedicated research attention. With aging, people with schizophrenia face the onset of age-related medical conditions, such as cognitive problems or physical decline, and require additional health care. Compared to people without serious mental illness who are aging, those with schizophrenia are also more likely to be economically disadvantaged, have less family support and have greater problems navigating the health care system. This chapter describes patterns of mental health service use among older persons with schizophrenia. The data presented are descriptive and are not meant to explain differences in patterns of care. Where possible, we present data separately for persons 55 years of age and older and those 65 years and older. The estimates of the size and characteristics of the older population treated in various settings and the costs of services are tentative due to limitations in existing national surveys. However, the descriptive data presented provide some benchmarks, help identify gaps in services and point to potential future health system needs.

Trends in the prevalence of schizophrenia among older people

The population of people with schizophrenia in later life is comprised of those who had first onset early in life and aged with the disorder, and a smaller group who have late-onset, defined as onset after the age of 40 [9]. Within the latter group, researchers and clinicians also distinguish between late-onset schizophrenia and very-late-onset schizophrenia-like psychosis, defined as onset after the age of 60 [9].

The first large-scale epidemiological study in the United States that tried to estimate the prevalence of schizophrenia in the community was the Epidemiologic Catchment Area (ECA) study conducted in the early 1980s, which estimated the prevalence of schizophrenia among persons 65 years and older at 0.3%; the comparable estimate for the total population was 1.5% [10]. The ECA showed no significant gender, race or ethnic differences in the estimated prevalence of schizophrenia among older persons.

While the ECA represented the first effort to provide national estimates of a wide variety of mental disorders, the data were limited by small sample sizes of people with schizophrenia, especially older people. Moreover, others have argued that the ECA underestimated the prevalence of schizophrenia in later life because the diagnostic criteria did not include schizophrenia with onset after the age of 45 and the ECA did not sample sufficiently in areas where elderly people with schizophrenia were likely to be living [11].

The most recent national survey in the US designed to provide estimates of the prevalence of mental disorders is the National Comorbidity Survey Replication (NCS-R) [12]. The researchers used a screening tool for detecting symptoms of non-affective psychoses (NAP), followed by a clinician rating of whether each endorsed symptom for a particular respondent was a possible, probable or unlikely symptom of a DSM disorder. Respondents who had a least one symptom of a possible or probable disorder were then administered a full diagnostic interview to determine diagnosis. Estimates derived from this research suggest that the lifetime prevalence of NAP is about 0.5% and the annual prevalence is about 0.3%. Those aged 60 years and older were estimated to have an annual prevalence of about 0.2%. Due to small sample sizes, the researchers were unable to provide estimates for schizophrenia specifically, although such disorders make up the majority of NAP cases. Moreover, due to small sample sizes, the researchers were unable to detect demographic differences in the prevalence of NAP.

Wu and colleagues used a wide range of administrative data from health insurance claims to derive estimates of the annual prevalence of schizophrenia in the US [13]. They estimated the overall annual prevalence of schizophrenia to be 0.54% for males and 0.49% for females. For those aged 65 years and older the estimates were 0.55% for men and 0.84% for women, with an overall annual prevalence in the elderly population of 0.71%. This may represent the lower bound of the true prevalence of schizophrenia because it only included people who have a diagnosis on claims data. However, most people with schizophrenia are likely to receive some treatment.

We estimate the prevalence of schizophrenia for two groups of older people: those 55 years and older and those 65 years and older. Assuming 0.71% is close to the true prevalence of schizophrenia, we estimate there were approximately 340 500 people in the United States 65 years and older living with schizophrenia in 2015. As the population of older Americans grows, so will the numbers of older people with schizophrenia. As shown in Figure 2.1, by 2030 the size of the population aged 65 and older with schizophrenia will have increased by more than 50%. By 2045 there will be more than 600 000 people aged 65 years or older with schizophrenia; by 2060 the estimate approaches 700 000. Of course, the numbers are even more striking when examining the prevalence for those aged 55 years and older; by 2060 the number will exceed one million.

As the population ages, older people will constitute a larger proportion of the total with schizophrenia. Wu and colleagues estimate the overall prevalence of diagnosed schizophrenia in the general population to be between 0.51 and 0.53%. Taking the lower bounds, in 2015 those aged 65 years and older comprised approximately 20% of the total population

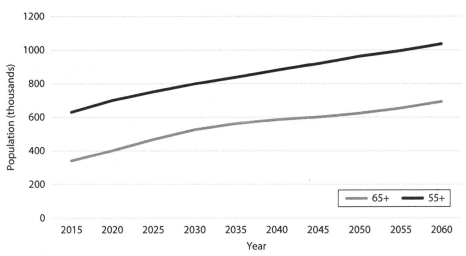

Figure 2.1 Estimated number of older people with schizophrenia in the United States, 2015–2060
Source: Estimates of the total population come from Census projected population on July 1 each year (US Census Bureau 2014)

with schizophrenia. By 2030 this will increase to 29%, and by 2060 fully one-third of people with schizophrenia will be 65 years and older and more than 50% will be 55 years or older. Policy and programs aimed at reducing the burden of schizophrenia will therefore need to increasingly target the specific needs and gaps in care of the elderly population.

The increase in the number of people with schizophrenia in later life will challenge the existing systems of care. Examination of current patterns of service utilization foreshadows the types of challenges that will be faced over the next few decades. The remainder of this chapter will review services in four areas: inpatient care, nursing home care, outpatient care and physical health care. The financing of mental health care for older adults with schizophrenia is also discussed.

The inpatient sector: psychiatric and general hospitals

Since the 1950s, the population of adults in psychiatric hospitals has dramatically decreased from more than 550 000 year-end residents at the end of 1955 to fewer than 40 000 currently [14]. Deinstitutionalization, the process of reducing the patient population cared for in psychiatric hospitals, had a particularly strong effect on patterns of mental health care for older people. As the number of residents in state psychiatric hospitals substantially declined from 1962 to 1972, the number of mentally ill elderly patients living in nursing homes increased at even a greater rate, suggesting that nursing homes were replacing psychiatric hospitals as the most common sites of institutional care [15].

Although psychiatric hospitals have a smaller role in the provision of mental health services than they once did, they remain an important sector of care, especially for patients with severe mental illnesses. In 2014, approximately 55% of adults 55 years and older who received mental health services in state psychiatric hospitals had a diagnosis of schizophrenia or a related condition [16]. Moreover, the number of admissions of patients 65 years and older to state hospitals slightly increased in the early 2000s indicating that psychiatric hospitals may be playing a larger role in providing services, although much of the increase appears to be in forensic beds [17].

As beds in psychiatric hospitals declined, general hospitals increasingly became the common site of care for mental disorders [18]. By 2004, about one-quarter of all stays among adults in community hospitals were for mental health conditions [19]. Care in general hospitals includes beds in psychiatric units as well as beds in general medical wards, often referred to as scatter beds. Psychiatric beds in general hospitals increased in the 1990s as beds in psychiatric hospitals declined. Between 1992 and 2002, for example, the number of stays for elderly Medicare beneficiaries with psychiatric diagnoses in long-term hospitals declined by over 50%, while stays in general hospitals increased [20]. The expansion in general hospitals was generally driven by more stays in psychiatric units rather than in scatter beds [20].

The most recent data about the size of the older population with schizophrenia receiving care in general hospitals are from the National Inpatient Sample (NIS) collected as part of the Healthcare Cost and Utilization Project (HCUP) [21]. The NIS is a probability sample of discharges from non-federal, short-term general and specialty hospitals across the United States. The NIS samples hospitals within geographic regions, and then draws a systematic sample of discharges from selected hospitals. The data were collected in 2014. Estimates are weighted to be nationally representative.

As shown in Table 2.1, in 2014 there were almost 40 000 discharges of patients aged 65 years or older from general hospitals with a primary diagnosis of schizophrenia, and almost 250 000 discharges for people with a diagnosis of schizophrenia listed anywhere on the record (non-primary diagnosis). Among those aged 55 years and older, there were just over 100 000 discharges with a primary diagnosis of schizophrenia and four times as many with an any-listed diagnosis. Discharges with a primary diagnosis of schizophrenia who were 65 years of age and older were less likely to be men (38.7%) than the general population of older adults treated in general hospitals (44.7%). People discharged with a primary diagnosis of schizophrenia were also younger than people discharged without a primary diagnosis of schizophrenia. For both age groups (those 55 and over and those 65 and over) the average length of stay was longest for those with a primary diagnosis of schizophrenia, about five days longer for 65 years and older and seven days longer for 55 years and older, compared with the total population of discharges in each of the respective age groups. Older patients with a primary diagnosis of schizophrenia were more likely to be treated in public hospitals than the general population; those 65 years and older were almost three times more likely to be treated in public general hospitals than the general population. There were strong race differences, particularly for persons 55 years and older, with just over 40% of discharges being non-white patients compared to about 25% for the total population of discharges in that age group. Finally, people hospitalized with schizophrenia came from more socioeconomically disadvantaged communities. For example, about 40% of discharges for persons with a primary diagnosis of schizophrenia were for people living in zip-codes where the median income was below $40 000, compared to 28% of all discharges.

In summary, while older patients with a primary diagnosis of schizophrenia make up only a small fraction of annual discharges from general hospitals, they have longer average lengths of stay compared to the total population of older patients. Discharges for persons with schizophrenia are also more likely to be non-white, female, economically disadvantaged and younger patients than the total population hospitalized.

Table 2.1 Characteristics of discharges from general hospitals of persons 55 years and older with a diagnosis of schizophrenia, 2014

	55 years and older			65 years and older		
	Principal diagnosis schizophrenia	Any schizophrenia	Total	Principal diagnosis schizophrenia	Any schizophrenia	Total
Number of discharges	101 939	428 675	17 270 707	39 940	246 275	12 327 770
Rate per 100 000 population	114.88	483.10	19 463.46	83.50	514.90	25 774.14
Length of stay (days)	12.26	8.25	5.23	10.50	7.88	5.27
% Male	46.98	47.00	46.72	38.73	41.70	44.7
% Medicare	64.09	73.06	71.92	85.42	89.24	89.24
% Public hospitals	13.76	12.55	11.23	30.64	11.87	10.63
% 85+	4.60	11.59	16.43	11.74	20.17	23.02
% Non-white	41.74	32.95	24.50	35.59	27.08	34.11
% Median zip-code income <$40 000	40.35	36.43	28.31	35.47	32.60	27.05

Source: Based on analysis from the Nationwide Inpatient Sample [21].

Nursing homes

People with serious mental illness are often discharged from inpatient psychiatric hospitals directly to other institutional settings, including nursing homes and rest homes: a process referred to as transinstitutionalization [22–25]. Nursing homes are ill-equipped to adequately address the care needs of people with schizophrenia or other serious mental illnesses [26], but community-based alternatives are not widely available and payment structures are not always in place to pay for this less-restrictive care [27]. Concern over the effects of transinstitutionalization has coincided with general concern over the safety and quality of US nursing homes [28]. In response to these concerns, the Omnibus Budget Reconciliation Act of 1987 (OBRA-87) was passed. Specific to mental health, the OBRA-87 mandated preadmission screening to ensure that only those in need of nursing home level care were admitted, and annual reviews of residents to screen for mental health problems and service needs. The OBRA-87 legislation has improved quality of care delivered in nursing homes [29], and reduced admissions to nursing homes among younger people with serious mental illness who could be better served in the community [30]. However, middle-aged and older adults with schizophrenia are still at greater risk of being admitted to nursing homes than their counterparts with no mental illness [31]. Many older adults with serious mental illness are classified as low-care status at nursing home admission, indicating that they may be able to live in less restrictive settings [32]. Once in a nursing home, most people with serious mental illness do not receive any care from a mental health provider [32].

The OBRA-87 legislation also mandated routine, standardized assessment of people living in CMS-certified nursing homes. These standardized resident assessments provide information on resident preferences, deficits in activities of daily living, diagnoses, cognitive status and overall health status. The data collected from these assessments are referred to as the Minimum Data Set (MDS). A current diagnosis of schizophrenia, including schizoaffective and schizophreniform disorders, is captured in the current version of the resident assessment (MDS, v.3.0, Section I). Using national MDS data from 2015, we identified 1 169 497 residents aged 65 or older without schizophrenia and 64 207 residents aged 65 or older with schizophrenia living in nursing homes. This population does not include people who were admitted to nursing homes for short, rehabilitation (post-hospitalization) stays.

As shown in Table 2.2, the population of people 55 years and over in nursing homes who have a diagnosis of schizophrenia is significantly younger than the total population of nursing home residents. While about 30% of the residents with a diagnosis of schizophrenia are 80 years or older, 70% of residents without schizophrenia are in this older age group. Nursing home residents with a diagnosis of schizophrenia are also significantly more likely to be African American (21%) compared to residents without schizophrenia (12%).

Residents with schizophrenia have less cognitive and physical impairment than residents without schizophrenia, although there is a significant amount of comorbidity within the population of people with schizophrenia. Of nursing home residents with schizophrenia, 40% have moderate or severe cognitive impairment, compared to 48% of residents without schizophrenia. On average, nursing home residents with schizophrenia require extensive or total support completing four activities of daily living, such as walking, dressing or eating; nursing home residents without schizophrenia require extensive or total support on five activities of daily living. Residents of nursing homes with a schizophrenia diagnosis had been in the facility longer than residents without schizophrenia. The average length of stay for older residents with schizophrenia was 2.5 years compared to 1.6 years for residents without schizophrenia.

Use of antipsychotics for long-stay nursing home residents with schizophrenia was high. Of residents with schizophrenia, 80% had received an antipsychotic medication in the last seven days; only 17% of residents without schizophrenia received antipsychotic medications. Antipsychotic medications are a primary component of medical treatment for schizophrenia. After the IOM report and the subsequent passage of OBRA in 1987, national policy shifted toward reducing the inappropriate use of antipsychotics to manage behavioral symptoms of dementia. There was some concern that the national focus on reducing inappropriate antipsychotic use in nursing homes would lead to undertreatment of people who had appropriate indications for receiving these medications, such as people with schizophrenia. While OBRA-87 successfully reduced inappropriate use of antipsychotics to treat behavioral symptoms of dementia [33], residents with appropriate indications for these medications are still receiving them at a high rate. The only measure of mental health service utilization in the MDS is whether or not a resident saw any type of mental health professional within the last week. On this variable, long-term nursing home residents 65 years and older with schizophrenia were only slightly more likely to have seen

Table 2.2 Characteristics of nursing home residents 55 years and older with and without schizophrenia (only long-stay residents, ≥90 days in facility), 2015

Resident characteristics	No schizophrenia diagnosis		Schizophrenia diagnosis		Total long-stay population	
	Aged 55+ (1 285 256)	Aged 65+ (1 169 497)	Aged 55+ (92 694)	Aged 65+ (64 207)	Aged 55+ (1 377 950)	Aged 65+ (1 233 704)
% Male	32.59	30.40	42.63	36.95	33.26	30.74
% 80+	63.98	70.31	20.70	29.89	61.07	68.21
% White	79.47	78.47	69.01	68.83	78.76	77.97
% Black	13.04	11.84	22.95	21.06	13.71	12.32
% Hispanic	5.04	4.91	6.16	6.10	5.11	4.98
% Moderate or severe cognitive impairment	46.38	48.31	35.16	40.38	45.63	47.90
Number of ADL impairments, mean (SD)	5.05 (3.1)	5.13 (3.0)	3.40 (3.3)	3.86 (3.3)	4.94 (3.1)	5.07 (3.1)
Years in facility, mean (SD)	1.62 (2.2)	1.62 (2.1)	2.46 (3.4)	2.55 (3.5)	1.67 (2.3)	1.67 (2.2)
% With any antipsychotics in last week	17.51	17.01	83.27	80.95	21.93	20.34
% Seen by mental health professional in last week	2.36	2.35	5.09	5.02	2.50	2.48

Source: Data from the Minimum Data Set, 2015

a mental health professional in the past week than nursing home residents without schizophrenia (5% and 2%, respectively). One reason for this may be that mental health professionals consult on behavioral issues related to dementia.

In summary, older people with schizophrenia living in nursing homes are more likely to be younger and non-white than nursing home residents without schizophrenia. People with schizophrenia have lived in the nursing home longer than those without schizophrenia, but have less cognitive and physical impairment than people without schizophrenia; 5% had seen a mental health professional within the past week and 80% were prescribed antipsychotics.

Outpatient care

Most care for older adults with schizophrenia is delivered in non-institutional settings. However, there has been very little research on the patterns of care in outpatient settings for these patients. Research focused on older people with any mental disorders suggests that they are less likely than their younger counterparts to receive mental health treatment [34]. Even among those with serious mental illness, older patients are much less likely to report receiving treatment than younger patients [35].

Medicare is the primary payer source of outpatient services for patients 65 years and over; thus, analyses of data based on Medicare claims provide some evidence of patterns of outpatient service use for this population. Lisa Dixon and her colleagues examined the use and costs of ambulatory services among a national sample of over 12 000 Medicare enrollees with a service claim associated with schizophrenia in 1991 [36]. They reported that Medicare enrollees of 65 years and older with a diagnosis of schizophrenia who used mental health ambulatory services had approximately 4.8 visits in the past year, including individual therapy, group therapy, family therapy or psychiatric somatotherapy (pharmacologic management with minimal psychotherapy). However, this research also indicates that even among those with Medicare, many people with schizophrenia did not receive services. Approximately 25% of Medicare enrollees with schizophrenia had no ambulatory claim for services in a year, and those over the age of 65 were less likely to have received services than younger adults. While the data do not include claims paid by other sources (e.g. Medicaid), the large percentage of people who do not have a Medicare claim for ambulatory services suggests that many older people with schizophrenia do not receive adequate treatment.

Physical health care

Schizophrenia is associated with higher risk of mortality; in a review of studies from around the world, Laursen, Nordentoft and Mortensen concluded that life expectancy for people with schizophrenia is about 20 years shorter than for the general population [37]. In a Medicaid cohort aged 20 to 64 in the United States, Olfson and colleagues found that over a seven-year period the death rate was about 3.5 times higher for persons with schizophrenia [38].

Because the frailest, most unhealthy people are the most likely to die young, those with schizophrenia who survive into later life are among the most resilient and healthy people with the disorder. That said, most studies find that older adults with schizophrenia have higher rates of many chronic diseases than their counterparts of the same age without schizophrenia. In part, this increased morbidity may be related to the side effects of long-term treatment for schizophrenia. Common antipsychotics carry increased risk of metabolic problems such as obesity, elevated cholesterol and diabetes [39]. Hendrie et al., in a large observational study of patients over the age of 65, found schizophrenia was associated with higher risk of hypothyroidism, heart failure, chronic obstructive pulmonary disease, congestive heart failure and dementia [40]. Moreover, excess mortality persisted in later life, with about a 25% percent increased risk of death even after controlling for health conditions, health behaviors and demographic characteristics.

In general, research suggests that people with schizophrenia may be undertreated for physical health problems, have lower rates of use of preventive care [41], and have higher rates of delayed or forgone health care [42]. In a national study, patients with psychotic disorders (defined as self-reported schizophrenia or other paranoid or delusional disorders) were less likely to have a usual source of primary care than those without a mental disorder. In addition, they were more likely to report that they were unable to get medical care, that care was delayed because of costs or that they were unable to get needed prescription medication [42].

Unfortunately, there are very few studies of the health care experiences of older people with schizophrenia. Research suggests that older adults with schizophrenia are more likely to be hospitalized [40] and to visit the physician [43] than those without schizophrenia. Despite this increased contact with the health care system, older patients with schizophrenia are less likely to get treatment for physical health problems than the general population. In a small community study, Vahia et al. found that people with hypertension or heart disease were less likely to receive treatment if they had schizophrenia [43]. In another small study, women with schizophrenia were less likely to receive gynecological services than their counterparts without the condition [44].

The need to better address comorbid mental and physical health problems, as well as common psychosocial needs, such as housing, has led to calls for collaborative care models of service delivery. Such models range from relatively modest changes in the way specialty mental health providers and primary care providers communicate, to fully integrated models where mental and physical health services are colocated and a variety of professionals from the health care and social service sectors work as a team to manage the needs of patients [45]. Evidence suggests that, in general, collaborative care models improve outcomes for patients with mental health disorders, although it is not clear which specific features of collaborative models are most important [45]. However, there is insufficient evidence about whether collaborative care models are effective for schizophrenia [46].

The most recent evolution of integrated care includes Patient Centered Medical Homes (PCMHs), Health Homes and Accountable Care Organizations (ACOs) [47]. PCMHs, funded through Medicare, are mainly designed in primary care settings. Health Homes are Medicaid funded and focus on patients with chronic conditions, including serious mental illness. ACOs are provider run, and are responsible for managing the costs and provision of services to a defined patient population. All three models are intended to improve the coordination of physical and mental health services, meet the holistic needs of patients, adhere to evidence-based practice standards and involve patients and their families in decision-making. Early evidence suggests that they hold promise for those with severe mental illness. In a study of a Medicaid enrollees in North Carolina, Domino et al. found that patients with severe mental illness enrolled in a primary-care-based medical home had less emergency room use, better adherence to medications and greater use of both primary and specialty mental health services [48]. While such models hold promise, it is too early to conclude whether they will begin to address the needs of the older population with schizophrenia. The reader will find more in-depth discussions of physical health issues and care models in Chapters 7 and 14 of this volume.

Financing

Schizophrenia is among the most costly conditions to manage over a lifetime, and costs of care increase with age and acquisition of other comorbid conditions [8]. As many people with schizophrenia have difficulty maintaining competitive employment during their working years [49], government insurance programs shoulder most of the economic burden of treating older adults with schizophrenia.

Almost 90% of people with schizophrenia have Medicaid or Medicare; over a quarter have both [50]. Most people with schizophrenia enter the Medicare program before the age of 65 by qualifying for Medicare through receipt of Social Security disability [51]. For this reason, Medicare insures around half of all people with schizophrenia [52]. The costs to the Medicare program are substantial. Feldman et al. estimate the cost to Medicare was about 80% higher for a person with schizophrenia compared to the general Medicare population, much of this cost associated with higher rates of hospitalization [51].

Medicaid is the primary payer for long-term nursing home services for people with schizophrenia. Largely because Medicaid payments for nursing home services are significantly less than private payments, people with schizophrenia are more likely to be admitted to lower-quality nursing homes (based on number of quality deficiencies) [53]. Medicaid recipients tend to be admitted to nursing homes with a greater concentration of Medicaid residents, fewer nurses per resident and higher hospitalization rates [54,55]. In states with higher Medicaid reimbursement rates, people with Medicaid reside in higher-quality nursing homes [56]. Increasing Medicaid reimbursement rates would positively impact the quality of care received by people with schizophrenia in nursing homes.

Policy changes that affect Medicaid or Medicare directly affect the care received by people with schizophrenia and the associated costs. Of particular importance to older adults with schizophrenia, in 2006 Medicare launched an outpatient drug benefit, known as Medicare Part D. Over 90% of Medicare recipients with schizophrenia qualify for the low-income subsidies, which means there are no premiums and only nominal copayments associated with obtaining outpatient prescription drugs through Part D [52]. While it seemed as though these policy changes would increase access to prescription drugs for people with schizophrenia, effects varied by state. People with schizophrenia living in states with historically generous Medicaid plans did not fare as well under the transition to Part D [57], and many people with schizophrenia experienced discontinuity of care during the transition [57,58].

Several policies enacted under the Patient Protection and Affordable Care Act (ACA) may also help older people with schizophrenia access health services [59]. These policies include: not allowing insurance discrimination based on pre-existing conditions; expanding Medicaid to the near poor; and listing mental health services as part of the essential benefits which health insurance plans must cover, similar to physical health conditions [59,60].

The ACA also strengthened parity in coverage between mental and physical health services [61]. While the Mental Health Parity and Addiction Equity Act of 2008 was applauded, it required parity in benefits only if mental health and substance use conditions were covered, thus creating an incentive not to cover these services. The ACA required that behavioral health be covered as part of the Medicaid expansion and in plans offered through individual marketplaces. The ACA also required behavioral health coverage to be at parity with physical health coverage. The Medicare Improvements for Patients and Providers Act (MIPAA) further extended parity in the Medicare population [62]. Prior to 2010, enrollees were required to pay a 50% copayment for mental health outpatient services, compared to a 20% copayment for physical health services. MIPPA phased out the gap so that by 2014 the copayment for both mental and health services was equal (20%).

Conclusions

The results highlight the fact that most older people with schizophrenia are not treated in institutional settings. However, elderly patients with schizophrenia are more likely to be admitted to institutional care at younger ages and, once admitted, have longer lengths of stay than the general population 65 years and older.

The results also point to high levels of unmet need in services for the older population with schizophrenia. This finding is consistent with other research that indicates that almost three-fifths of adults with severe psychiatric disorders do not receive specialty mental health services in a year [30]. It is somewhat surprising, however, that among a population that has insurance, many people with schizophrenia still do not receive services. This applies to the nursing home population, where most people with schizophrenia receive antipsychotic medications but do not receive other mental health services. It also applies to the outpatient population, where more than a third of the population had no claims for mental health services [36].

The data used are limited both by the types of information collected and by small sample sizes, which make it impossible to do extensive sub-group analyses. In particular, the sample sizes of race and ethnic sub-groups with schizophrenia are too small to permit meaningful analyses. There are older persons with schizophrenia receiving care in other settings not covered in this review, including residential care, Veterans Administration hospitals and nursing homes, jails and prisons, adult day care centers and so on. Unfortunately, we lack the data to sufficiently explore the characteristics and types of services received by the elderly treated in these settings.

As the size of the older population increases in the coming decades, it is likely that meeting the needs of those with schizophrenia will be even more difficult. On the one hand, there have been several policy changes that are encouraging: the movement towards mental health parity in the Medicare and Medicaid programs, Medicaid expansions under the ACA, the implementation of medical homes and the emphasis on community services that emerged after the Olmstead decision may facilitate older people with schizophrenia in getting the physical, mental and social services that they need as they age. On the other hand, there are also discouraging signals, including reductions in inpatient capacity, both in general and psychiatric hospitals, and the inappropriate placement and lower-quality care of patients with serious mental illness in nursing homes. Cost pressures in public programs that largely fund care for people with schizophrenia will only grow. The challenges remain formidable. Demographic changes will continue to push researchers and policy-makers to better understand and address the service needs of older adults with schizophrenia.

Acknowledgment

4T32 HS000011 AHRQ "National Research Service Award".

References

1. C. Hjorthoj, A. E. Sturup, J. J. McGrath, et al. Years of potential life lost and life expectancy in schizophrenia: a systematic review and meta-analysis. *Lancet Psychiatry* 2017;**4**:295–301.

2. K. Berry and C. Barrowclough. The needs of older adults with schizophrenia: implications for psychological interventions. *Clinical Psychology Review* 2009;**29**(1):68–76.

3. C. I. Cohen and GAP Committee on Aging. Practical geriatrics: directions for research and policy on schizophrenia and older adults: summary of the GAP committee report. *Psychiatric Services* 2000;**51**(3):299–302.

4. C. I. Cohen, P. D. Meesters and J. Zhao. New perspectives on schizophrenia in later life: implications for treatment, policy, and research. *Lancet Psychiatry* 2015;**2**(4):340–50.

5. H. A. Whiteford, L. Degenhardt, J. Rehm, et al. Global burden of disease attributable to mental and substance use disorders: findings from the Global Burden of Disease Study 2010. *Lancet* 2013;**382**(9904):1575–86.

6. H. Y. Chong, S. L. Teoh, D. B. Wu, et al. Global economic burden of schizophrenia: a systematic review. *Neuropsychiatric Disease and Treatment* 2016;**12**:357–73.

7. M. Cloutier, M. S. Aigbogun, A. Guerin, et al. The economic burden of schizophrenia in the United States in 2013. *Journal of Clinical Psychiatry* 2016;**77**(6):764–71.

8. S. J. Bartels, R. E. Clark, W. J. Peacock, et al. Medicare and Medicaid costs for schizophrenia patients by age cohort compared with costs for depression, dementia, and medically ill patients. *American Journal of Geriatric Psychiatry* 2003;**11**(6):648–57.

9. R. Howard, P. V. Rabins, M. V. Seeman, et al. Late-onset schizophrenia and very-late-onset schizophrenia-like psychosis: an international consensus. *American Journal of Psychiatry* 2000;**157**(2):172–8.

10. S. J. Keith, D. A. Regier and D. S. Rae. Schizophrenic disorders. In *Psychiatric Disorders in America: The Epidemiologic Catchment Area Study*, ed L. N. Robins and D. A. Regier. New York: Free Press, 1991, 33–52.

11. B. W. Palmer, S. C. Heaton and D. V. Jeste. Older patients with schizophrenia: challenges in the coming decades. *Psychiatric Services* 1999;**50**(9):1178–83.

12. R. C. Kessler, H. Birnbaum, O. Demler, et al. The prevalence and correlates of non-affective psychosis in the National Comorbidity Survey Replication (NCS-R). *Biological Psychiatry* 2005;**58**(8):668–76.

13. E. Q. Wu, L. Shi, H. Birnbaum, et al. Annual prevalence of diagnosed schizophrenia in the USA: a claims data analysis approach. *Psychological Medicine* 2006;**36**(11):1535–40.

14. D. Mechanic, D. D. McAlpine and D. A. Rochefort. *Mental Health and Social Policy: Beyond Managed Care*. Boston, MA: Pearson Education, 2014.

15. R. G. Frank. The creation of Medicare and Medicaid: the emergence of insurance and markets for mental health services. *Psychiatric Services* 2000;**51**(4):465–8.

16. Substance Abuse and Mental Health Services Administration, Center for Behavioral Health Statistics and Quality. Mental Health Annual Report: 2014. National Use of Mental Health Services. HHS Publication No.17-5033, 2017.

17. R. W. Manderscheid, J. E. Atay and R. A. Crider. Changing trends in state psychiatric hospital use from 2002 to 2005. *Psychiatric Services* 2009;**60**(1):29–34.

18. D. Mechanic, D. D. McAlpine and M. Olfson. Changing patterns of psychiatric inpatient care in the United States, 1988–1994. *Archives of General Psychiatry* 1998;**55**(9):785–91.

19. P. Owens, M. Myers, A. Elixhauser, et al. *Care of Adults with Mental Health and Substance Abuse Disorders in US Community Hospitals, 2004*. HCUP Fact Book No. 10. Rockville, MD: Agency for Healthcare Research and Quality, 2007.

20. D. R. Hoover, A. Akincigil, J. D. Prince, et al. Medicare inpatient treatment for elderly non-dementia psychiatric illnesses 1992–2002; length of stay

and expenditures by facility type. *Administration and Policy in Mental Health and Mental Health Services Research* 2008;**35**(4):231–40.

21. Agency for Healthcare Research and Quality. Healthcare Cost and Utilization Project (HCUP), Nationwide Inpatient Sample (NIS), 2011.

22. N. W. Bowersox, B. J. Szymanski and J. F. McCarthy. Associations between psychiatric inpatient bed supply and the prevalence of serious mental illness in Veterans Affairs nursing homes. *American Journal of Public Health* 2013;**103**(7):1325–31.

23. J. Avorn, P. Dreyer, K. Connelly, et al. Use of psychoactive medication and the quality of care in rest homes: findings and policy implications of a statewide study. *New England Journal of Medicine* 1989;**320**(4):227–32.

24. J. M. Kruzich. The chronically mentally ill in nursing homes: issues in policy and practice. *Health and Social Work* 1986;**11**(1):5–14.

25. L. J. Schmidt, A. M. Reinhardt and R. L. Kane. The mentally ill in nursing homes: new back wards in the community. *Archives of General Psychiatry* 1977;**34**(6):687–91.

26. W. E. Reichman, A. C. Coyne, S. Borson, et al. Psychiatric consultation in the nursing home: a survey of six states. *American Journal of Geriatric Psychiatry* 1998;**6**(4):320–7.

27. R. I. Freedman and A. Moran. Wanderers in a promised land: the chronically mentally ill and deinstitutionalization. *Medical Care* 1984;**22**(12 Suppl):S1–60.

28. Institute of Medicine. *Improving the Quality of Care in Nursing Homes*. Washington, DC: The National Academies Press, 1986.

29. C. Hawes, V. Mor, C. D. Phillips, et al. The OBRA-87 nursing home regulations and implementation of the Resident Assessment Instrument: effects on process quality. *Journal of the American Geriatrics Society* 1997;**45**(8):977–85.

30. D. Mechanic and D. D. McAlpine. Use of nursing homes in the care of persons with severe mental illness: 1985 to 1995. *Psychiatric Services* 2000;**51**(3):354–8.

31. A. O. Andrews, S. J. Bartels, H. Xie, et al. Increased risk of nursing home admission among middle aged and older adults with schizophrenia. *American Journal of Geriatric Psychiatry* 2009;**17**(8):697–705.

32. D. G. Shea, P. A. Russo and M. A. Smyer. Use of mental health services by persons with a mental illness in nursing facilities: initial impacts of OBRA87. *Journal of Aging and Health* 2000;**12**(4):560–78.

33. M. D. Llorente, E. J. Olsen, O. Leyva, et al. Use of antipsychotic drugs in nursing homes: current compliance with OBRA regulations. *Journal of the American Geriatrics Society* 1998;**46**(2):198–201.

34. P. S. Wang, M. Lane, M. Olfson, et al. Twelve-month use of mental health services in the United States: results from the National Comorbidity Survey Replication. *Archives of General Psychiatry* 2005;**62**(6):629–40.

35. B. E. Karlin, M. Duffy and D. H. Gleaves. Patterns and predictors of mental health service use and mental illness among older and younger adults in the United States. *Psychological Services* 2008;**5**(3):275.

36. L. Dixon, A. Lyles, C. Smith, et al. Use and costs of ambulatory care services among Medicare enrollees with schizophrenia. *Psychiatric Services* 2001;**52**(6):786–92.

37. T. M. Laursen, M. Nordentoft and P. B. Mortensen. Excess early mortality in schizophrenia. *Annual Review of Clinical Psychology* 2014;**10**:425–48.

38. M. Olfson, T. Gerhard, C. Huang, et al. Premature mortality among adults with schizophrenia in the United States. *JAMA Psychiatry* 2015;**72**(12):1172–81.

39. D. C. Henderson. Schizophrenia and comorbid metabolic disorders. *Journal of Clinical Psychiatry* 2004;**66**:11–20.

40. H. C. Hendrie, W. Tu, R. Tabbey, et al. Health outcomes and cost of care among older adults with schizophrenia: a 10-year study using medical records across the continuum of care. *American Journal of Geriatric Psychiatry* 2014;**22**(5):427–36.

41. O. Lord, D. Malone and A. J. Mitchell. Receipt of preventive medical care and medical screening for patients with mental illness: a comparative analysis. *General Hospital Psychiatry* 2010;**32**(5):519–43.

42. D. W. Bradford, M. M. Kim, L. E. Braxton, et al. Access to medical care

among persons with psychotic and major affective disorders. *Psychiatric Services* 2008;**59**(8):847–52.

43. I. V. Vahia, S. Diwan, A. O. Bankole, et al. Adequacy of medical treatment among older persons with schizophrenia. *Psychiatric Services* 2008;**59**(8):853–9.

44. L. A. Lindamer, A. Bailey, W. Hawthorne, et al. Gender differences in characteristics and service use of public mental health patients with schizophrenia. *Psychiatric Services* 2003;**54**(10):1407–9.

45. M. Butler, R. L. Kane, D. McAlpine, et al. Integration of mental health/substance abuse and primary care. *AHRQ Evidence Report* 2008;**173**:1–362.

46. S. Reilly, C. Planner, L. Gask, et al. Collaborative care approaches for people with severe mental illness. *Cochrane Database of Systematic Reviews* 2013(11):CD009531.

47. Y. Bao, L. P. Casalino and H. A. Pincus. Behavioral health and health care reform models: patient-centered medical home, health home, and accountable care organization. *Journal of Behavioral Health Services and Research* 2013;**40**(1):121–32.

48. M. E. Domino, R. Wells and J. P. Morrissey. Serving persons with severe mental illness in primary care-based medical homes. *Psychiatric Services* 2015;**66**(5):477–83.

49. R. Rosenheck, D. Leslie, R. Keefe, et al. Barriers to employment for people with schizophrenia. *American Journal of Psychiatry* 2006;**163**(3):411–7.

50. E. Khaykin, W. W. Eaton, D. E. Ford, et al. Health insurance coverage among persons with schizophrenia in the United States. *Psychiatric Services* 2010;**61**(8):830–4.

51. R. Feldman, R. A. Bailey, J. Muller, et al. Cost of schizophrenia in the Medicare program. *Population Health Management* 2014;**17**(3):190–6.

52. Y. Zhang, S. H. Baik and J. P. Newhouse. Use of intelligent assignment to Medicare Part D plans for people with schizophrenia could produce substantial savings. *Health Affairs* 2015;**34**(3):455–60.

53. Y. Li, X. Cai and P. Cram. Are patients with serious mental illness more likely to be admitted to nursing homes with more deficiencies in care? *Medical Care* 2011;**49**(4):397–405.

54. M. Rahman, D. C. Grabowski, P. L. Gozalo, et al. Are dual eligibles admitted to poorer quality skilled nursing facilities? *Health Services Research* 2014;**49**(3):798–817.

55. M. Rahman, D. C. Grabowski, O. Intrator, et al. Serious mental illness and nursing home quality of care. *Health Services Research* 2013;**48**(4):1279–98.

56. V. Mor, A. Gruneir, Z. Feng, et al. The effect of state policies on nursing home resident outcomes. *Journal of the American Geriatrics Society* 2011;**59**(1):3–9.

57. J. M. Madden, A. S. Adams, R. F. LeCates, et al. Changes in drug coverage generosity and untreated serious mental illness: transitioning from Medicaid to Medicare Part D. *JAMA Psychiatry* 2015;**72**(2):179–88.

58. J. C. West, J. E. Wilk, D. S. Rae, et al. First-year Medicare Part D prescription drug benefits: medication access and continuity among dual eligible psychiatric patients. *Journal of Clinical Psychiatry* 2010;**71**(4):400–10.

59. K. Beronio, S. Glied and R. Frank. How the Affordable Care Act and Mental Health Parity and Addiction Equity Act greatly expand coverage of behavioral health care. *Journal of Behavioral Health Services and Research* 2014;**41**(4):410–28.

60. H. H. Goldman. Will health insurance reform in the United States help people with schizophrenia? *Schizophrenia Bulletin* 2010;**36**(5):893–4.

61. J. Bartlett and R. Manderscheid. What does mental health parity really mean for the care of people with serious mental illness? *Psychiatric Clinics of North America* 2016;**39**(2):331–42.

62. L. Ostrow and R. Manderscheid. Medicare mental health parity: a high potential change that is long overdue. *Journal of Behavioral Health Services and Research* 2010;**37**(3):285–90.

Assessment and Diagnosis of Psychotic Symptoms in Older Adults

Michael Reinhardt, M.D., Dina Ghoneim, M.D.,
Tessa Murante D.O., Eric Nelson, Paulina Vargas,
and Shifra Mincer

Introduction

Both DSM-5 and the World Health Organization require the presence of hallucinations – without insight into their nature, delusions, or both, for the operational diagnosis of psychosis [1]. Conceptually, both systems understand psychosis to comprise an impairment in reality testing. For certain diagnoses in DSM-5, disorganized thinking or speech can replace hallucinations and delusions in the diagnosis of a psychotic disorder, when it is accompanied by grossly disorganized behavior, catatonia (with schizophrenia, schizophreniform, brief psychotic, and schizoaffective disorders) and/or negative symptoms (with schizophrenia, schizophreniform, and schizoaffective disorders). Moreover, the disorganized thought must be so severe as to impair effective communication. The prevalence of psychotic symptoms in older adults varies widely depending on setting, with estimates ranging from 1% to 63% [2–4]. Despite the concise definition of psychosis provided by DSM-5, the clinical phenomenology and treatment of psychosis in older adults vary considerably, depending on the underlying etiology. Given the multitude of potential etiologies for psychosis – both primary psychiatric illnesses and psychotic disorders secondary to other medical conditions – and the clear limitations and potential adverse effects of available pharmacological treatments, accurate assessment and diagnosis of psychosis is essential. The principal aims of this chapter will be to examine the prevalence of psychotic symptoms and disorders, describe the different types of psychotic disorders in older adults, offer some insight into distinguishing between the disorders, and provide an overview of treatment strategies.

Epidemiology

Community studies

Population studies report the prevalence of psychotic symptoms in non-demented older adults to range from 1% to 13.4%, with a median value of 3.6% [4]. Most studies have been conducted in Western countries, but studies in Malaya and Brazil found comparable, albeit slightly higher, rates of 5.2% and 9.1%, respectively [5,6]. In the United States, Cohen et al. reported substantial racial differences among older adults in Brooklyn, New York: blacks were three times more likely to report psychotic symptoms than whites [7].

As described below, rates of psychotic symptoms are much higher in various psychiatric disorders, sometimes exceeding over 80% of cases, e.g., delirium, Lewy body dementia.

Various risk factors have been found to be associated with psychosis in later life, including advanced age, sensory impairment, social isolation, paranoid personality, structural brain abnormalities, cognitive dysfunction, poor physical health, depression, negative life events, and impaired functioning [4,5]. The association of psychotic symptoms with depression found in several studies suggested that psychotic symptoms may be a manifestation of distress in many people and not necessarily benign phenomena [7].

Clinical epidemiology

Psychotic symptoms can be broadly grouped into two categories: primary psychiatric disorders and psychotic disorders due to another condition (secondary psychotic disorders). The minority of psychotic symptoms in late life are the direct effect of primary psychiatric illness (approximately two-fifths) while the majority are attributable to other medical conditions (approximately three-fifths) [2,8–10]. It is of critical importance to follow the diagnostic hierarchy of psychiatric illness; that is, first assume the presence of another medical etiology before concluding a psychiatric illness is present. Sixty percent of psychosis presentations in older adults are attributable to such pre-existing medical conditions, including major neurocognitive disorders (dementias), delirium, and substance use. The remaining 40% of psychosis presentations are attributable to primary psychiatric illnesses, including bipolar and major depressive disorders with psychotic features, and schizophrenia-spectrum illnesses. (In an earlier article, we referred to all the etiologies of psychotic disorders as the six "Ds": Disease, Delirium, Drugs, Dementia, Depression and bipolar disorder, and Delusions and schizophrenia-spectrum disorders [10].) Table 3.1 [2,8–11] outlines the relative contribution of these etiologies to the presentation of psychosis in the elderly.

The lifetime risk for developing a psychotic disorder is 23%, but the prevalence varies with place of residence [2,10,12]. In community-dwelling adults without major neurocognitive disorders who are aged sixty-five and older the prevalence is somewhere between 0

Table 3.1 Relative contribution of various etiological factors to psychosis in elderly people

Etiology	Relative contribution
Primary Disorders	
Major depressive disorder	33%
Bipolar disorder	5%
Delusions and schizophrenia-spectrum disorders	4%
Delusional disorder	2%
Schizophrenia	1%
Schizoaffective disorder	1%
Secondary Disorders	
Major neurocognitive disorder (dementia)	40%
Medical disease	7%
Delirium	7%
Drug toxicity (substance use and medications)	4%

and 4% compared to 5–15% for adults in geriatric inpatient units, and a prodigious 63% among adult nursing home residents [2,3,13].

That being said, recorded prevalence rates of psychosis in adults may be falsely low. Individuals may be reluctant to report such symptoms or have poor insight into their nature. Although the use of collateral informants could minimize these factors, it is rarely employed. In addition, older adults may be less likely to meet the strict diagnostic criteria for psychosis, although they may have subthreshold disorders that are often associated with impaired functioning and distress.

Current prevalence numbers are also limited by the period of data collection. Longitudinal data would provide a more accurate picture of the course and extent of psychotic symptoms and disorders in older adults.

Diagnosis, assessment, and treatment

Preliminary issues

While ideally the principle of Occam's razor can simplify multiple medical diagnoses into one, older adults often do present with multiple comorbidities. It is therefore not unusual for an older adult to present with a new psychotic disorder in addition to an already exist-ing medical disorder. For example, a person with schizophrenia may develop Alzheimer's disease; people with dementia are more prone to develop delirium. Furthermore, these comorbid psychotic disorders may have a transformative impact on typical presentations. For example, a person with schizophrenia who develops Alzheimer's disease may initially exhibit more bizarre symptoms than those typically seen in most dementias [14]. As the Alzheimer's disease progresses, however, the person may come to resemble the more typi-cal dementia patient.

A second diagnostic conundrum occurs when psychotic symptoms are prodromes of neurocognitive disorders. The presence of psychotic symptoms confers a 2.5- to 3.5-fold risk of developing a dementia syndrome; between 18.5% and 58% of non-demented patients with new-onset psychotic symptoms develop dementia approximately 5 years after the initial diagnosis [6]. Thus, a diagnosis of a primary psychotic disorder in the context of new onset psychotic symptoms must be viewed as a provisional diagnosis.

Examination and laboratory assessment

In theory, primary psychiatric illness should never be diagnosed pending exclusion of causation by another medical condition or substance, because treatment may vary broadly based on etiology. However, as noted above, sometimes diagnoses may change over time as more symptoms of a secondary disorder manifest themselves. Because there are numer-ous potential etiologies for psychosis in the elderly, the evaluation of these symptoms requires a comprehensive geriatric assessment. Risk factors for psychosis in the elderly include a decline in cognition, sensory impairment (hearing and vision), co-occurring medical or psychiatric conditions, high medication burden, alterations in pharmacody-namics/kinetics, and age-related neuroanatomic and neurochemical changes [10].

Due to the high probability of cognitive impairment, whenever feasible, available history should be corroborated by collateral informants with attention paid to the time course of illness, antecedent factors (social, financial, physical stressors), temporal-ity of psychotic symptoms (if any), and modifiable physical and environmental factors that may worsen psychosis. Such factors include hydration status, the presence of pain, constipation or diarrhea, urinary/bowel incontinence, nutritional status, fatigue, impairments of vision and/or hearing, and environmental stimulation. The evaluation should also consider history of recent falls (potential head injuries), acute medical conditions, other psychiatric symptoms (depression/anxiety), and changes in medications (adverse effects or drug–drug interactions) [10].

While there are no pathognomonic signs to differentiate psychosis caused by psychiatric illness from that caused by another physiological condition, there are some characteristics that may serve to distinguish the latter from the former: acuity of onset (days to weeks), age of onset, visual hallucinations without the presence of auditory hallucinations, presence or absence of past psychiatric or family history, symptoms that are worse than expected or resistant to treatment, symptoms occurring after a change in personality, symptoms occurring in conjunction with a medical disease known to cause psychotic symptoms, cognitive abnormalities, and medication/substance use or abuse [10]. Additionally, it is important to differentiate between psychosis and agitation (a nonspecific term referring to aggression, combativeness, shouting, hyperactivity, and disinhibition). While the literature often clusters these two symptoms together, the distinction is important for patients with neurocognitive disorders because available pharmacological treatments may be moderately effective for agitation, whereas they are only minimally effective for psychosis [15].

Laboratory and radiologic testing should be undertaken to assist in the diagnostic process. Although the approach to diagnostic testing must be tailored to the individual patient, it often includes comprehensive metabolic panels, complete blood count with differential, thyroid stimulating hormone level, vitamin B12 level, rapid plasmin reagin test, urinalysis, and toxicology. Further screens for infectious etiologies (e.g., HIV screening, blood cultures) or autoimmune conditions may be done as clinically indicated. Neuroimaging is generally indicated for new-onset psychotic disorders, while EEG and polysomnography should be considered on a case-by-case basis [10].

The differential diagnosis for psychosis in the elderly is outlined in Table 3.2.

Specific disorders

Delirium

The diagnosis of delirium is established through observation of an acute change in mental status. This change in mental status is characterized by a fluctuating deficit in attention, with changes in cognition that are not better explained by another neurocognitive disorder [11]. The diagnosis of delirium remains reliant on clinical acumen, despite multiple efforts to establish diagnostic biomarkers [16,17]. Behavioral symptoms are very common during delirium, including hallucinations and delusions, sleep disturbances, aberrant behavior, and affective lability [16,18]. In particular, hallucinations and delusions are common in delirium, with prevalence rates ranging from 40 to 70% for hallucinations and from 24 to 79% for delusions [19–21]. As the diagnosis of delirium may be mistaken for other conditions, including major neurocognitive disorders, depression, and psychotic spectrum illnesses, a careful and comprehensive assessment of the patient's history, including collateral history, is imperative. Families and caregivers should be interviewed regarding baseline cognitive status and any formal assessment of baseline cognitive status

Table 3.2 The differential diagnosis and differentiation of psychotic disorders in the elderly

Diagnosis	Criteria (selections from [11])	Time course
Delirium	• Fluctuating attention and awareness • Disturbance of cognition (new) • Not explained by a pre-existing neurocognitive disorder	Hours to days
Mild neurocognitive disorder	• Decline from premorbid function in at least one or more cognitive domains • Cognitive deficit does not interfere with independence or daily activity • Cognitive deficit is not due to delirium or better explained by another disorder	Months to years
Major neurocognitive disorder	• Significant decline in cognition and performance in at least one cognitive domain • Deficits interfere with everyday life • Cognitive deficit is not due to delirium or better explained by another disorder • Underlying etiology is specified	Months to years
Delusional disorder[a,b]	• One delusion, non-bizarre • Does not meet criteria for schizophrenia • Limited affective symptoms • Minimally impaired psychosocial functioning	>1 month to years
Brief psychotic disorder[a]	• Similar diagnostic criteria to schizophrenia, excepting duration • Psychosocial dysfunction must be present	Days to 1 month
Schizophreniform disorder[a,b]	• Psychosocial functioning not necessarily impaired	1 to 6 months
Schizophrenia[a,b]	• At least two of the following: delusions, hallucinations, disorganized thought, disorganized or catatonic behavior, negative symptoms	>6 months
Late-onset schizophrenia[a,b]	• Meets criteria for schizophrenia • Age of onset >40	>6 months
Very-late-onset schizophrenia-like psychosis[a,b]	• Meets criteria for schizophrenia • Age of onset >60	>6 months
Schizoaffective disorder[a]	• Delusions or hallucinations ≥ 2 weeks without a mood episode • Depression or mania must be present for the majority of a person's illness	>6 months
Substance- or medication-induced psychotic disorder[b]	• Hallucinations or delusions present • Psychosis directly related to the mechanism of a substance or medication	Hours to years
Psychotic disorder secondary to other medical condition[a,b]	• Hallucinations or delusions present • Psychosis directly related to the pathophysiology of the other medical condition	Months to years

[a]Symptoms cannot be better explained by substance use, another medical condition, or another mental disorder [2]
[b]Social and/or occupational dysfunction must be present

should be obtained. The timeline of change of mental status is a major indicator of delirium, i.e., hours to days rather than weeks to months or years for other conditions. Mental health treatment history, including standardized screening instruments for psychosis and depression, should be utilized whenever possible, as should standardized assessment of cognition at the time of evaluation [16,17]. Laboratory and diagnostic testing should be aimed at uncovering the underlying etiology of the delirium and frequently include neuroimaging and electroencephalography in addition to routine laboratory and radiologic testing for metabolic derangements and infectious etiologies [16,17].

To aid in diagnosis, several standardized instruments have been validated for use across multiple populations, including the Confusion Assessment Method (CAM), the CAM-S, which allows for measurement of severity and tracking response to treatment, the Four "A"s test, the 3-Minute Diagnostic Assessment, and the Family Confusion Assessment Method, which is reliant on caregivers and family for history [18,22–25].

Various "motor subtypes" of delirium have been observed. These motor subtypes include hyperactive, hypoactive, mixed, and non-motor variants [26,27]. These entities differ by presentation and are of clinical relevance, as morbidity and mortality rates vary amongst them. A recent study by Morandi and colleagues estimated 21.5% of delirium presentations are consistent with hyperactive delirium, 38.5% with hypoactive delirium, 27.3% with mixed hypoactive/hyperactive delirium, and 12.7% with non-motor delirium [27]. While both hypoactive and hyperactive delirium are associated with psychotic symptoms, hypoactive delirium is often overlooked in clinical settings and is notable for increased rates of morbidity and mortality, while hyperactive delirium has been linked to better detection, improved outcomes, and increased use of antipsychotic medications when compared to the hypoactive subtype [28].

Prevention of delirium or its timely diagnosis and treatment is of vital importance. It has been well established that delirium is a harbinger for longer hospital stays, declines in cognition and function, increased mortality and morbidity, and increased rates of institutionalization [28]. Multiple meta-analyses have confirmed the clinical utility and cost-effectiveness of various preventive strategies [17]. These include early mobilization, adequate hydration, sleep enhancement, orientation to time and place, therapeutic activities such as reminiscence (for cognitive stimulation), and hearing and vision optimization by using hearing and vision aids, as needed [17].

Regarding treatment, a recent Cochrane meta-analysis indicated that there is currently no good evidence to recommend the routine use of antipsychotics or other pharmacotherapies for the treatment of delirium in the elderly [29]. Due to the lack of high quality evidence for their benefit, antipsychotic medications are recommended only in cases of severe agitation, distress, or threats to the safety of the patient or those around them, and they should be administered for the shortest requisite duration. Their routine use is not supported at this time [17,29].

Dementia

Older adults with dementia (major neurocognitive disorders) comprise the largest group of patients with psychotic symptoms in later life. Indeed, approximately 40% experience either delusions or hallucinations during the course of their illness [10,30]. Psychotic symptoms in dementia are associated with worse cognitive and functional outcomes, increased rates of institutionalization, higher morbidity and mortality, and increased caregiver burnout [30,31]. These poorer outcomes in the context of dementia and psychosis emphasize the importance of accurate diagnosis and treatment of these illnesses.

The diagnosis of a major neurocognitive disorder, according to the DSM-5, is established by having a significant deficit in at least one cognitive domain and impairment in social or occupational functioning that is not better explained by another mental or physical condition, including delirium; for Alzheimer's disease, the memory/learning domain and one other domain must be impaired [11]. Neurocognitive disorders typically evolve over the course of months to years. Comprehensive geriatric assessment, neuropsychological testing, caregiver/family history, neuroimaging and laboratory testing for the reversible causes of dementia and potential etiologies for psychosis, as noted previously in this chapter, are vital. Final diagnosis should be withheld until all potentially reversible etiologies of cognitive decline have been identified and remedied. Family/caregiver history is valuable for reporting symptoms, functional decline, and the onset of illness – all of which are difficult to accurately elicit from the patient.

The presence of hallucinations and delusions varies across the different etiologies of major neurocognitive disorders and throughout the course of these illnesses. In Alzheimer's disease, the prevalence of hallucinations, dependent on the population sampled, ranges from 4 to 76%, while delusions are present in 16–70%. In major vascular neurocognitive disorder, the prevalence of hallucinations is similar to that found in Alzheimer's disease; however, the prevalence of delusions is relatively lower. Lewy body disease presents with three types of psychotic symptoms: hallucinations (predominantly visual, 25–83% prevalence), delusions (13–75% prevalence), and misidentification syndromes (29–50%). While visual hallucinations (most common) that occur in the context of Parkinson's disease are frequently benign with retained insight, those that occur in major neurocognitive disorder due to Parkinson's disease may be more complex in nature, distressing, and with loss of insight [10].

Psychotic symptoms that occur during Alzheimer's disease are perhaps the best categorized. Visual hallucinations are most common, followed by auditory hallucinations; perceptual disturbances in other modalities occur less frequently. The most common delusional beliefs in Alzheimer's disease are delusions of theft, loss, infidelity, persecution, and the belief that one's home is not one's own; misidentifications may also occur, such as the "mirror sign" (believing it is a stranger rather than oneself in the mirror) [10]. Temporally, delusions typically occur relatively early in the illness and hallucinations later. The literature suggests that hallucinations and delusions may represent distinct clinical, genetic, and pathophysiological processes, and that psychotic symptoms in Alzheimer's disease may have a differential effect on outcomes; the presence of hallucinations may denote a worse prognosis than the presence of delusions [31,32]. A more recent longitudinal study by Connors et al. found that both delusions and hallucinations contributed equally to morbidity and mortality in Alzheimer's disease [33].

With regard to the treatment of psychotic symptoms occurring in the course of neurocognitive disorders, the most recent expert guidelines unanimously recommend non-pharmacologic over pharmacologic management, due to the potential for morbidity and mortality related to pharmacologic treatment [15].

Non-pharmacologic approaches for psychosis in dementia

In general, non-pharmacologic approaches to psychosis in dementia should be first line. The American Psychiatric Association's guidelines (2016) state that pharmacologic treatment is indicated only if non-pharmacologic management has failed and/or the presenting symptoms cause significant distress to either the patient or the caregiver. If psychosis or agitation is associated with a potential danger to oneself or others, pharmacologic management may be first line [15].

The available evidence for non-pharmacologic management is strongest for approaches to the caregiver, including caregiver education, problem-solving regarding behavioral symptoms, and caregiver support. All these methods have shown significant reduction in neuropsychiatric symptoms in study subjects [34,35]. Adult day programs and environmental approaches that address over- and understimulation, excessive noise, lack of activity, and lack of routine have all shown a positive effect. Music therapy has also been shown to be effective in reducing aggression/agitation. Approaches with limited or inconsistent evidence include cognitive training, reminiscence therapy, validation therapy, acupuncture, aromatherapy, and light therapy [15,35–38].

Pharmacological approaches for psychosis in dementia

Cholinesterase inhibitors and memantine

There is some evidence that cognitive enhancing medications, in addition to their modest benefits for slowing cognitive decline, may improve overall neuropsychiatric symptoms, including psychosis, although improvement in psychosis in controlled studies has been inconsistent [39,40]. The benefits may be more pronounced for cholinesterase inhibitors in major neurocognitive disorder with Lewy bodies, and for major neurocognitive disorders due to Parkinson's disease than in other neurocognitive illnesses [41]. Several studies have found similar results for memantine in regard to reduction of overall neuropsychiatric symptom burden and psychosis; however, this was not replicated in a subsequent, larger, randomized controlled trial [42–47].

Antipsychotics for treatment of psychosis in dementia

Antipsychotic medications are used broadly for the treatment of dementia-related psychosis in the United States, despite none of these medications being officially approved by the FDA for this use. This widespread use of antipsychotics occurs despite a black box warning and mounting evidence for potential harm when using these medications for dementia-related psychosis [48]. Agitation, psychosis, and aggression are the symptom domains most likely to be improved by antipsychotic treatment; violence, caregiver distress, and patient distress may all be improved, as may quality of life, with these treatments [15]. Most studies have been conducted with second-generation antipsychotics; there are limited data available for first-generation antipsychotics in this population, as well as a paucity of data on comparative efficacy between first- and second-generation psychotics [15]. The literature suggests that side effect profiles are generally more favorable for second-generation antipsychotics versus first-generation [15].

The relatively modest benefits of antipsychotics are dramatically tempered by the increasing evidence for potential adverse effects, up to and including mortality. Meta-analyses have confirmed an increased risk of mortality for second-generation antipsychotics in treating these symptoms, with an estimated increase in mortality risk of 1 in 100 to 1 in 50 [49,50]. This response seems to be dose-dependent and highest during initiation of treatment (the first 120 days), with a smaller risk sustained throughout the treatment course [15]. The mortality risk remains controversial, and several prospective studies have found no increased risk for mortality in dementia patients [51]. Due to the potential risk associated with the use of these medications, current guidelines recommend an attempt at tapering and discontinuation within four months of treatment initiation. If symptoms of psychosis recur, the guidelines allow for the resumption of treatment.

Major neurocognitive disorder due to Parkinson's disease and major neurocognitive disorder with Lewy bodies present treatment challenges because of their high potential for severe adverse effects. Quetiapine was a first-choice antipsychotic treatment followed by clozapine if side effects developed with quetiapine, or if it was ineffective. More recently a new agent, pimavanserin, which is a 5HT2A inverse agonist, was approved for use with psychosis associated with Parkinson's disease [52,53]. This drug is being evaluated for alleviation of psychotic symptoms in AD, Lewy body dementia, and in schizophrenia.

For those patients who require antipsychotic medications, either due to distress or dangerous behaviors, recommended dosing ranges include [54,55]:

- Risperidone 0.25–1.5 mg
- Olanzapine 2.5–10 mg
- Quetiapine 12.5–200 mg
- Aripiprazole 2.5–12.5 mg

Antidepressants

Very little data exists on the use of antidepressants for psychosis and agitation in dementia [56]. Of the studies that do exist, only two found in the Cochrane database show some benefit of sertraline and citalopram on neuropsychiatric symptoms of dementia. Even so, the overall quality of evidence in these two studies is poor [56–58]. The Effect of Citalopram on Agitation in Alzheimer's Disease trial (CiTAD trial), a randomized, placebo-controlled, double-blind study with 186 participants, demonstrated that subjects who received citalopram showed significant improvement in overall neuropsychiatric measures and caregiver distress compared to placebo [59].

There is a paucity of investigations comparing antidepressant medications to antipsychotics in the treatment of psychosis in dementia; however, one study found that citalopram is as effective as risperidone [58]. Presumably, antidepressants would be better tolerated than antipsychotics and have fewer side effects. The use of citalopram in the CitAD trial yielded concerns about worsening of cognition and QT prolongation [59]. In a 2011 meta-analysis, there was no difference in withdrawal from studies due to adverse events between antipsychotics and SSRIs [56].

Psychotic disorders due to another medical condition

The diagnosis of psychotic disorders due to another medical condition should be thoroughly considered prior to the diagnosis of a primary psychotic disorder. This diagnosis is established through the presence of delusions or hallucinations that may be directly attributed to the pathophysiological process of a medical condition and cannot occur solely during the course of delirium. Assessment of the patient should proceed along the algorithm described previously in this chapter, including a comprehensive geriatric assessment with appropriate diagnostic testing based on history and physical examination. The potential diagnoses that have been linked to psychosis are myriad, including metabolic, infectious, neoplastic, and endocrine etiologies. Treatment of these conditions should proceed first with stabilization of the medical condition etiologically linked to the psychotic symptoms. If psychotic symptoms are severe and distressing, treatment with antipsychotic medications may be warranted. Time-limited treatment with minimum-necessary dosing should be the rule. According to expert consensus, the choice of antipsychotic should be based on each patient's individual history and medical comorbidities [10,60].

Substance/medication-induced psychotic disorder

Due to the large number of substances that may cause psychosis and the high prevalence of exposure to such substances in the elderly, clinical suspicion for substance/medication-induced psychotic disorders should always be high. This diagnosis is established when delusions and/or hallucinations are present and may be directly, temporally, and plausibly linked to a substance intoxication/withdrawal or exposure to a medication [61]. Multiple substances are considered to cause psychosis during intoxication, including alcohol, cannabis and its derivatives, hallucinogens, inhalants, sedatives/hypnotics, and stimulants [61]. Furthermore, alcohol and sedatives/hypnotics are linked to psychosis during withdrawal [61]. The most commonly implicated medications in these conditions are dopamine agonists, anticholinergics, cimetidine, corticosteroids, digoxin, antiarrhythmics, and immunotherapies, particularly interferon [62]. At the time of publication there are no controlled studies on the treatment of substance/medication-induced psychotic disorders in the elderly. Evidence-based treatments (psychotherapeutic and pharmacologic) for substance-use disorders should be used with the goal of obtaining remission from substance use. As with psychotic disorders due to another medical condition, antipsychotic medications may be used in the context of severe, distressing, or dangerous symptoms. Antipsychotic medication should be dose- and time-limited, with choice of antipsychotic based on an individual's medical comorbidities and the features of his or her illness.

Schizophrenia-spectrum disorders

Schizophrenia

The diagnosis of schizophrenia is established according to DSM-5 criteria. It requires the presence of a disturbance lasting at least six months with two or more of the following symptoms actively present for at least one month: delusions, hallucinations, disorganized speech, grossly disorganized or catatonic behavior, and/or negative symptoms [61]. These diagnostic criteria hold for both early- and late-onset schizophrenia, though the International Late-onset Schizophrenia Group has proposed subdividing the disorder into distinct categories based on age of onset. Early-onset schizophrenia is defined as schizophrenia that occurs before the age of 40, while late-onset schizophrenia is defined as illness with onset between the ages of 40 and 60, and very-late-onset schizophrenia-like psychosis is defined as disease that occurs after the age of 60 [63]. The subcategorization of schizophrenia into these groups is clinically important due to phenomenological differences and varied treatment needs. Most (75–80%) of schizophrenia cases in late life are early onset, with only 20–25% being late onset, and an incidence of only 7.5 in 100 000 accounting for very-late-onset schizophrenia-like-psychosis [64].

There are some clinical and phenomenological differences in the subtypes of schizophrenia in later life. Older adults with early-onset schizophrenia experience a mild cognitive impairment at the onset of their illness, but appear to undergo otherwise normal cognitive aging. Psychosocial functioning tends to improve with age as symptoms of psychosis and hospitalization rates decline. Conversely, these individuals experience accelerated physical aging with increased medical and psychiatric comorbidities, and decreased life expectancy when compared to healthy controls. Age of onset does not appear to affect the increased rates of mortality observed in older adults with schizophrenia. Furthermore, there are increased rates of depression and suicide in older adults with schizophrenia [65].

The extent to which late-onset schizophrenia differs from the early-onset disorder is a disputed area among investigators. In general, late-onset schizophrenia has been found to be different from early-onset schizophrenia in various respects: women are more likely to be affected than men, there is reduced incidence of hallucinations, delusions, and disorganization, there is a lower dose requirement for antipsychotics, there are increased persecutory-type delusions, hallucinations in other sensory modalities (visual, tactile, olfactory) are more commonly reported than auditory hallucinations, and there are increased sensory impairments [66–69].

Very-late-onset schizophrenia-like psychosis appears to be less heritable and is characterized by a higher prevalence in women than either early-onset or late-onset schizophrenia, higher prevalence of partition persecutory delusions, and decreased prevalence of thought disorder and negative symptoms. Higher prevalence of neurologic abnormalities, however, has been found in some studies [63].

A more detailed discussion about early- and late-onset schizophrenia is found in Chapter 4.

Treatment

There is limited literature on treatments for schizophrenia patients over the age of 65. A 2012 Cochrane review found no studies meeting quality criteria for a meaningful review [70]. In older patients with early-onset schizophrenia, the majority of available data have demonstrated some evidence for the use of risperidone and olanzapine [51,71]. Though limited, there is also some evidence for the use of clozapine for treatment-resistant elderly patients [72]. Another study demonstrated the superiority of paliperidone over placebo in patients over 65 [73].

Antipsychotic dosing for elderly patients with schizophrenia is often lower than in younger patients [10]. For late-onset schizophrenia, starting doses of antipsychotics should be 25% of a typical adult dose with maintenance doses of 25–50% of young adult doses. Similarly, patients over 65 years of age who have early-onset schizophrenia can often be maintained at lower antipsychotic doses (50–75% of typical adult doses) [10]. A recent study supporting this clinical experience in dosing ranges has been conducted in which an antipsychotic dose reduction of up to 40% in patients with late-life schizophrenia yielded evidence that D2/D3 receptor occupancy therapeutic windows were lower in elderly patients (50–60% receptor occupancy in older patients as compared to 65–80% receptor occupancy in younger patients) [74].

Clinical experience and consensus guidelines support the use of the following antipsychotics (with dose ranges) for late-life schizophrenia [60]:

- Risperidone 1.25–3.5 mg
- Quetiapine 100–300 mg
- Olanzapine 7.5–15 mg
- Aripiprazole 15–30 mg

Chapter 13 in this volume provides an extensive review of pharmacological approaches to psychotic disorders.

Non-pharmacological management of schizophrenia in late-life schizophrenia

When possible, non-pharmacological interventions for schizophrenia should be first line or used concomitantly with pharmacotherapy. Recent years have brought advances in evidence-based methodology in this population group. The overall benefits of these approaches include short-term improvements in community living skills/functioning, self-efficacy, and negative symptom burden [75–80].

Chapter 14 provides an overview of various non-pharmacological approaches in schizophrenia.

Schizoaffective disorder

While there is a paucity of studies available on schizoaffective disorder in older adults, the extant data consistently found schizoaffective disorder to be epidemiologically and clinically more akin to schizophrenia than bipolar disorder. Meesters and coauthors estimated the 12-month prevalence of schizoaffective disorder in adults over the age of 60 to be 0.14% [81]. In contrast to older people with schizophrenia, those with schizoaffective disorder have increased treatment resistance, risk of suicide, and severity of illness [82]. Those patients with the depressive type of schizoaffective disorder may be at higher risk for suicide than those with the bipolar type [83].

Studies on treatment of schizoaffective disorder are minimal, in both young and older patients. Patients with schizoaffective disorder have been included in studies on schizophrenia in later life [51]. As an extrapolation from treatment of younger patients, recommendations include starting with low doses of antipsychotic medication (increasing slowly as needed), along with careful use of mood stabilizers and antidepressants at the lowest effective dose [10].

Delusional disorder

Delusional disorder is diagnosed according to DSM-5 by the presence of non-bizarre delusions without prominent hallucinations, lasting one month or longer [84]. Prevalence of delusional disorder in the elderly is estimated at 0.03%, with a slight female predominance and impaired social functioning, but with minimal change to cognition, personality, or occupational function [85,86].

The treatment of delusional disorder is not well investigated. Despite the older age of onset for this disorder (middle or late adulthood), there are no specific studies for the treatment of delusional disorder in patients over 65. A review of the literature on younger patients reveals that risperidone and olanzapine are the most widely used treatments for the disorder, with some limited evidence for their efficacy [87]. Risperidone and olanzapine have been found to be as effective as pimozide, once thought to be the first-line treatment for delusional disorder [87].

Major depressive disorder with psychotic features

Major depressive disorder (MDD) is a common disorder in adults aged 55 and over, with prevalence estimates ranging from 4 to 7% [88–90]. In people 65 and over, the National Comorbidity Survey Replication found 12-month prevalence rates of 2.6% and a lifetime prevalence rate of 9.8% [90]. In the DSM-5, psychosis in MDD is denoted by a diagnostic specifier, "with psychotic features" that may be further categorized using the specifiers "with mood [congruent] psychotic features" or "with mood [incongruent] psychotic features" [11]. The former is described as delusions and hallucinations that are "consistent with the typical depressive themes of personal inadequacy, guilt, disease, death, nihilism, or deserved punishment". Mood incongruent features are classified as delusions or hallucinations that do not involve the aforementioned themes or that contain a mixture of mood-incongruent and mood-congruent themes.

Elderly patients with depression are more likely to have psychotic features and exhibit treatment resistance, a factor that may be related to the increased cerebrovascular risk in this population [91]. A recent study identified that baseline cerebrovascular risk score was an independent risk factor for treatment resistance in the elderly [92]. Furthermore, in both elderly and younger patients, there is some evidence that SSRIs and TCAs are less effective for depression with psychotic features, whereas ECT is more or equally effective in treatment of psychotic depression as compared to non-psychotic depression [93]. For these reasons, electroconvulsive therapy should be considered early in treatment, particularly in the frail elderly [94,95].

While there are no specific studies in the elderly, there is evidence that a combination of treatment with antipsychotic and antidepressant medications is superior to monotherapy with either treatment, in randomized controlled trials and by expert consensus, and this is reflected in most international guidelines [96,97]. The few randomized controlled trials that have been conducted in this area demonstrate efficacy for the following combination therapies: olanzapine with sertraline (over monotherapy with olanzapine) and olanzapine with fluoxetine (over placebo and monotherapy with olanzapine) [98,99].

Bipolar disorder

In DSM-5, both bipolar I and bipolar II disorders have psychotic specifiers. It is also important to note that psychotic symptoms may be present during manic, hypomanic, or depressive episodes [11]. As with major depressive disorder, psychoses are defined by the presence of hallucinations or delusions. Likewise, they are classified as "congruent" or "incongruent." The former consists of hallucinations or delusions that are "typical manic themes of grandiosity, invulnerability, etc., but may also include themes of suspiciousness or paranoia, especially with respect to others' doubts about the individual's capacities, accomplishments, and so forth" [11]. Incongruent psychotic symptoms contain hallucinations or delusions that do not involve these themes or that contain a mixture of mood-incongruent and mood-congruent themes. An important diagnostic consideration is that late-onset bipolar illness is often secondary to a medical/neurological disease or may be drug-induced.

There are few available studies on treatment of older patients with bipolar disorder. A recent study, the GERI-BD trial (treatment of bipolar mania in older adults study), found that divalproex and lithium were well-tolerated and efficacious; lithium treatment, however, resulted in a greater reduction of mania scores [100]. The use of lithium in the elderly, despite its superior efficacy in classic mania, often prompts concerns about adverse effects; however, an administrative database study found no differences in acute care utilization and medical comorbidity in elderly patients with bipolar disorder who were treated with lithium, as compared to divalproex or atypical antipsychotics, suggesting that lithium does not lead to worsened acute health outcomes [101]. Clearly, further studies will need to be conducted to further delineate the benefits and risks of these medications in patients over 65.

Regarding the use of antipsychotics, all second-generation antipsychotics (except clozapine) are indicated for psychosis in the setting of acute mania, although evidence to guide use in geriatric populations is limited [102]. In studies that included and specifically assessed older patients with acute mania, the superiority of olanzapine monotherapy over divalproex monotherapy was noted [102]. Additionally, quetiapine was found to be more effective than placebo in the treatment of mania for patients of all ages, demonstrating superior efficacy in older patients as compared to younger patients [103]. There is also evidence from a small, prospective open-label trial (N = 15) suggesting that asenapine may be effective for older patients with acute mania [104].

Conclusion

1. Psychotic disorders are very common with a lifetime prevalence of nearly 25%, with risk increasing with advanced age. Point prevalence varies with settings, ranging from 5–63% percent. Prevalence rates of psychotic symptoms in older adults in the general community have ranged from 1 to 13.4%, with a median value of 3.6%.

2. Psychotic disorders can be divided into those primary disorders (two-fifths of cases) that are due to the direct effect of a psychiatric disorder and secondary disorders (three-fifths of cases) that are caused by a non-psychiatric condition. Dementia is the most common cause of psychoses (40% of cases).

3. The mnemonic "Six Ds" can be used to remember the principal causes of psychotic disorders: Disease, Delirium, Drugs, Dementia, Depression and mania, and Delusions and schizophrenia-spectrum disorders.

4. Whenever possible, primary psychiatric illness should never be diagnosed pending exclusion of causation by another medical condition or substance as treatment may vary broadly based on etiology, although sometimes it is difficult to initially identify underlying medical or neurological causes.

5. Diagnostic concerns in older adults include the possibility of a second psychotic disorder arising alongside an existing psychotic disorder. Importantly, secondary disorders may initially resemble a primary disorder.

6. While there are no pathognomonic signs to differentiate psychosis caused by psychiatric illness from that caused by another physiological condition, there are some characteristics that may serve to distinguish the latter from the former: acuity of onset (days to weeks), atypical age of onset, visual hallucinations without auditory hallucinations, lack of past psychiatric or family history, severe or treatment-resistant symptoms, symptoms occurring after a change in personality, symptoms occurring in conjunction with a medical disease, cognitive abnormalities, and medication/substance abuse. Research is needed to develop more biological and clinical assessment tools that can enhance diagnostic accuracy.

7. There are very few controlled studies evaluating pharmacological treatment for any of the psychotic disorders in later life. Most treatment guidelines have been developed through expert consensus panels. Antipsychotics are most commonly

used, but there is concern regarding increased morbidity and mortality in older patients. Novel agents such as pimavanserin, which is a 5HT2A inverse agonist, may have utility beyond their current use for psychosis in Parkinson's disease.

8. Whenever possible, psychosocial interventions should be tried initially, and medication should be used only when the former has failed or when symptoms are so severe that they present a danger to the patient or other people.

References

1. Arciniegas, D.B., Psychosis. *Continuum: Lifelong Learning in Neurology*, 2015. **21**(3 Behavioral Neurology and Neuropsychiatry): p. 715.

2. Holroyd, S. and S. Laurie, Correlates of psychotic symptoms among elderly outpatients. *International Journal of Geriatric Psychiatry*, 1999. **14**(5): p. 379–84.

3. Karim, S. and E.J. Byrne, Treatment of psychosis in elderly people. *Advances in Psychiatric Treatment*, 2005. **11**: p. 286–96.

4. Sigström, R., I. Skoog, S. Sacuiu, et al., The prevalence of psychotic symptoms and paranoid ideation in non-demented population samples aged 70–82 years. *International Journal of Geriatric Psychiatry*, 2009. **24**(12): p. 1413–19.

5. Subramaniam, M., E. Abdin, J. Vaingankar, et al., Prevalence of psychotic symptoms among older adults in an Asian population. *International Psychogeriatrics*, 2016. **28**(7): p. 1211–20.

6. Soares, W.B., S.R.I. Ribeiz, D.P. Bassitt, M.C. De Oliveira, and C.M.C. Bottino, Psychotic symptoms in older people without dementia from a Brazilian community-based sample. *International Journal of Geriatric Psychiatry*, 2015. **30**(5): p. 437–45.

7. Cohen, C.I., C. Magai, R. Yaffee, and L. Walcott-Brown, Racial differences in paranoid ideation and psychoses in an older urban population. *American Journal of Psychiatry*, 2004. **161**(5): p. 864–71.

8. Manepalli, J.N., M. Gebretsadik, J. Hook, and G. Grossberg, Differential diagnosis of the older patient with psychotic symptoms. *Primary Psychiatry*, 2007. **14**(8): p. 55–62.

9. Webster, J. and G.T. Grossberg, Late-life onset of psychotic symptoms. *American Journal of Geriatric Psychiatry*, 1998. **6**(3): p. 196–202.

10. Reinhardt, M.M. and C.I. Cohen, Late-life psychosis: diagnosis and treatment. *Current Psychiatry Reports*, 2015. **17**(2): p. 1.

11. American Psychiatric Association, *Diagnostic and Statistical Manual of Mental Disorders (DSM-5®)*. 2013, Arlington, VA: American Psychiatric Association.

12. Christenson, R. and D. Blazer, Epidemiology of persecutory ideation in an elderly population in the community. *American Journal of Psychiatry*, 1984. **141**(9): p. 1088–91.

13. Östling, S., K. Bäckman, M. Waern, et al., Paranoid symptoms and hallucinations among the older people in Western Europe. *International Journal of Geriatric Psychiatry*, 2013. **28**(6): p. 573–9.

14. Ciompi, L., Catamnestic long-term study on the course of life and aging of schizophrenics. *Schizophrenia Bulletin*, 1980. **6**(4): p. 606.

15. American Psychiatric Association, *The American Association of Psychiatry Practice Guideline on the Use of Antipsychotics to Treat Agitation or Psychosis in Patients with Dementia*. 2016, Arlington, VA: American Psychiatric Association.

16. Inouye, S.K., R.G.J. Westendorp, and J.S. Saczynski, Delirium in elderly people. *Lancet*, 2014. **383**(9920): p. 911–22.

17. Oh, E.S., T.G. Fong, T.T. Hshieh, et al., Delirium in older persons: advances in diagnosis and treatment. *Journal of the American Medical Association*, 2017. **318**(12): p. 1161–74.

18. Inouye, S.K., C.H. van Dyck, C.A. Alessi, et al., Clarifying confusion: the confusion assessment method: a new method for detection of delirium. *Annals of Internal Medicine*, 1990. **113**(12): p. 941–8.

19. Boettger, S. and W. Breitbart, Phenomenology of the subtypes of delirium: phenomenological differences between hyperactive and hypoactive delirium. *Palliative and Supportive Care*, 2011. **9**(2): p. 129–35.

20. Meagher, D.J., M. Moran, B. Raju, et al., Phenomenology of delirium: assessment of 100 adult cases using standardised measures. *British Journal of Psychiatry*, 2007. **190**: p. 135–41.

21. Webster, R. and S. Holroyd, Prevalence of psychotic symptoms in delirium. *Psychosomatics*, 2000. **41**(6): p. 519–22.

22. Inouye, S.K., C.M. Kosar, D. Tommet, et al., The CAM-S: development and validation of a new scoring system for delirium severity in 2 cohorts. *Annals of Internal Medicine*, 2014. **160**(8): p. 526–33.

23. Bellelli, G., A. Morandi, D.H.J. Davis, et al., Validation of the 4AT, a new instrument for rapid delirium screening: a study in 234 hospitalised older people. *Age and Ageing*, 2014. **43**(4): p. 496–502.

24. Marcantonio, E.R., L.H. Ngo, M. O'Connor, et al., 3D-CAM: derivation and validation of a 3-minute diagnostic interview for CAM-defined delirium: a cross-sectional diagnostic test study. *Annals of Internal Medicine*, 2014. **161**(8): p. 554–61.

25. Steis, M.R., L. Evans, K.B. Hirschman, et al., Screening for delirium using family caregivers: convergent validity of the Family Confusion Assessment Method and interviewer-rated confusion assessment method. *Journal of the American Geriatrics Society*, 2012. **60**(11): p. 2121–6.

26. Lipowski, Z., *Delirium: Acute Confusional States*. 1990, New York: Oxford University Press, p. 97.

27. Morandi, A., S.G. Di Santo, A. Cherubini, et al., Clinical features associated with delirium motor subtypes in older inpatients: results of a multicenter study. *American Journal of Geriatric Psychiatry*. **25**(10): p. 1064–71.

28. Witlox, J., L.S.M. Eurelings, J.F.M. de Jonghe, et al., Delirium in elderly patients and the risk of postdischarge mortality, institutionalization, and dementia: a meta-analysis. *Journal of the American Medical Association*, 2010. **304**(4): p. 443–51.

29. Siddiqi, N., J.K. Harrison, A. Clegg, et al., Interventions for preventing delirium in hospitalised non-ICU patients. *Cochrane Database of Systematic Reviews*, 2016: CD005563.

30. Ropacki, S.A. and D.V. Jeste, Epidemiology of and risk factors for psychosis of Alzheimer's disease: a review of 55 studies published from 1990 to 2003. *American Journal of Psychiatry*, 2005. **162**(11): p. 2022–30.

31. Scarmeas, N., J. Brandt, M. Albert, et al., Delusions and hallucinations are associated with worse outcome in Alzheimer disease. *Archives of Neurology*, 2005. **62**(10): p. 1601–8.

32. Murray, P.S., S. Kumar, M.A. Demichele-Sweet, and R.A. Sweet, Psychosis in Alzheimer's disease. *Biological Psychiatry*, 2014. **75**(7): p. 542–52.

33. Connors, M.H., D. Ames, M. Woodward, and H. Brodaty, Psychosis and clinical outcomes in Alzheimer disease: a longitudinal study. *American Journal of Geriatric Psychiatry*. **26**(3): p. 304–13.

34. Kales, H.C., L.N. Gitlin, and C.G. Lyketsos, Assessment and management of behavioral and psychological symptoms of dementia. *British Medical Journal*, 2015. **350**: p. h369.

35. Brodaty, H. and C. Arasaratnam, Meta-analysis of nonpharmacological interventions for neuropsychiatric symptoms of dementia. *American Journal of Psychiatry*, 2012. **169**(9): p. 946–53.

36. Clare, L., R.T. Woods, E.D. Moniz Cook, M. Orrell, and A. Spector, Cognitive rehabilitation and cognitive training for early-stage Alzheimer's disease and vascular dementia. *Cochrane Database of Systematic Reviews*, 2003. (4): CD003260.

37. Forbes, D., I. Culum, A.R. Lischka, et al., Light therapy for managing cognitive, sleep, functional, behavioural, or psychiatric disturbances in dementia. *Cochrane Database of Systematic Reviews*, 2009(4): CD003946.

38. Thorgrimsen, L., T.P.H. Birks, L.M. Thorgrimsen, et al., Aroma therapy for dementia. *Cochrane Database of Systematic Reviews*, 2003(3): CD003150.

39. Rodda, J., S. Morgan, and Z. Walker, Are cholinesterase inhibitors effective in the management of the behavioral and psychological symptoms of dementia in Alzheimer's disease? A systematic review of randomized, placebo-controlled trials of donepezil, rivastigmine and galantamine. *International Psychogeriatrics*, 2009. 21(5): p. 813–24.

40. Trinh, N.H., J. Hoblyn, S. Mohanty, and K. Yaffe, Efficacy of cholinesterase inhibitors in the treatment of neuropsychiatric symptoms and functional impairment in Alzheimer disease: a meta-analysis. *Journal of the American Medical Association*, 2003. 289(2): p. 210–16.

41. Rolinski, M., C. Fox, I. Maidment, and R. McShane, Cholinesterase inhibitors for dementia with Lewy bodies, Parkinson's disease dementia and cognitive impairment in Parkinson's disease. *Cochrane Database of Systematic Reviews*, 2012(3): CD006504.

42. Cumbo, E. and L.D. Ligori, Differential effects of current specific treatments on behavioral and psychological symptoms in patients with Alzheimer's disease: a 12-month, randomized, open-label trial. *Journal of Alzheimer's Disease*, 2014. 39(3): p. 477–85.

43. Gauthier, S., H. Loft, and J. Cummings, Improvement in behavioural symptoms in patients with moderate to severe Alzheimer's disease by memantine: a pooled data analysis. *International Journal of Geriatric Psychiatry*, 2008. 23(5): p. 537–45.

44. Lachaine, J., C. Beauchemin, A. Crochard, and S. Bineau, The impact of memantine and cholinesterase inhibitor initiation for Alzheimer disease on the use of antipsychotic agents: analysis using the Regie de l'Assurance Maladie du Quebec Database. *Canadian Journal of Psychiatry*, 2013. 58(4): p. 195–200.

45. Gauthier, S., Y. Wirth, and H.J. Mobius, Effects of memantine on behavioural symptoms in Alzheimer's disease patients: an analysis of the Neuropsychiatric Inventory (NPI) data of two randomised, controlled studies. *International Journal of Geriatric Psychiatry*, 2005. 20(5): p. 459–64.

46. Wilcock, G.K., C.G. Ballard, J.A. Cooper, and H. Loft, Memantine for agitation/aggression and psychosis in moderately severe to severe Alzheimer's disease: a pooled analysis of 3 studies. *Journal of Clinical Psychiatry*, 2008. 69(3): p. 341–8.

47. McShane, R., A. Areosa Sastre, and N. Minakaran, Memantine for dementia. *Cochrane Database of Systematic Reviews*, 2006(2): CD003154.

48. Jeste, D.V., D. Blazer, D. Casey, et al., ACNP White Paper: update on use of antipsychotic drugs in elderly persons with dementia. *Neuropsychopharmacology*, 2008. 33(5): p. 957–70.

49. Schneider, L.S., K. Dagerman, and P.S. Insel, Efficacy and adverse effects of atypical antipsychotics for dementia: meta-analysis of randomized, placebo-controlled trials. *American Journal of Geriatric Psychiatry*, 2006. 14(3): p. 191–210.

50. Schneider, L.S., K.S. Dagerman, and P. Insel, Risk of death with atypical antipsychotic drug treatment for dementia: meta-analysis of randomized placebo-controlled trials. *Journal of the American Medical Association*, 2005. 294(15): p. 1934–43.

51. Jeste, D.V., Y. Barak, S. Madhusoodanan, F. Grossman, and G. Gharabawi, International multisite double-blind trial of the atypical antipsychotics risperidone and olanzapine in 175 elderly patients with chronic schizophrenia. *American Journal of Geriatric Psychiatry*, 2003. 11(6): p. 638–47.

52. Cummings, J., S. Isaacson, R. Mills, et al., Pimavanserin for patients with Parkinson's disease psychosis: a randomised, placebo-controlled phase 3 trial. *Lancet*, 2014. **383**(9916): p. 533–40.

53. Fox, S.H., Pimavanserin as treatment for Parkinson's disease psychosis. *Lancet*, 2014. **383**(9916): p. 494–6.

54. Maher, A.R., M. Maglione, S. Bagley, et al., Efficacy and comparative effectiveness of atypical antipsychotic medications for off-label uses in adults: a systematic review and meta-analysis. *Journal of the American Medical Association*, 2011. **306**(12): p. 1359–69.

55. Meeks, T.W. and D.V. Jeste, Beyond the black box: what is the role for antipsychotics in dementia? *Current Psychiatry*, 2008. **7**(6): p. 50–65.

56. Seitz, D.P., N. Adunuri, S.S. Gill, et al., Antidepressants for agitation and psychosis in dementia. *Cochrane Database of Systematic Reviews*, 2011(2): CD008191.

57. Finkel, S.I., J.E. Mintzer, M. Dysken, et al., A randomized, placebo-controlled study of the efficacy and safety of sertraline in the treatment of the behavioral manifestations of Alzheimer's disease in outpatients treated with donepezil. *International Journal of Geriatric Psychiatry*, 2004. **19**(1): p. 9–18.

58. Pollock, B.G., B.H. Mulsant, J. Rosen, et al., A double-blind comparison of citalopram and risperidone for the treatment of behavioral and psychotic symptoms associated with dementia. *American Journal of Geriatric Psychiatry*, 2007. **15**(11): p. 942–52.

59. Porsteinsson, A.P., L.T. Drye, B.G. Pollock, et al., Effect of citalopram on agitation in Alzheimer disease: the CitAD randomized clinical trial. *Journal of the American Medical Association*, 2014. **311**(7): p. 682–91.

60. Alexopoulos, G.S., J.E. Streim, and D. Carpenter, Commentary: expert consensus guidelines for using antipsychotic agents in older patients. *The Journal of Clinical Psychiatry*, 2004. **65**(suppl 2): p. 100–2.

61. American Psychiatric Association, *Diagnostic and Statistical Manual of Mental Disorders (DSM-5®)*. 2013, Arlington, VA: American Psychiatric Association.

62. Brunelle, S., M.G. Cole, and M. Elie, Risk factors for the late-onset psychoses: a systematic review of cohort studies. *International Journal of Geriatric Psychiatry*, 2012. **27**(3): p. 240–52.

63. Howard, R., P.V. Rabins, M.V. Seeman, and D.V. Jeste, Late-onset schizophrenia and very-late-onset schizophrenia-like psychosis: An international consensus. *American Journal of Psychiatry*, 2000. **157**(2): p. 172–8.

64. Stafford, J., R. Howard, and J.B. Kirkbride, The incidence of very late-onset psychotic disorders: a systematic review and meta-analysis, 1960-2016. *Psychological Medicine*, 2017: p. 1–2.

65. Cohen, C.I., P.D. Meesters, and J. Zhao, New perspectives on schizophrenia into later life: Implications for treatment, policy, and research. *Lancet Psychiatry*, 2015. **2**(4): p. 340–50.

66. Palmer, B.W., F.S. McClure, and D.V. Jeste, Schizophrenia in late life: findings challenge traditional concepts. *Harvard Review of Psychiatry*, 2001. **9**(2): p. 51–8.

67. Vahia, I.V., B.W. Palmer, C. Depp, et al., Is late-onset schizophrenia a subtype of schizophrenia? *Acta Psychiatrica Scandinavica*, 2010. **122**(5): p. 414–26.

68. Iglewicz, A., T.W. Meeks, and D.V. Jeste, New wine in old bottle: late-life psychosis. *Psychiatric Clinics of North America*, 2011. **34**(2): p. 295–318.

69. Howard, R., O. Almeida, and R. Levy, Phenomenology, demography and diagnosis in late paraphrenia. *Psychological Medicine*, 1994. **24**(02): p. 397–410.

70. Essali, A. and G. Ali, Antipsychotic drug treatment for elderly people with late-onset schizophrenia. *Cochrane Database of Systematic Reviews*, 2012. (2): CD004162.

71. Marriott, R.G., W. Neil, and S. Waddingham, Antipsychotic medication for elderly people with schizophrenia.

Cochrane Database of Systematic Reviews, 2006(1): CD005580.

72. Suzuki, T., G. Remington, H. Uchida, et al., Management of schizophrenia in late life with antipsychotic medications: a qualitative review. *Drugs and Aging*, 2011. **28**(12): p. 961–80.

73. Tzimos, A., V. Samokhvalov, M. Kramer, et al., Safety and tolerability of oral paliperidone extended-release tablets in elderly patients with schizophrenia: a double-blind, placebo-controlled study with six-month open-label extension. *American Journal of Geriatric Psychiatry*, 2008. **16**(1): p. 31–43.

74. Graff-Guerrero, A., T.K. Rajji, B.H. Mulsant, et al., Evaluation of antipsychotic dose reduction in late-life schizophrenia: a prospective dopamine D2/3 receptor occupancy study. *JAMA Psychiatry*, 2015. **72**(9): p. 927–34.

75. Granholm, E., J.R. McQuaid, F.S. McClure, et al., A randomized, controlled trial of cognitive behavioral social skills training for middle-aged and older outpatients with chronic schizophrenia. *American Journal of Psychiatry*, 2005. **162**(3): p. 520–9.

76. Granholm, E., J.R. McQuaid, F.S. McClure, et al., Randomized controlled trial of cognitive behavioral social skills training for older people with schizophrenia: 12-month follow-up. *Journal of Clinical Psychiatry*, 2007. **68**(5): p. 730–7.

77. Patterson, T.L., J. Bucardo, C.L. McKibbin, et al., Development and pilot testing of a new psychosocial intervention for older Latinos with chronic psychosis. *Schizophrenia Bulletin*, 2005. **31**(4): p. 922–30.

78. Patterson, T.L., B.T. Mausbach, C. McKibbin, et al., Functional Adaptation Skills Training (FAST): A randomized trial of a psychosocial intervention for middle-aged and older patients with chronic psychotic disorders. *Schizophrenia Research*, 2006. **86**(1-3): p. 291–9.

79. Bartels, S.J., S.I. Pratt, K.T. Mueser, et al., Long-term outcomes of a randomized trial of integrated skills training and preventive healthcare for older adults with serious mental illness. *American Journal of Geriatric Psychiatry*, 2014. **22**(11): p. 1251–61.

80. Mueser, K.T., S.I. Pratt, S.J. Bartels, et al., Randomized trial of social rehabilitation and integrated health care for older people with severe mental illness. *Journal of Consulting and Clinical Psychology*, 2010. **78**(4): p. 561–73.

81. Meesters, P.D., L. Haan, H.C. Comijs, et al., Schizophrenia spectrum disorders in later life: prevalence and distribution of age at onset and sex in a Dutch catchment area. *American Journal of Geriatric Psychiatry*, 2012. **20**(1): p. 18–28.

82. Post, F., Schizo-affective symptomatology in late life. *British Journal of Psychiatry*, 1971. **118**(545): p. 437–45.

83. Baran, X.Y. and R.C. Young, Bipolar and depressive types of schizoaffective disorder in old age. *American Journal of Geriatric Psychiatry*, 2006. **14**(4): p. 382–3.

84. Kendler, K.S., Demography of paranoid psychosis (delusional disorder): a review and comparison with schizophrenia and affective illness. *Archives of General Psychiatry*, 1982. **39**(8): p. 890–902.

85. Maher, B., Delusional thinking and cognitive disorder. *Integrative Physiological and Behavioral Science*, 2005. **40**(3): p. 136–46.

86. Maglione, J.E., I.V. Vahia, and D.V. Jeste, Schizophrenia spectrum and other psychotic disorders. In *The American Psychiatric Publishing Textbook of Geriatric Psychiatry*, ed. D.C. Steffens, D.G. Blazer, and M.E. Thakur, 2015.

87. Mews, M.R. and A. Quante, Comparative efficacy and acceptability of existing pharmacotherapies for delusional disorder: a retrospective case series and review of the literature. *Journal of Clinical Psychopharmacology*, 2013. **33**(4): p. 512–19.

88. Byers, A.L., K. Yaffe, K.E. Covinsky, et al., High occurrence of mood and anxiety disorders among older adults: The National Comorbidity Survey Replication. *Archives of General Psychiatry*, 2010. **67**(5): p. 489–96.

89. Luppa, M., C. Sikorski, T. Luck, et al., Age- and gender-specific prevalence of depression in latest-life: systematic review and meta-analysis. *Journal of Affective Disorders*, 2012. **136**(3): p. 212–21.

90. Kessler, R.C., P. Berglund, O. Demler, et al., Lifetime prevalence and age-of-onset distributions of DSM-IV disorders in the national comorbidity survey replication. *Archives of General Psychiatry*, 2005. **62**(6): p. 593–602.

91. Brodaty, H., G. Luscombe, G. Parker, et al., Increased rate of psychosis and psychomotor change in depression with age. *Psychological Medicine*, 1997. **27**(5): p. 1205–13.

92. Bingham, K.S., E.M. Whyte, B.S. Meyers, et al., Relationship between cerebrovascular risk, cognition, and treatment outcome in late-life psychotic depression. *American Journal of Geriatric Psychiatry*, 2015. **23**(12): p. 1270–5.

93. Nelson, E.B., Psychotic depression: beyond the antidepressant/antipsychotic combination. *Current Psychiatry Reports*, 2012. **14**(6): p. 619–23.

94. Andreescu, C., B.H. Mulsant, A.J. Rothschild, et al., Pharmacotherapy of major depression with psychotic features: what is the evidence? *Psychiatric Annals*, 2006. **36**(1): p. 31–8.

95. Geduldig, E.T. and C.H. Kellner, Electroconvulsive therapy in the elderly: new findings in geriatric depression. *Current Psychiatry Reports*, 2016. **18**(4): p. 40.

96. Wijkstra, J., J. Lijmer, H. Burger, et al., Pharmacological treatment for psychotic depression. *Cochrane Database of Systematic Reviews*, 2015(7): p. CD004044.

97. Leadholm, A.K., A.J. Rothschild, W.A. Nolen, et al., The treatment of psychotic depression: is there consensus among guidelines and psychiatrists? *Journal of Affective Disorders*, 2013. **145**(2): p. 214–20.

98. Meyers, B.S., A.J. Flint, A.J. Rothschild, et al., A double-blind randomized controlled trial of olanzapine plus sertraline vs olanzapine plus placebo for psychotic depression. *Archives of General Psychiatry*, 2009. **66**(8): p. 838–47.

99. Rothschild, A.J., D.J. Williamson, M.F. Tohen, et al., A double-blind, randomized study of olanzapine and olanzapine/fluoxetine combination for major depression with psychotic features. *Journal of Clinical Psychopharmacology*, 2004. **24**(4): p. 365–73.

100. Young, R.C., B.H. Mulsant, M. Sajatovic, et al., GERI-BD: a randomized double-blind controlled trial of lithium and divalproex in the treatment of mania in older patients with bipolar disorder. *American Journal of Psychiatry*, 2017. **174**(11): p. 1086–93.

101. Rej, S., C. Yu, K. Shulman, et al., Medical comorbidity, acute medical care use in late-life bipolar disorder: a comparison of lithium, valproate, and other pharmacotherapies. *General Hospital Psychiatry*, 2015. **37**(6): p. 528–32.

102. Sajatovic, M. and P. Chen, Geriatric bipolar disorder. *Psychiatric Clinics of North America*, 2011. **34**(2): p. 319–33.

103. Sajatovic, M., J.R. Calabrese, and J. Mullen, Quetiapine for the treatment of bipolar mania in older adults. *Bipolar Disorder*, 2008. **10**(6): p. 662–71.

104. Sajatovic, M., P. Dines, E. Fuentes-Casiano, et al., Asenapine in the treatment of older adults with bipolar disorder. *International Journal of Geriatric Psychiatry*, 2015. **30**(7): p. 710–19.

A Comparison of Early- and Late-Onset Schizophrenia

Dina Ghoneim, M.D.

Introduction

The conceptualization of late-onset schizophrenia has evolved over time: at times unrecognized as a diagnostic possibility (as in DSM-III, which stipulated that schizophrenia could not be diagnosed after the age of 45 years); at other times explicitly identified as a distinct subtype of schizophrenia (as in DSM-III-R). In DSM-IV and -5, uncertainty regarding its diagnostic status continued. Is it the same illness as earlier onset schizophrenia, a specific subtype of schizophrenia with distinct diagnostic features, or a different illness altogether? As it stands, no age specifiers are mentioned for diagnosing schizophrenia in DSM-5 [1]. This shifting conceptualization consensus likely reflects the following factors: (1) the heterogeneity of this disorder and (2) a dearth of research on the topic.

A consensus statement issued by the International Late-Onset Schizophrenia Group in 2000, has, in contrast to DSM-5, attempted to define late-onset schizophrenia in order to help delineate any differences or similarities it may have to earlier-onset forms of schizophrenia. The group proposed the following definitions [2]:

1. Late-onset schizophrenia: age of onset between 40 and 60
2. Very-late-onset schizophrenia-like-psychosis: age of onset after 60.

These definitions have been useful primarily for furthering research, but, as will be detailed further below, may have a clinical and/or prognostic utility as well. In this chapter we will use the terms late-onset schizophrenia (LOS) and very-late-onset schizophrenia-like-psychosis (VLOSLP) as defined above. Early-onset schizophrenia (EOS) will be used to refer to a patient who has developed the disorder prior to the age of 40 years.

Demographics

Despite the dearth of information on late-onset schizophrenia, the disorder is surprisingly common. Those who have an onset after age 40 years make up nearly a quarter of those diagnosed with this disorder [3]. No reviewed studies report prevalence figures for onset of schizophrenia after the age of 60. Most studies in this age group instead report prevalence rates of non-affective psychosis, most of which are caused by dementia or delirium.

Patients with LOS are more likely to have higher levels of education than those with EOS. Patients with VLOSLP have education levels that are on average intermediate to EOS patients and LOS patients, although these differences may be a function of increasing educational requirements with time in many countries and not a reflection of overall functioning. Additionally, more patients with LOS have had successful work histories and been married than those with EOS. In a similar manner, VLOSLP patients also demonstrated higher rates of marriage than those with EOS [4]. In contrast, mortality rates may be higher in patients with VLOSLP in comparison to older patients with EOS, perhaps due to higher rates of medical comorbidities and accidents [5].

The gender difference between EOS and LOS has been a consistent demographic distinction that has been replicated and reported multiple times. LOS patients encompass a much higher proportion of female patients compared to EOS. In VLOSLP, the predominance of women is even more pronounced. The reasons for these gender differences are not entirely clear. It is believed that estrogen plays a protective role in the development of schizophrenia due to its mild antidopaminergic effects and that its decline during menopause unmasks some women's inherent vulnerability to schizophrenia (this is known as the "estrogen theory") [6]. Indeed, estrogen has been demonstrated to increase blood flow to the brain, protect against amyloid plaques, and act as a neurotrophic factor [6]. Results of using estrogen as an adjunct to antipsychotic medication have been mixed [7,8], while more recently introduced selective estrogen receptor modulators may also hold some promise [9]. Additionally, the estrogen theory does not provide an explanation for males who develop LOS or for women who, despite having the benefit of estrogen, develop schizophrenia before the age of 40. Moreover, it is theoretically possible that men develop biological and/or psychosocial protection against schizophrenia as they grow older.

Clinical presentation

Positive and negative symptoms

Most studies have found that patients with LOS did not differ significantly from those with EOS regarding severity of positive symptoms [10]. Overall, positive symptoms in the LOS population are more likely to be characterized by well-organized delusions, persecutory delusions, visual or tactile hallucinations, and auditory hallucinations with running commentary [2,11]. Earlier studies have noted that patients with LOS present with a higher proportion of the paranoid subtype and with lower negative symptom severity [2,12,13]. However, a large recent study that collected data on 854 persons with schizophrenia aged 40 and above found no difference in negative symptom severity or in paranoid subtype prevalence [14]. Overall, symptom presentation in EOS and LOS was more similar than different.

VLOSLP, on the other hand, differs from EOS symptom presentation in more apparent ways. Persecutory delusions and auditory hallucinations remain common at presentation [15], but positive symptoms are more likely to include visual and tactile hallucinations, as well as somatic delusions [5]. This finding, however, has not been replicated in all studies [4]. Additionally, in contrast to EOS, positive symptoms in the VLOSLP group have been found to be less severe and less florid at presentation, whereas the EOS group reported at illness onset having a greater variety of hallucinations, delusions, and behavioral disturbances, as well as more delusions of reference, grandiosity, and influence [4]. Most studies demonstrated an absence or lower rate of formal thought disorder in the VLOSLP population [16–18], although, again, this was not a universal finding [4,15]. Negative symptoms are considered to be very rare in VLOSLP [2]. Historically, the diagnosis of

VLOSLP has been less well-defined due to the diagnostic uncertainty, partially caused by an increased proportion of medical illnesses, delirium, and neurodegenerative conditions in the population over the age of 60 years.

Cognition

Both EOS and LOS present with cognitive deficits. Most studies have reported that, as in EOS, cognitive deficits in LOS generally remain stable over time [10,12,19]. There is less consensus on the nature and severity of these cognitive deficits. Some studies have reported less severe cognitive deficits in LOS as compared to EOS [12,20]; others have found no differences in severity [13,14,21]. A 2009 study by Rajji et al. reported that relatively preserved cognitive areas in patients with LOS included arithmetic, digit symbol coding, and vocabulary [22]. In contrast, patients with LOS tended to do worse than those with EOS in the following categories: attention (auditory and visual), verbal fluency, global measures of cognition, IQ, and visuospatial construction. Other studies found relatively higher scores among patients with LOS in comparison to EOS patients on tests of flexibility/abstraction and learning [12,14], as well as verbal memory and processing speed [14]. Of note, after correcting for duration of illness, differences in flexibility/abstraction and verbal memory were found to be non-significant, although processing speed remained significantly better [14]. In general, conflicting findings in regard to cognition may be due to confounding caused by differences in duration of illness, education, premorbid intellect, and comorbid diseases [11].

Cognition in VLOSLP is a controversial domain, as conversion to dementia in the longer run has been reported in various studies [23]. There have been several studies suggesting that the symptoms thought to be those of very-late-onset schizophrenia are prodromes of dementia. The risk for dementia may be three times that of their age peers [23,24] and one study found that roughly one-half of patients had developed dementia on five-year follow-up [25]. Whether this propensity to develop dementia shows a true characteristic of this subtype or suggests initial misdiagnosis is under debate. Cognitive impairments in VLOSLP differ from those seen in patients with Alzheimer's disease, as in VLOSLP learning capacity is preserved [2]. The early course of frontotemporal dementia can be very difficult to discern from VLOSLP. In clinical practice VLOSLP should be regarded as a diagnosis by exclusion that can only be made after more common causes of cognitive deterioration (like delirium and dementia) have been sufficiently ruled out. Often, follow-up of the patient for a longer period of time is needed to reach a firmer diagnosis of VLOSLP.

Insight into etiology

Neuropathology and neuroimaging studies

Hahn and colleagues' review of neuroimaging studies that compared EOS and LOS patients found differences in eight out of ten studies, but across studies these were not consistent [26]. Brain MRIs in patients with LOS in comparison to EOS patients typically show no significant differences in white matter hyperintensities, strokes, tumors, or atrophy [12,27]. Additionally, both EOS and LOS patients have been characterized by reductions in some medial temporal region volumes, reductions in the anterior superior temporal gyri [28], and reductions in corpus callosum volume [29]. One study suggested that a distinguishing feature between LOS and EOS is the presence of larger thalamic and ventricular volumes in LOS [30].

A diffusion tensor imaging (DTI) study measuring fractional anisotropy (a proxy measure for white matter integrity) in 20 patients with LOS demonstrated significant reductions of white matter integrity in the left parietal lobe and the right posterior cingulum in comparison to age-matched controls [31]. This study was not able to demonstrate correlations between fractional anisotropy and clinical measures (like PANSS scores, antipsychotic dose, or duration of illness). Similar DTI findings were not found in previous studies of early-onset schizophrenia [32]. While studies of this type need to be replicated, it does point to further evidence of possible neuroanatomical differences between LOS and EOS.

There are very few high-quality neuroimaging studies in VLOSLP. A DTI study of 14 VLOSLP patients found no differences in fractional anisotropy compared to normal age-matched controls [33].

Genetics/heritability

Most family studies that involved patients with LOS suffer from methodological shortcomings [2], but there is evidence that the relatives of VLOSLP patients have a lower morbid risk for schizophrenia than EOS relatives [34]. As the genetic basis of schizophrenia is being explored, genetic targets have been identified as potential mediators of age of onset. One of these targets, a 32-base-pair deletion in CCR5, a chemokine receptor gene, has been identified as correlating with age of onset (as approximated by age of first psychiatric hospitalization) [35]. It is speculated that CCR5, a chemokine receptor that binds several chemokines and retroviruses, may be involved as a potential inflammatory mediator of schizophrenia onset.

The role of inflammation

Because of the association of autoimmune disease and infections with schizophrenia, there has been increasing interest in identifying the role of inflammation in the pathophysiology of schizophrenia [36]. One prospective population study demonstrated that an elevated level of C-reactive protein (CRP), a proxy measure for inflammation, was associated with a 6–11 times greater risk of developing schizophrenia in mid to late life [37]. Again, new studies will be needed to replicate and further explore this association.

The role of sensory deficits

More than two decades ago, Jeste reported an association between sensory deficits (worse corrected vision and hearing) and LOS [38]. With regard to hearing impairment, later studies have put this finding in doubt as being specific for LOS [39] and the association may more likely reflect problems with access to care than be an etiological factor in the development of LOS.

Treatment

The clinical consensus is that patients with LOS and VLOSLP may respond well to anti-psychotics. However, very little specific research has been done in this area. LOS and VLOSLP patients typically require lower doses than both younger patients and older patients with EOS [10,12]. A 2012 Cochrane review of antipsychotic treatment for elderly patients with LOS revealed only one small randomized, double-blind study with little valuable data [40]. Open studies of typical and atypical antipsychotic agents in LOS and VLOSLP patients have shown favorable results in 50% or more of participants [41]. Non-pharmacological treatments have not been specifically investigated in LOS or VLOSLP.

Summary

Both LOS and VLOSLP present a diagnostic challenge to clinicians and researchers. The diagnosis is complicated by the considerable number of conditions that can be associated with delusions and hallucinations in the elderly, including mood disorders, medical disorders, delirium, dementia, medication use, and sensory deficits. Furthermore, the nosological position of VLOSLP is still under debate. Despite these challenges, the literature suggests a range of meaningful differences between EOS, LOS, and VLOSLP that deserve further investigation. These differences are summarized in Table 4.1:

Table 4.1

	Age of Onset	Gender	Symptoms	Cognition	Treatment
Early-onset schizophrenia (EOS)	<40 years	M > F (before age 30)	↑Severity of positive symptoms ↑Variety of positive symptoms ↑Delusions of reference and grandiosity	Deficits at presentation generally stable over time	Higher doses of antipsychotics may be required Non-pharmacological treatments effective
Late-onset schizophrenia (LOS)	40–60 years	F > M	Like EOS	Deficits at presentation generally stable over time	↓Doses of antipsychotics may be effective Non-pharmacological treatments not investigated
Very-late-onset schizophrenia-like psychosis (VLOSLP)	>60 years	F ≫ M	↑Visual/tactile hallucinations ↑Somatic delusions ↓Severity of positive symptoms ↓Formal thought disorder	↑Cognitive decline over time in a significant minority	↓↓Doses of antipsychotics may be effective Non-pharmacological treatments not investigated

References

1. American Psychiatric Association. *Diagnostic and Statistical Manual of Mental Disorders*, 5th edn. Arlington, VA: American Psychiatric Association, 2013.

2. Howard R, Rabins PV, Seeman MV, Jeste DV; The International Late-Onset Schizophrenia Group. Late-onset schizophrenia and very-late-onset schizophrenia-like psychosis: an international consensus. *Am J Psychiatry*. 2000;157(2):172–8. Consensus Development Conference Research Support, Non-U.S. Gov't Review.

3. Jeste DV, Lanouette NM, Vahia IV. Schizophrenia and paranoid disorders. In: Blazer DG, Steffens DC, eds., *Textbook of Geriatric Psychiatry*, 4th edn. Washington, DC: American Psychiatric Press, 2009: 317–31.

4. Girard C, Simard M. Elderly patients with very late-onset schizophrenia-like psychosis and early-onset schizophrenia: cross-sectional and retrospective clinical findings. *Open J Psychiatry*. 2012;2:305–16.

5. Talaslahti T, Alanen HM, Hakko H, et al. Patients with very-late-onset schizophrenia-like psychosis have higher mortality than elderly patients with earlier onset schizophrenia. *Int J Geriatr Psychiatry*. 2015;30(5):453–9.

6. Seeman MV. The role of estrogen in schizophrenia. *J Psychiatry Neurosci*. 1996;21(2):123–7.

7. Chua WL, de Izquierdo SA, Kulkarni J, Mortimer A. Estrogen for schizophrenia. *Cochrane Database Syst Rev*. 2005;(4):CD004719.

8. Kulkarni J, Gavrilidis E, Wang W, et al. Estradiol for treatment-resistant schizophrenia: a large-scale randomized-controlled trial in women of child-bearing age. *Mol Psychiatry*. 2015;20(6):695–702.

9. Kulkarni J, Gavrilidis E, Gwini SM, et al. Effect of adjunctive raloxifene therapy on severity of refractory schizophrenia in women: a randomized clinical trial. *JAMA Psychiatry*. 2016;73(9):947–54.

10. Palmer BW, Bondi MW, Twamley EW, et al. Are late-onset schizophrenia spectrum disorders neurodegenerativ conditions? Annual rates of change on two dementia measures. *J Neuropsychiatry Clin Neurosci*. 2003;15(1):45–52.

11. Maglione JE, Thomas SE, Jeste DV. Late-onset schizophrenia: do recent studies support categorizing LOS as a subtype of schizophrenia? *Curr Opin Psychiatry*. 2014;27(3):173–8.

12. Jeste DV, Symonds LL, Harris MJ, et al. Nondementia nonpraecox dementia praecox? Late-onset schizophrenia. *Am J Geriatr Psychiatry*. 1997;5(4):302–17.

13. Jeste DV, Harris MJ, Krull A, et al. Clinical and neuropsychological characteristics of patients with late-onset schizophrenia. *Am J Psychiatry*. 1995;152(5):722–30.

14. Vahia IV, Palmer BW, Depp C, et al. Is late-onset schizophrenia a subtype of schizophrenia? *Acta Psychiatr Scand*. 2010;122:414–426.

15. Girard C, Simard M. Clinical characterization of late- and very late-onset first psychotic episode in psychiatric inpatients. *Am J Geriatr Psychiatry*. 2008;16(6):478–87.

16. Köhler S, van der Werf M, Hart B, et al. Evidence that better outcome of psychosis in women is reversed with increasing age of onset: a population-based 5-year follow-up study. *Schizophr Res*. 2009;113(2):226–32.

17. Hassett, A. A descriptive study of first presentation psychosis in old age. *Aus NZ J Psychiatry*. 1999;33(6):814–24.

18. Reeves S, Stewart R, Howard R. Service contact and psychopathology in very-late-onset schizophrenia-like psychosis: the effects of gender and ethnicity. *Int J Geriat Psychiatry*. 2002;17:473–9.

19. Heaton RK, Gladsjo JA, Palmer BW, et al. Stability and course of neuropsychological deficits in schizophrenia. *Arch Gen Psychiatry*. 2001;58(1):24–32.

20. Rajji TK, Mulsant BH. Nature and course of cognitive function in late-life schizophrenia: a systematic review. *Schizophr Res*. 2008;102(1):122–40.

21. Heaton R, Paulsen JS, McAdams LA, et al. Neuropsychological deficits in schizophrenics: relationship to age, chronicity, and dementia. *Arch Gen Psychiatry.* 1994;51(6):469–76.

22. Rajji TK, Ismail Z, Mulsant BH. Age at onset and cognition in schizophrenia: meta-analysis. *Br J Psychiatry.* 2009;195(4):286–93.

23. Kørner A, Lopez AG, Lauritzen L, Andersen PK, Kessing LV. Late and very-late first-contact schizophrenia and the risk of dementia – a nationwide register based study. *Int J Geriatr Psychiatry* 2009;24:61–7.

24. Lagodka A, Robert P. Is late-onset schizophrenia related to neurodegenerative processes? A review of literature. *Encephale* 2009;35:386–93.

25. Brodaty H, Sachdev P, Koschera A, Monk D, Cullen B. Long-term outcome of late-onset schizophrenia: 5-year follow-up study. *Br J Psychiatry* 2003;183:213–9.

26. Hahn C, Lim HK, Lee CU. Neuroimaging findings in late-onset schizophrenia and bipolar disorder. *J Geriatr Psychiatry Neurol* 2014;27:56–62.

27. Rivkin P, Kraut M, Barta P, et al. White matter hyperintensity volume in late-onset and early-onset schizophrenia. *Int J Geriat Psychiatry.* 2000;15:1085–9.

28. Barta PE, Powers RE, Aylward EH, et al. Quantitative MRI volume changes in late onset schizophrenia and Alzheimer's disease compared to normal controls. *Psychiat Res Neuroim.* 1997;68(2):65–75.

29. Sachdev P, Brodaty H. Quantitative study of signal hyperintensities on T_2-weighted magnetic resonance imaging in late-onset schizophrenia. *Am J Psychiatry.* 1999:156(12):1958–67.

30. Corey-Bloom J, Jernigan T, Archibald S, Harris MJ, Jeste DV. Quantitative magnetic resonance imaging of the brain in late-life schizophrenia. *Am J Psychiatry.* 1995;152(3):447–9.

31. Chen L, Chen X, Liu W, et al. White matter microstructural abnormalities in patients with late-onset schizophrenia identified by a voxel-based diffusion tensor imaging. *Psychiat Res Neuroim.* 2013;212(3):201–7.

32. Kubicki M, Styner M, Bouix S, et al. Reduced interhemispheric connectivity in schizophrenia: tractography based segmentation of the corpus callosum. *Schizophr Res.* 2008;106(2–3):125–31.

33. Jones DK, Catani M, Pierpaoli C, et al. A diffusion tensor magnetic resonance imaging study of frontal cortex connections in very-late-onset schizophrenia-like psychosis. *Am J Ger Psychiatr.* 2005;13(12):1092–9.

34. Howard R, Graham C, Sham P, et al. A controlled family study of late-onset non-affective psychosis (late paraphrenia). *Br J Psychiatry.*1997;170:511–14.

35. Rasmussen HB, Timm S, Wang AG, et al. Association between the CCR5 32-bp deletion allele and late onset of schizophrenia. *Am J Psychiatry.* 2006;163(3):507–11.

36. Benros ME, Nielsen PR, Nordentoft M, et al. Autoimmune diseases and severe infections as risk factors for schizophrenia: a 30-year population-based register study. *Am J Psychiatry.* 2011;168(12):1303–10.

37. Wium-Andersen MK, Ørsted DD, Nordestgaard BG. Elevated C-reactive protein associated with late- and very-late-onset schizophrenia in the general population: a prospective study. *Schizophrenia Bull.* 2014;40(5):1117–27.

38. Jeste DV. Late-onset schizophrenia. *Int J Geriat Psychiatry.* 1993;8:283–5.

39. Linszen MM, Brouwer RM, Heringa SM, Sommer IE. Increased risk of psychosis in patients with hearing impairment: Review and meta-analyses. *Neurosci Biobehav Rev.* 2016;62:1–20.

40. Essali A, Ali G. Antipsychotic drug treatment for elderly people with late-onset schizophrenia. *Cochrane Database Syst Rev.* 2012;(2):CD004162.

41. Scott J, Greenwald BS, Kramer E, Shuwall M. Atypical (second generation) antipsychotic treatment response in very late-onset schizophrenia-like psychosis. *Int Psychogeriatr.* 2011;23:742–48.

Chapter

5

Biological Changes in Older People with Schizophrenia

Michael B. Centorino, M.D. and Susan K. Schultz, M.D.

Introduction

Age-related biologic changes in schizophrenia will continue to increase in importance as we witness marked growth in the older population over the next few decades. Within the mental health discipline, the additive effects of age-related biologic changes and medical comorbidity superimposed on chronic schizophrenia may pose significant treatment challenges. This chapter will review these challenges, addressing key questions, such as:

1. How do age-related brain changes affect people with schizophrenia?
2. What have we learned from post-mortem studies about neurodegenerative processes in schizophrenia?
3. Do the probable neurodevelopmental abnormalities in schizophrenia predispose to accelerated brain aging or neurodegeneration?
4. What has recent research in neuroimaging, genetics and biomarkers of aging offered in understanding the course of schizophrenia?
5. How do the effects of chronic medication exposure influence the biologic features of schizophrenia in later life?

We will address some of the fundamental issues as well as highlight gaps that offer opportunities for future research.

Neuroimaging in schizophrenia

Several decades ago, studies using computed tomography (CT) led the way in establishing schizophrenia as an illness associated with neurobiologic abnormalities that are discernible early in the illness, if not premorbidly. Initial brain imaging studies in schizophrenia demonstrated an increase in the ventricle-to-brain ratio (VBR), suggesting a deficit of cerebral tissue relative to CSF volume [1–3]. Interestingly, this is precisely the same finding reported among early CT studies of Alzheimer's disease, i.e., an increased VBR distinguishes patients from comparison subjects [4–6]. These similarities reflect the fact that VBR is a non-specific measure that may be influenced by any number of pathogenic processes that serve to either increase ventricular volume or reduce tissue volumes. However, the presence of brain abnormalities early in life among persons with schizophrenia does raise the possibility of neurodevelopmental abnormalities that predispose to age-related deterioration.

Neuroimaging studies in young adults with schizophrenia have discerned specific features that appear to have prognostic meaning. For example, enlarged ventricles have been associated with negative symptoms, as well as a greater likelihood of cognitive impairment and greater impairment in premorbid functioning [7–9]. Early studies of morphometric measures in schizophrenia among older individuals have also shown a relationship between enlarged ventricles and a poor outcome, including a greater likelihood of progressive cognitive decline and more severe negative symptoms in later life [10–12]. In contrast to early imaging studies using CT, magnetic resonance imaging (MRI) allows for better delineation between gray and white matter and cerebrospinal fluid through superior resolution capabilities. Non-elderly adults with schizophrenia have demonstrated reduced tissue volumes in a variety of regions, including frontal and temporal cortices, the amygdala, thalamus and hippocampus [13]. In contrast, studies of schizophrenia with onset in later life have reported a greater variety of non-specific structural changes, such as increased deep white matter hyperintensities [14]. The area of white matter changes has emerged as a key feature of age-related changes among those with schizophrenia, using new methods, as discussed later in this chapter.

Recent techniques in brain imaging analysis have allowed researchers to look carefully at differences in anatomic measures reflecting brain maturation to determine if differences during brain development leading to the onset of schizophrenia have an influence not only on illness onset but on brain health and outcomes over the lifespan. Overall, the conceptualization of the illness has included a prenatal vulnerability, perhaps genetic, that predisposes to abnormal brain maturation, which ultimately leads to the onset of psychotic symptoms in early adulthood. This conceptualization has been termed the "two hit" hypothesis of schizophrenia that has also set the stage for trying to understand how this scenario may affect adult brain function and risk of changes with advanced age. An intriguing study examined the question of whether there is evidence for accelerated brain aging in schizophrenia based on standardized morphometric measures known to reflect anatomic aging relative to healthy controls [15]. The study utilized a machine-learning-based MRI assessment that could examine the difference between chronological and neuroanatomic age among patient groups. In a young-to-mid-life sample of patients with schizophrenia derived from multiple centers, it was shown that brain aging was significantly more advanced, based on neuroanatomic MRI measures, relative to healthy controls. However, this study also observed that other groups of people with mental illness, e.g., major depression, showed a similar morphometric pattern of advanced aging, but to a lesser extent than observed with schizophrenia. This study is significant in its ability to detect these differences within the lifespan of the illness, even in a sample that excluded subjects typically considered "older," i.e., 65 years or older.

Other recent studies have focused on schizophrenia and included individuals up to the age of 65 years. For example, a study by Cropley and colleagues observed that progressive brain changes occurred across the lifespan with volume loss in gray matter occurring in the first decades of illness, with evidence in later life of white matter deterioration suggesting a pattern of accelerated aging [16]. This study included adults with schizophrenia across the adult age range, including up to 65 years. These findings support the premise of a vulnerability to age-related changes in the brain in persons with schizophrenia. The underlying mechanisms that induce these changes remain an active area of research, in many ways complicated by the interactions between the disease itself and lifestyle factors and medication exposure effects, discussed later in this chapter.

Functional imaging across the lifespan in schizophrenia

Functional imaging may provide answers to some of the more complex questions regarding changes in neural activity over a lifetime in schizophrenia. Functional neuroimaging allows the exploration of relationships between cognitive tasks and regional brain activity. Early work used single photon emission computed tomography (SPECT) and positron emission tomography (PET), which was pivotal in first discerning the functional changes associated with the illness. However, functional magnetic resonance imaging (fMRI) has emerged as the most common means of examining brain function in mental illness due to the ability to examine brain functional tasks most readily. Along with the advantage of avoiding exposure to radiation, fMRI also allows for testing multiple cognitive tasks in one experimental session. Across all methods, functional neuroimaging studies have demonstrated both early-onset abnormalities and probable later-life vulnerabilities among patients with schizophrenia. Multiple early imaging studies demonstrated reduced activity in frontal regions in schizophrenia that appear to increase with age [17–20].

Reductions in frontal lobe activity may relate directly to the expression of negative symptoms, such as avolition or anhedonia. Further, if poor frontal activation is inherent to schizophrenia and aging of the brain also may result in less efficient frontal activity, there may be an additive effect across the lifespan. This notion is consistent with clinical descriptions of schizophrenia in later life, i.e., negative symptoms may persist or worsen with age, in contrast to psychotic symptoms, which may improve [21]. Age-related worsening of brain function may be mediated by white matter aging, observed by Cropley and colleagues to be potentially accelerated in the context of schizophrenia [16]. Another recent study examined how functional brain activity may be affected by white matter dysfunction using fMRI to examine neural connectivity [22]. It was demonstrated that compared to healthy subjects, patients with schizophrenia have reduced efficiency of brain networks involved in higher-order cognitive function, including the cingulo-opercular and fronto-parietal networks.

Genetic influences on the life course of schizophrenia

Cognitive dysfunction is considered a core feature of schizophrenia that is often observable prior to the first episode of psychosis, although there may be remarkable variation across individuals with the illness. Research addressing a possible genetic component underlying cognitive dysfunction in schizophrenia has been an important area of study, although there are few studies that have examined how genetic influences affect age-related cognitive change in schizophrenia. Among young to mid-life patients, researchers have investigated the relationship of cognitive function and multiple common genetic polymorphisms with potential to impair cognition in schizophrenia [23]. In general, the results have been varied. This variability may be due to several factors that encompass the severity of illness at the time, sample demographics and assessment measures. Furthermore, it is possible that the cumulative effect of multiple allelic variations is more important than any single variant. Consequently, polygenic influences have been an emerging area of recent study.

For example, recent work has highlighted several functional enzymes that have been identified as having an impact on cognition function through distinct mechanisms. Among these functional enzymes is catechol-O-methyltransferase (COMT) which is responsible for the degradation of catecholamines, such as dopamine and norepinephrine. A common variant of COMT, 158Val/Met, results in an increase in dopamine in the synapse in the presence of the Met allele. This genetic variation is particularly meaningful for schizophrenia although it has potential implications for cognitive function in all persons. COMT is particularly active in the prefrontal cortex, which is important for patients with schizophrenia, given that low dopamine concentrations in the prefrontal cortex have been associated with poorer cognitive performance [24]. It has been hypothesized that carrying the Met allele is protective against cognitive dysfunction in schizophrenia due to an increase in dopamine availability [25]. Results to date remain uncertain in terms of age-related cognitive decline in later life; however, Met allele carriers have been shown to perform better in cognitive assessments in several studies of non-elderly patients that include schizophrenia participants as well as healthy controls [25].

To return to the concept of polygenic influences affecting cognition through different mechanisms, a common variant studied in multiple disorders at cognitive risk is the apolipoprotein E (APOE) variant. APOE is a plasma lipoprotein involved in synaptic signaling and plasticity, the most studied APOE variants are epsilon-2, -3 and -4, with APOE epsilon-4 being associated with cognitive dysfunction across most conditions, although its role in schizophrenia and cognitive aging remains unclear [26,27]. Some studies have suggested deficits in executive function among patients with bipolar affective disorder with the APOE epsilon-4 allele, but studies that have included patients with schizophrenia have not identified an effect of the APOE epsilon-4 allele [28]. To better evaluate polygenic influences, a "risk score" may be calculated by examining the alleles across several loci and estimating the effect size of each allele associated with a specific disease trait such as cognition. This "polygenic risk score" sums these trait-associated alleles together in a way that may help to understand the multiple genetic contributions to clinical outcomes. Along these lines, one interesting longitudinal study examined genotypes of middle-aged and older adults from a community-based representative sample participating in the Health and Retirement Study [29]. This analysis involved older adults who had no psychiatric illness, but the investigators applied the polygenic risk alleles thought to be associated with cognitive function in schizophrenia to see if they had an effect in a general population. They observed that these polygenic risk alleles were associated with general modest decline when the sample was examined over a longitudinal period, particularly in attention and spatial working memory. However, when another set of polygenic risk alleles that have been associated with Alzheimer's disease was examined in this sample, there was a greater effect on cognition. These findings suggest that the genetic influences affecting cognitive function over time in schizophrenia are likely to be distinct from those associated with dementia. Overall, the evidence from histopathology, clinical studies and polygenic risk analyses appears to show that persons with schizophrenia have their own distinct trajectory of age-related brain changes into later life [30].

Biomarkers of aging in schizophrenia

Schizophrenia has been associated with accelerated medical morbidity and earlier mortality for a number of reasons, largely relating to cardiovascular disease. One biomarker of interest that is related to the metabolic syndrome, vascular disease and mortality is high sensitivity C-reactive protein (hs-CRP). This biomarker is known to predict accelerated morbidity in community samples as well as in patients with schizophrenia, and it may be exacerbated by lifestyle factors such as poor diet and smoking. One study has examined the biomarker hs-CRP among patients with schizophrenia or schizoaffective disorder relative to a comparison sample to determine whether the presence of schizophrenia was associated with a higher level even after controlling for demographic and lifestyle factors that may influence the results. It was found that hs-CRP levels were significantly higher in schizophrenia and the elevated levels were associated with female gender, more severe negative symptoms and greater medical comorbidity. When the hs-CRP biomarker was compared to other biomarkers of poor health risk, including fasting glucose, hemoglobin A1c and BMI, it was observed that elevated hs-CRP was associated with deleterious elevations in these biomarkers as well. However, there was no relationship between hs-CRP and age or cognitive impairment. Consequently this evidence shows that there are biomarkers present that predict accelerated aging from a medical comorbidity standpoint, but longitudinal studies into later life and advanced aging remain to be done to determine the long-term effects on brain function in schizophrenia [31].

Another study using biomarkers was conducted in a large Danish cohort that compared men with psychiatric hospitalizations to the rest of the cohort to examine both biomarkers associated with disease risk as well as early mortality. Men were divided into different types of psychiatric illness, including schizophrenia, substance use and affective disorders. It was observed that elevations in hs-CRP, IL-6 and IL-18 were present in the groups with psychiatric illness. However, other markers, including IL-10, TNF-alpha and IFN-gamma, were not different in the psychiatric groups relative to others in the cohort. When mortality by the age of 55 years was examined in this cohort, the groups with psychiatric disorder had elevated rates, with the highest risk for early mortality seen in those with substance-use disorders, followed by those with schizophrenia [32]. Other studies examining inflammatory markers have suggested that there are elevations in TNF-alpha and IL-6 levels in schizophrenia patients. Implications for accelerated disease were also suggested by the finding that these elevations were associated with greater depression and comorbid physical illnesses. Like many studies, there has not yet been longitudinal follow-up into advanced aging, as the mean age of the sample in this analysis was 48.1 years [33]. Overall, these biomarkers consistently suggest a risk of accelerated aging, but full implications for longevity in schizophrenia will remain to be studied as some in this population advance toward the oldest-old range.

One biomarker that has emerged to suggest a dynamic marker of aging is that of telomere length. It is known that variations in telomere length are the result of a wide range of genetic and environmental interactions that are likely to be relevant to aging in many contexts as well as schizophrenia. One study examined telomere length in adults with schizophrenia and noted that shorter telomere length, representing poorer health, was associated with individuals with schizophrenia relative to controls. However, there was no difference in telomere length between the patients and their unaffected siblings, reflecting the possible presence of a genetic influence that mediates this particular aging biomarker. Further work by the same group has shown that reduced telomere length is associated with reduced gray matter brain volumes and poor memory performance, yet the implications for possible decline with advanced aging remain to be characterized [34–35].

Complicating the analysis of biomarkers in schizophrenia, as well as genetic risk factors, is the lack of clarity and specificity of the diagnosis itself, despite many decades of nosologic studies and extensive biologically focused research. New approaches, such as the Research Domain Criteria (RDoC) proposed by the National Institute of Mental Health (NIMH) have challenged the field to re-evaluate traditional diagnostic boundaries in favor of circuitry or molecular-based measures. Along these lines, one group has used a large biomarker panel (neuropsychological, stop signal, saccadic control and auditory stimulation paradigms) across a large sample comprising groups across the psychotic disorders spectrum as well as healthy comparison subjects [36]. This broad approach was able to identify three neurobiologically distinct psychosis biotypes that did not respect clinical diagnosis boundaries that would have categorized the sample by schizophrenia, schizoaffective or bipolar disorder with psychosis in general clinical practice. These differential biomarker patterns across biotypes may help identify specific subgroups within a broader spectrum of psychosis that have differential risk for age-related changes across the lifespan. For example, the biomarker pattern suggesting the most severe illness, biotype 1, might identify patients who are often inpatients or treated in longer-term settings, while persons with biotype 2 or 3 may be more likely to be managed in the community. Longer-term outcomes relative to biologic aging may be driven by factors that reside outside of information suggested by current diagnostic categories.

Neuropathologic studies of schizophrenia

In view of the previous discussion regarding neuroimaging abnormalities with aging in schizophrenia, one would expect that persons with schizophrenia would similarly show marked differences from healthy subjects in histological findings on postmortem evaluation. This is indeed the case, however this literature is perhaps more mixed and complex than the imaging literature discussed above. Despite extensive antemortem diagnostic assessments and rigorous postmortem analyses, there remains no clear neuropathologic change seen in postmortem examination of elderly patients with long-term schizophrenia [37]. Similarly, a variety of other studies have been unable to demonstrate significant differences in patients with schizophrenia on postmortem evaluation despite notable antemortem cognitive deficits [38–40]. Studies of postmortem changes in persons with schizophrenia have been less often utilized in recent decades to address aging in schizophrenia due to the advent of newer imaging technologies that provide more information regarding cellular changes. However, one relatively recent study has investigated whether chronic schizophrenia is associated with glial changes in the dorsolateral prefrontal cortex, superior temporal gyrus and the anterior cingulate gyrus. This study demonstrated a specific increase in the numerical density of microglia in the temporal and frontal cortices of chronic schizophrenics, which was not related to aging. This was interpreted to reflect fundamental differences in cortical neuropil architecture in schizophrenia [41].

While the support for abnormalities in neuropil architecture has been mixed in recent years, there is emerging evidence for abnormal microglial activation that may induce inflammation, with deleterious effects across the lifespan [42–44]. Overall there appears to be support for early abnormalities in cytoarchitecture and neuronal number in schizophrenia that have a distinct trajectory over the lifespan, influenced by multiple factors, including microglial activation, that contribute to greater functional losses with aging in schizophrenia when compared to unaffected individuals [45]. While the role of microglial activation inherent to the disease is likely a main risk factor for age-related changes, it has interestingly been suggested that antipsychotic medication may have an ameliorative effect of reducing cytokine activity in this context [46]. The implications of antipsychotic treatment are discussed further below, focusing on recent studies that have been less encouraging due to cumulative side effect risks.

Effects of long-term antipsychotic exposure

The confounding influence of chronic medication adds a layer of complexity to an already complex situation. In view of the widespread availability of antipsychotic medications for many decades, a large cohort of patients with schizophrenia entering late life have received consistent antipsychotic medication throughout the course of their nearly life-long illness, opening research opportunities less obfuscated by older treatment modalities. Chronic use of antipsychotic medication has both advantages and disadvantages, but is certainly preferable to its historical predecessors of insulin coma, institutionalization, physical restraints, hydrotherapy and prefrontal leucotomy.

The advent of conventional dopamine-antagonist antipsychotic medication in the mid-twentieth century ushered in an era of substantial symptom reduction and better social functioning, as well as a host of its own adversities, from extrapyramidal side effects (EPS) to tardive dyskinesia (TD). While newer antipsychotic medications were largely designed to avoid these problems, their use has been associated with a worrisome progressive increase in the rate of metabolic syndrome, including abdominal obesity, insulin resistance and hypertension. These adversities, in part, have led to reports of 75% of patients discontinuing both conventional and newer-generation antipsychotic medications within 18 months of treatment [47,48].

When considering the combination of long-term effects of dopamine antagonism on motor systems that lead to abnormal movements, as well as the metabolic effects of medications, it is likely that the chronic use of antipsychotic medication may accelerate a number of physiologic parameters that induce accelerated aging. This chapter will review the two primary clinical concerns relating to long-term antipsychotic exposure. The first of these is the chronic effect of dopamine receptor blockade and the consequences in terms of abnormal movements. The second is the complex issue of metabolic syndrome, which is increasingly recognized as a public health problem.

Interactions of aging and antipsychotic associated movement disorders

The term tardive dyskinesia (TD) emerged in the 1960s, referring to the delayed onset of involuntary movements. However, spontaneous, involuntary, TD-like movements have been described in 5–10% of persons suffering from psychotic disorders since long before the advent of antipsychotics, and moreover, spontaneous orofacial dyskinesia can develop in 1–8% of older adults [49]. There are several theories on the nature and origin of TD. The historic model involved the induction of dopamine hypersensitivity secondary to chronic blockade, although early on it was evident that dopamine hypersensitivity did not entirely account for the problem [50]. It may be attributable to a number of factors, ranging from an imbalance in dopaminergic and cholinergic systems, as well as potentially noradrenergic or GABA-ergic dysfunction; excitotoxicity has also been postulated [51].

While there has been comparatively less attention given to TD in research over recent years, there is little evidence that it has disappeared as a problem. TD continues to show an estimated annual incidence of 3–5%, increasing linearly for the first 4–5 years of antipsychotic exposure [48,52] and afterwards, yielding a rate of approximately 25% at 5 years, 49% after 10 years and 68% after 25 years [49]. Among the elderly, TD annual rates have been estimated between 2.5% and 13.6% [53]. Among older psychiatric outpatients (mean age of 65.5 years) treated with an average dose equivalent to 150 mg of chlorpromazine, reported rates of TD are strikingly 3–5 times higher than in younger patients; this older group demonstrated a cumulative incidence of 20–26% at 1 year, 30–52% at 2 years and 42–60% at 3 years, despite generally being prescribed lower doses [52,54].

Later work has suggested that the occurrence of TD in older adults does not differ between those treated with conventional and newer-generation antipsychotic medication [55]. The hazard ratio within this older population for developing TD is reported as 1.13 per 10 000 mg cumulative chlorpromazine-equivalent dose, and 1.28 per 100 mg of mean chlorpromazine equivalent daily dose [55].

As noted above, the shift in prescribing from typical to atypical antipsychotics has not reduced the occurrence of TD as much as initially hoped, as there is conflicting evidence between either no improvement or a decrease in TD incidence from approximately 5.5% in typical antipsychotic medication to a range between 5.9% and 0.8% in atypical antipsychotic medication within the first five years of treatment [55–57]. There have been attempts to separate "probable" TD (lesser severity and time-limited duration) from "persistent" TD (longer-lasting and more severe), in which reports show no difference in the incidence of "persistent" TD between antipsychotic classes, but a lower rate of "probable" TD with atypical antipsychotic medication, and that while overall TD rates were similar, severe TD was more likely to be caused by first-generation antipsychotics [42]. In older adults, the risk of "probable" TD is reported as 7% with second-generation, and 23% with first-generation antipsychotics [58].

Possibly due to the expectation of newer atypical (also termed "second-generation") antipsychotics reducing the symptoms of cogwheel rigidity, bradykinesia and tremor, patients on atypical antipsychotics are 30 times less likely to be prescribed adjunctive anticholinergic medication compared to those on conventional (i.e., "first-generation") antipsychotics, despite equivalent rates of EPS (5–10%) across antipsychotic classes. Extrapyramidal side effects, most commonly appearing as "parkinsonian" symptoms, may be particularly problematic in late life, most likely due to subcortical degenerative changes, as well as decreased physiologic clearance of medication [59–60]. Furthermore, with normal aging, there is a reduction in dopaminergic tone across brain regions that may underlie vulnerabilities to these adverse effects, as well as potentially the decline in cognitive performance associated with aging [61].

Brain aging and medication exposure may have unique interactions on dopaminergic function over time. For example, it has been reported that among patients with schizophrenia, those who developed TD showed reduced density of dopaminergic receptor terminals, while those that did not develop TD did not show the same reduction in density [62]. In terms of brain changes over a lifetime, some studies have suggested that specific brain morphologic changes may be related to medication use. Findings primarily focused on the basal ganglia structures include both structural enlargement and increased functional activity [63–66].

Studies addressing the potential genetic mediators of TD and metabolic syndrome have not yet been replicated sufficiently and consequently do not inform treatment strategies at this time. In general, treatment interventions for abnormal movements in schizophrenia have encompassed a wide range of compounds over the years with no clearly effective treatment emerging with consistency. These include amantadine, clonazepam, gingko biloba, levetiracetam, melatonin, piracetam, propranolol, resveratrol, branched-chain amino acids, omega-3 fatty acids, vitamin B6, vitamin E, zonisamide and tetrabenazine [50]. More recently, valbenazine, a selective monoamine transporter 2 inhibitor, similar in mechanism to tetrabenazine, has been shown to improve the symptoms of TD [67]. Though valbenazine has not been tested in the geriatric population, the aforementioned tetrabenazine has been used clinically for some time for a variety of conditions that induce abnormal movements. Tetrabenazine has been associated with drowsiness, depression and akathisia and has shown an increased risk of parkinsonism when prescribed to geriatric patients [68].

In summary, there are a number of established risk factors for the development of TD. These include higher doses of antipsychotics, in terms of both daily quantity and cumulative lifetime exposure, signs of EPS initially upon exposure to antipsychotic use, and older age at the time of first exposure. However, while there might be some evidence that severe cases of TD are uncommon in the current era of predominant use of second-generation agents, the overall problem in clinical practice has not changed dramatically and perhaps has become less of a focus of care relative to new problems related to advanced aging and the metabolic syndrome as discussed below.

The relationship of metabolic syndrome and increasing age in schizophrenia

Metabolic syndrome, including insulin resistance, hypertension, hyperlipidemia and visceral adiposity, has presented significant clinical challenges across the population, but particularly in patients with schizophrenia. Metabolic syndrome is a concern due to its cumulative impact on the aging process and difficulties in achieving successful management in the context of a chronic psychotic disorder. Given that metabolic syndrome is in part iatrogenic due to the influence of medication, this provides an opportunity to intervene through close medication management, but also offers a significant challenge since medications most often cannot be avoided entirely. The overall rate of metabolic syndrome is 32.5% for persons with schizophrenia, while the highest rate has been reported with clozapine (51.9%), distantly followed by olanzapine (28.2%) and risperidone (27.9%); the lowest prevalence is 20.2% among patients receiving no medications at all [69]. The affinity for both histaminergic (H1) and serotonergic (5-HT2c) receptor blockade is associated with the bulk of variance in weight gain between antipsychotics. In addition, antipsychotic-induced weight gain has been shown to be heritable [69].

It has long been observed that people with chronic psychotic disorders have been at greater risk of earlier mortality from all causes. However, recent data have suggested a particular concern related to the metabolic syndrome. For example, a risk of cardiovascular disease, with consequent strokes and premature mortality, has been documented in persons with schizophrenia and related psychotic disorders [70]. Along these lines, the Framingham Study data demonstrated that the 10-year risk for coronary heart disease, including angina, myocardial infarction, and cardiac death, is elevated by 79% among persons with schizophrenia [71].

The brain effects of conditions related to the metabolic syndrome, such as obesity, are key to determining how they may manifest in the context of mental illness. For example, neuroinflammation resulting from obesity has been shown to have deleterious effects on the hypothalamus, cortex, brainstem and amygdala [72]. In addition to associations with reduced brain volume, neuroinflammation is associated with cognitive dysfunction (including learning, memory and attention deficits), reduced levels of brain-derived neurotrophic factor, altered glutamatergic signaling and impaired insulin regulation, as well as the maintenance of obese phenotypes [72].

Maintaining a normal weight may be especially difficult when prescribed adipogenic medication, and losing weight in the context of serious mental illness poses many challenges. Modest weight loss responses have been shown for omega-3 fatty acid and folate supplementation, metformin, topiramate and behavioral therapy [73], but ultimately, obesity prevention appears to be the most prudent strategy. First-episode patients with schizophrenia are more sensitive to antipsychotic side effects (e.g., akathisia, weight gain) and have higher response rates, suggesting that trying agents less associated with weight gain may be particularly advantageous for first-episode or antipsychotic-naïve patients. Careful selection and close monitoring of medications may be of substantial benefit in reducing the chances of a lifetime of problematic medication changes.

Conclusions

In reflecting on the current state of biologic aging in the context of schizophrenia, there have been many influences that have collectively broadened the spectrum of relevant issues. Early research in past decades has suggested an earlier mortality from all causes in schizophrenia, but the population at the time included individuals who experienced the onset of illness prior to the widespread availability of medications in the context of chronic hospitalizations. In contrast, in the last several decades there has been remarkable progress toward community-based programs and more medication options. Together, these factors have contributed to greater longevity and less severe effects of aggressive medication management with first-generation antipsychotics. However, the trade-off has been an increase in the long-term effects of chronic mental illness and aging, including metabolic syndrome complications. Adjusting our care practices to this new landscape is prudent to reduce the risk of accelerated brain aging among patients with schizophrenia.

References

1. Johnstone E.C., C.D. Frith, T.J. Crow, J. Husband, L. Kreel. Cerebral ventricular size and cognitive impairment in chronic schizophrenia. *Lancet* 308: 924–6, 1976.

2. Weinberger D.R., E.F. Torrey, A.N. Neophytides. Lateral cerebral ventricular enlargement in chronic schizophrenia. *Arch Gen Psychiatry* 36: 735–39, 1979.

3. Pearlson G.D., D.J. Garbacz, R.H. Tompkins, et al. Lateral cerebral ventrical size in late onset schizophrenia. In *Schizophrenia and Aging*, ed. N. E. Miller, Cohen, G.D. New York: Guilford: 246–248, 1987.

4. De Leon M.J., S.H. Ferris, A.E. George, et al. Computed tomography evaluations of brain-behavior relationships in senile dementia of the Alzheimer's type. *Neurobiol Aging* 1: 69–79, 1980.

5. Naeser M.A., C. Gebhardt, H.L. Levine. Decreased computerized tomography numbers in patients with presenile dementia: detection in patients with otherwise normal scans. *Arch Neurol* 37: 401–9, 1980.

6. Veroff A.E., G.D. Pearlson, H.S. Ahn. CT scan and neuropsychological correlates of Alzheimer's disease and Huntington's disease. *Brain Cogn* 1(2): 177–84, 1982.

7. Seno H., M. Shibata, A. Fujimoto, et al. Computed tomographic study of aged schizophrenic patients. *Psychiatry Clin Neurosci* 51(6): 373–7, 1997.

8. Putnam, K.M., P.D. Harvey. Cognitive impairment and enduring negative symptoms: a comparative study of geriatric and nongeriatric schizophrenia patients. *Schizophr Bull* 26(4): 867–78, 2000.

9. Harvey M.P., P.J. Moriarty, J.I. Friedman, et al. Differential preservation of cognitive functions in geriatric patients with lifelong chronic schizophrenia: less impairment in reading compared with other skill areas. *Biol Psychiatry* 47(11): 962–8, 2000.

10. Rossi A., M. Bustini, P. Prosperini, et al. Neuromorphological abnormalities in schizophrenic patients with good and poor outcome. *Acta Psychiatr Scand* **101**(2): 161–6, 2000.

11. Tandon R., J.R. DeQuardo, S.F. Taylor, et al. Phasic and enduring negative symptoms in schizophrenia: biological markers and relationship to outcome. *Schizophr Res* **45**(3): 191–201, 2000.

12. Mathalon D.H., E.V. Sullivan, K.O. Lim, A. Pfefferbaum. Progressive brain volume changes and the clinical course of schizophrenia in men: a longitudinal magnetic resonance imaging study. *Arch Gen Psychiatry* **58**(2): 148–57, 2001.

13. Pearlson G.D., L. Marsh. Structural brain imaging in schizophrenia: a selective review. *Biol Psychiatry* **46**: 627–49, 1999.

14. Keshavan M.S., B.H. Mulsant, R.A. Sweet, et al. MRI changes in schizophrenia in late life: a preliminary controlled study. *Psych Res* **60**: 117–23, 1996.

15. Koutsouleris, N., C. Davatzikos, S. Borgwardt, et al. Accelerated brain aging in schizophrenia and beyond: a neuroanatomical marker of psychiatric disorders. *Schizophr Bull* **40**(5): 1140–53, 2014.

16. Cropley V.L., P. Klauser, R.K. Lenroot, et al. Accelerated gray and white matter deterioration with age in schizophrenia. *Am J Psychiatry* **174**(3): 286–295, 2017.

17. Andreasen N.C., K. Rezai, R. Alliger, et al. Hypofrontality in neuroleptic naïve patients and in patients with chronic schizophrenia: assessment with xenon 133 single-photon emission computed tomography and the Tower of London. *Arch Gen Psychiatry* **49**(12): 943–58, 1992.

18. Buchsbaum M.S., E.A. Hazlett. Functional brain imaging and aging in schizophrenia. *Schizophr Res* **27**(2-3): 129–41, 1997.

19. Goldstein P.C., G.G. Brown, A. Marcus, J.R. Ewing. Effects of age, neuropsychological impairment and medication on regional cerebral blood flow in schizophrenia and major affective disorder. *Henry Ford Hosp Med J* **38**(4): 202–6, 1990.

20. Dupont L.P., P.P. Lehr, G. Lamoureaux, et al. Preliminary report: cerebral blood flow abnormalities in older schizophrenic patients. *Psychiatry Res* **55**(3): 121–30, 1994.

21. Harvey P.D., J. Lombardi, M. Leibman, et al. Cognitive impairment and negative symptoms in geriatric chronic schizophrenia patients: a follow-up study. *Schizophr Res* (**22**): 223–31, 1996.

22. Sheffield J.M., G. Repovs, M.P. Harms, et al. Evidence for accelerated decline of functional brain network efficiency in schizophrenia. *Schizophr Bull* **42**(3): 753–61, 2015.

23. Snitz, B.E., A.W. Macdonald, C.S. Carter. Cognitive deficits in unaffected first-degree relatives of schizophrenia patients: a meta-analytic review of putative endophenotypes. *Schizophr Bull* **32**(1): 179–94, 2006.

24. Fallon S.J., C.H. Williams-Gray, R.A. Barker, A.M. Owen, A. Hampshire. Prefrontal dopamine levels determine the balance between cognitive stability and flexibility. *Cerebral Cortex* **23**(2): 361–9, 2013.

25. Ira E., M. Zanoni, M. Ruggeri, P. Dazzan, S. Tosato. COMT, neuropsychological function and brain structure in schizophrenia: a systematic review and neurobiological interpretation. *J Psychiatry Neurosci* **38**(6): 366–80, 2013.

26. Niizato K., K. Genda, R. Nakamura, S. Iritani, K. Ikeda. Cognitive decline in schizophrenics with Alzheimer's disease: a mini-review of neuropsychological and neuropathological studies. *Prog Neuro-Psychopharmacol Biol Psychiatry* **25**(7): 1359–66, 2001.

27. Thabit H., S.M. Kennelly, A. Bhagarva, et al. Utilization of Frontal Assessment Battery and Executive Interview 25 in assessing for dysexecutive syndrome and its association with diabetes self-care in elderly patients with type 2 diabetes mellitus. *Diabetes Res Clin Pract* **86**(3): 208–12, 2009.

28. Joober R., G. Rouleau, E. Fon, et al. Apolipoprotein E genotype in schizophrenia. *Am J Med Genet* **67**(2): 235, 1996.

29. Liebers D.T., M. Pirooznia F. Seiffudin, et al. Polygenic risk of schizophrenia and cognition in a population-based survey of older adults. *Schizophr Bull* **42**(4): 984–91, 2016.

30. Mullins N., N. Perroud, R. Uher, et al. Genetic relationships between suicide attempts, suicidal ideation and major psychiatric disorders: a genome-wide association and polygenic scoring study. *Am J Med Genet B, Neuropsychiatric Genet* **165B**(5): 428–37, 2014.

31. Joseph J., C. Depp, A.S. Martin, et al. Associations of high sensitivity C-reactive protein levels in schizophrenia and comparison groups. *Schizophr Res* **168** (1–2): 456–60, 2015.

32. Osler M., E. Rostrup, M. Nordentoft, et al. Influence of early life characteristics on psychiatric admissions and impact of psychiatric disease on inflammatory biomarkers and survival: a Danish cohort study. *World Psychiatry* **14**(3): 364–5, 2015.

33. Lee E.E., S. Hong, A.S. Martin, L.T. Eyler, D.V. Jeste. Inflammation in schizophrenia: cytokine levels and their relationships to demographic and clinical variables. *Am J Geriatr Psychiatry* **25**(1): 50–61, 2017.

34. Czepielewski L.S., R. Massuda, B. Panizzutti, et al. Telomere length and CCL11 levels are associated with gray matter volume and episodic memory performance in schizophrenia: evidence of pathological accelerated aging. *Schizophr Bull* **44**(1): 158–67, 2018.

35. Czepielewski L.S., R. Massuda, B. Panizzutti, et al. Telomere length in subjects with schizophrenia, their unaffected siblings and healthy controls: evidence of accelerated aging. *Schizophr Res* **174**(1–3): 39–42, 2016.

36. Clementz B.A., J.A. Sweeney, J.P. Hamm, et al. Identification of distinct psychosis biotypes using brain-based biomarkers. *Am J Psychiatry* **173**(4): 373–84, 2016.

37. Arnold, S.E., J.Q. Trojanowski, R.E. Gur, et al. Absence of neurodegeneration and neural injury in the cerebral cortex in a sample of elderly patients with schizophrenia. *Arch Gen Psychiatry* **55**(3): 225–32, 1998.

38. Arnold S.E., J.Q. Trojanowski. Cognitive impairment in elderly schizophrenia: a dementia (still) lacking distinctive histopathology. *Schizophr Bull* **22**(1): 5–9, 1996.

39. Baldessarini R.J., J.D. Hegarty, E.D. Bird, F.M. Benes. Meta-analysis of postmortem studies of Alzheimer's disease-like neuropathology in schizophrenia. *Am J Psychiatry* **154**(6): 861–3, 1997.

40. Dwork A.J., E.S. Susser, J. Keilp, et al. Senile degeneration and cognitive impairment in chronic schizophrenia. *Am J Psychiatry* **155**(11): 1536–43, 1998.

41. Radewicz K., L.J. Garey, S.M. Gentleman, et al. Increase in HLA-DR immunoreactive microglia in frontal and temporal cortex of chronic schizophrenics. *J Neuropathol Exp Neurol* **59**(2): 137–50, 2000.

42. Najjar S., D.M. Pearlman. Neuroinflammation and white matter pathology in schizophrenia: systematic review. *Schizophr Res* **161**(1): 102–12, 2015.

43. Volk D.W. Role of microglia disturbances and immune-related marker abnormalities in cortical circuitry dysfunction in schizophrenia. *Neurobiol Dis* **99**: 58–65, 2017.

44. Laskaris L.E., M.A. Di Biase, I. Everall, et al. Microglial activation and progressive brain changes in schizophrenia. *Br J Pharmacol* **173**(4): 666–80, 2016.

45. Bakhshi K., S.A. Chance. The neuropathology of schizophrenia: a selective review of past studies and emerging themes in brain structure and cytoarchitecture. *Neuroscience* **303**: 82–102, 2015.

46. Obuchowicz Bielecka-Wajdman, A.M., M. Paul-Samojedny, M. Nowacka. Different influence of antipsychotics on the balance between pro- and anti-inflammatory cytokines depends on glia activation: an in vitro study. *Cytokine* **94**: 37–44, 2017.

47. Lieberman J.A., T.S. Stroup, J.P. McEvoy, et al. Effectiveness of antipsychotic drugs

in patients with chronic schizophrenia. *N Engl J Med* 353(12): 1209–23, 2005.

48. Jones P.B., T.R. Barnes, L. Davies, et al. Randomized controlled trial of the effect on quality of life of second- vs first-generation antipsychotic drugs in schizophrenia: Cost Utility of the Latest Antipsychotic Drugs in Schizophrenia Study (CUtLASS 1). *Arch Gen Psychiatry* 63(10): 1079–87, 2006.

49. Lerner P.P., C. Miodownik, V. Lerner. Tardive dyskinesia (syndrome): current concept and modern approaches to its management. *Psychiatry Clin Neurosci* 69(6): 321–34, 2015.

50. Gerlach J. Prevention/treatment of tardive dyskinesia. *Acta Psychiatr Scand Suppl* 291: 117–28, 1981.

51. Lencz T., A.K. Malhotra. Pharmacogenetics of antipsychotic-induced side effects. *Dialogues Clin Neurosci* 11(4): 405–15, 2009.

52. Woerner M.G., C.U. Correll, J.M. Alvir, et al. Incidence of tardive dyskinesia with risperidone or olanzapine in the elderly: results from a 2-year, prospective study in antipsychotic-naïve patients. *Neuropsychopharmacology* 36(8): 1738–46, 2011.

53. Woerner M.G., J.M. Alvir, B.L. Saltz, et al. Prospective study of tardive dyskinesia in the elderly: rates and risk factors. *Am J Psychiatry* 155(11): 1521–8, 1998.

54. Jeste D.V., M.P. Caligiuri, J.S. Paulsen, et al. Risk of tardive dyskinesia in older patients: a prospective longitudinal study of 266 outpatients. *Arch Gen Psychiatry* 52(9): 756–65, 1995.

55. Lee P.E., K. Sykora, S.S. Gill, et al. Antipsychotic medications and drug-induced movement disorders other than parkinsonism: a population-based cohort study in older adults. *J Am Geriatr Soc* 53(8): 1374–9, 2005.

56. Woerner M.G., C.U. Correll, J.M. Alvir, et al. Incidence of tardive dyskinesia with risperidone or olanzapine in the elderly: results from a 2-year, prospective study in antipsychotic-naïve patients.

Neuropsychopharmacology 36(8): 1738–46, 2011.

57. Kinon B.J., S. Kollack-Walker, D. Jeste, et al. Incidence of tardive dyskinesia in older adult patients treated with olanzapine or conventional antipsychotics. *J Geriatr Psychiatry Neurol* 28(1): 67–79, 2015.

58. O'Brien A. Comparing the risk of tardive dyskinesia in older adults with first-generation and second-generation antipsychotics: a systematic review and meta-analysis. *Int J Geriatr Psychiatry* 31(7): 683–93, 2016.

59. Byne W., C. Stamu, L. White, et al. Prevalence and correlates of parkinsonism in an institutionalized population of geriatric patients with chronic schizophrenia. *Int J Geriatr Psychiatry* 15(1): 7–13, 2000.

60. Dubovsky, S.I., A.N. Dubovsky. Geriatric neuropsychopharmacology. In *Textbook of Geriatric Neuropsychiatry*, ed. Dubovsky S.L., R. Buzan, Washington DC: The American Psychiatric Press: 800–1, 2000.

61. Volkow N.D., J. Logan, J.S. Fowler, et al. Association between age-related decline in brain dopamine activity and impairment in frontal and cingulate metabolism. *Am J Psychiatry* 157: 75–80, 2000.

62. Seeman P., M. Tinazzi. Loss of dopamine neuron terminals in antipsychotic-treated schizophrenia; relation to tardive dyskinesia. *Prog Neuropsychopharmacol Biol Psychiatry* 44: 178–83, 2013.

63. Miller D.D., N.C. Andreasen, D.S. O'Leary, et al. Effect of antipsychotics on regional cerebral blood flow measured with positron emission tomography. *Neuropsychopharmacology* 17(4): 230–40, 1997.

64. Gur, R.E., V. Maany, P.D. Mozley, et al. Subcortical MRI volumes in neuroleptic-naive and treated patients with schizophrenia. *Am J Psychiatry* 155(12): 1711–17, 1998.

65. Corson P.W., P. Nopoulos, D.D. Miller, S. Arndt, N.C. Andreasen. Change in basal ganglia volume over 2 years in patients with schizophrenia: typical versus atypical

neuroleptics. *Am J Psychiatry* **156**(8): 1200–4, 1999.

66. Lang D.J., L.C. Kopala, R.A. Vandorpe, et al. An MRI study of basal ganglia volumes in first-episode schizophrenia patients treated with risperidone. *Am J Psychiatry* **158**(4): 625–31, 2001.

67. Hauser R.A., S.A. Factor, S.R. Marder, et al. KINECT 3: a phase 3 randomized, double-blind, placebo-controlled trial of valbenazine for tardive dyskinesia. *Am J Psychiatry* **174**(5): 476–84, 2017.

68. Kenney C., C. Hunter, J. Jankovic. Long-term tolerability of tetrabenazine in the treatment of hyperkinetic movement disorders. *Mov Disord* **22**(2): 193–7, 2007.

69. Lett T.A., T.J. Wallace, N.I. Chowdhury, et al. Pharmacogenetics of antipsychotic-induced weight gain: review and clinical implications. *Mol Psychiatry* **17**(3): 242–66, 2012.

70. Mitchell A.J., D. Vancampfort, K. Sweers, et al. Prevalence of metabolic syndrome and metabolic abnormalities in schizophrenia and related disorders: a systematic review and meta-analysis. *Schizophr Bull* **39**(2): 306–18, 2013.

71. Jin H., D. Folsom, A. Sasaki, et al. Increased Framingham 10-year risk of coronary heart disease in middle-aged and older patients with psychotic symptoms. *Schizophr Res* **125**(2–3): 295–9, 2011.

72. Guillemot-Legris O., G.G. Muccioli. Obesity-induced neuroinflammation: beyond the hypothalamus. *Trends Neurosci* **40**(4): 237–53, 2017.

73. Gohlke J.M., E.J. Dhurandhar, C.U. Correll, et al. Recent advances in understanding and mitigating adipogenic and metabolic effects of antipsychotic drugs. *Front Psychiatry* **28**(3):62, 2012.

Cognitive Functioning in Older Adults with Schizophrenia

Tarek K. Rajji, M.D., F.R.C.P.C.

Schizophrenia typically emerges during early adulthood and people often end up living with this illness for most of their lives. Notwithstanding the shorter lifespan that these people continue to experience, the prevalence of schizophrenia among older adults is close to its prevalence among the general population [1–3]. Thus, as the general population continues to age, the number of older people living with schizophrenia will continue to grow.

Cognitive impairment is considered a core dimension in schizophrenia and it is present in most people living with this illness [4]. Cognitive impairment starts to reveal itself in many individuals before the full manifestation of the illness, which is consistent with the neurodevelopmental nature of schizophrenia, including its associated cognitive deficits [5]. These cognitive deficits tend to increase in magnitude around the onset of the illness, but then in general and over the course of adulthood, they remain stable in magnitude. However, late in life and in particular after the fifth and sixth decades of life, the course of these cognitive deficits remains to be fully characterized. During these later stages of the illness, patients with schizophrenia are likely to experience different trajectories, with some individuals going into remission from the illness, some experiencing rapid exacerbation and decline in overall function, and others remaining relatively stable and only experiencing aging-related decline in function. This mixture of trajectories is likely to apply to cognition as well. Given that the burden of schizophrenia in later life increases significantly due to the functional impairments that these patients experience [6,7] and that cognitive deficits associated with schizophrenia continue to be among the strongest predictors of function in late life [8–10], disentangling the trajectories of cognition among older patients with schizophrenia will have a significant impact on providing care for this population.

This chapter describes the current understanding of cognition and its course in older patients with schizophrenia, and the factors that could predict different trajectories, and then summarizes the studies that have tested cognitive and functional enhancement interventions in this population.

Longitudinal studies

Towards the characterization of cognitive trajectories in late-life schizophrenia, several research groups conducted longitudinal cohort studies using retrospectively or prospectively collected data.

Using diagnostic criteria of paraphrenia, Roth reported in 1955 on 46 patients whom he followed up for 3–4.5 years. They were all aged 60 or above and had an age at onset over 45 [11]. During the follow-up period, only one of these patients developed dementia. In contrast, and using similar diagnostic criteria, Holden reported that 13 out of 37 patients with paraphrenia and an onset after the age of 50 developed dementia during a follow-up period of up to three years [12].

More recent studies using current diagnostic criteria also reported various trajectories. Among older and chronically institutionalized patients, the literature supports an accelerated cognitive decline, though slower than in older patients with Alzheimer's dementia, for example at a rate of 1 point/year on the Mini-Mental State Examination (MMSE) [13] in contrast to 3 points/year in Alzheimer's dementia. Further, this accelerated decline seems to become evident after the age of 65 despite having lived with schizophrenia since early adulthood. Finally, this decline was evident after a follow-up period of at least two years and typically longer [14–21].

In contrast, older community-dwelling patients with schizophrenia seem to experience relative cognitive stability compared to age-matched healthy comparator groups. This relative stability of cognition was evident not only among those who developed schizophrenia in later life (i.e. after the age of 45), but also among those who lived with schizophrenia for most of their adult life, i.e., similar to the chronically institutionalized patients (e.g. [22–24]).

However, other clinical characteristics limit a comparison between the community- and institution-based studies. The community-based studies tended to have short follow-up periods with a maximum of three years. They also tended to focus on patients in their mid-fifties rather than their sixties or seventies as with institution-based studies. In fact, longer follow-up studies and studies that reported on older community-dwelling patients did observe an accelerated cognitive decline despite the small sample sizes in these studies [25–27].

Another critical difference between these two types of studies is that institutionalized patients have severe cognitive impairment at baseline with MMSE scores in the low teens, in contrast to typical MMSE scores in the twenties among community-dwelling patients. This baseline cognitive impairment is likely the major reason behind their chronic institutionalization. It also suggests that institutionalized patients have a lower cognitive reserve that prevents them from coping with aging-related cognitive decline and predisposes them to accelerated cognitive decline [28].

Notwithstanding these differences between community- and institution-based studies, the accelerated decline observed in the latter could also be due to the institutionalization itself. The limited social engagement and relatively impoverished environment that patients living in institutions experience could contribute to their poor cognitive reserve and decline [29]. Thus, the diverse trajectories of cognition in older patients with schizophrenia could be masked by the effect of institutionalization, even if poor cognitive and clinical functioning are among the factors that lead to chronic institutionalization of these patients.

This diversity in trajectories is supported by a large and relatively long community-based study (mean follow-up: 3.5 years) of persons with schizophrenia aged 40 and above. The authors found three groups of individuals: those who remain stable and represent 50% of the sample, those who slowly decline and represent 40% of the sample and those who rapidly decline and represent 10% of the sample [30]. Importantly, residential status was a strong predictor in differentiating the patients who remain stable from those who decline [31]. More recently, a longitudinal study (mean follow-up: 52 months) of 103 community-dwelling persons with schizophrenia aged 60 and over supported the heterogeneity model of cognitive trajectories [31]. The authors found 19% of people were "rapid decliners", 19% were "rapid improvers" and 62% remained fairly stable.

Finally, at a population level, one relatively recent large Danish epidemiological study demonstrated that individuals with schizophrenia experience twice the risk of developing dementia compared to those without schizophrenia [32]. This finding supports accelerated aging; however, the study also demonstrates the various demographic and clinical characteristics that largely modify this risk, suggesting again that there are diverse groups of older patients with schizophrenia with varied trajectories.

Profile of cognitive impairment in older adults with schizophrenia

Older adults with schizophrenia have been shown to be cognitively impaired on measures of global cognition, e.g., MMSE [13], the Dementia Rating Scale (DRS) [33] or the Repeatable Battery for the Assessment of Neuropsychological Status (RBANS) [34], irrespective of whether they were community-dwellers or chronically institutionalized (MMSE [35–45], DRS [38,42,46–50], RBANS [51]).

Beyond global cognition, the profile of deficits across the various cognitive domains has been described in general for both residential settings, although in more detail for community-dwelling patients, given that the severity of impairment among the institutionalized patients prevents the administration of detailed cognitive testing.

Executive dysfunction has been consistently described among older and community-dwelling patients with schizophrenia, using composite measures of executive function [38,40,44,45,52,53]. In addition, executive dysfunction has been described using individual measures of cognitive flexibility, problem solving and clustering [35,43,54]. The severity of these impairments did not depend on whether the onset of schizophrenia was early (before the age of 40) or later in life [38,43,55].

Consistent impairments have also been described in visuospatial ability, in both community-dwelling and institutionalized patients [37,39,43,48,53,54]. Interestingly, the severity of these deficits does not seem to depend on residential status [48], suggesting that some domains may remain less impaired, even in severe forms of schizophrenia.

Impairments in verbal fluency have also been consistently described among institutionalized [37,56] and community-dwelling patients [45,57] and, similar to executive dysfunction, they do not vary based on age at onset [38,43,55].

Dysfunctional information processing has been considered by some to be a core cognitive dysfunction in schizophrenia underlying a generalized deficit that manifests itself in other cognitive domains [58]. Consistently, older patients, especially those living in the community, exhibit impairments in psychomotor information processing speed compared to healthy individuals [38,52,55]. Further, and consistent with the hypothesis that impairments in information processing are core impairments, they do not differ based on age at onset [38,55].

Memory deficits have been described in both encoding and recall, among institutionalized as well as community-dwelling patients [36–38,40,43,44,47,48,52–54]. In contrast to other cognitive domains, residential status does seem to have an impact on the severity of memory impairment, as institutionalized patients have been shown to be more impaired than community-dwellers [48]. This differential effect of residence is consistent with a dementia-like trajectory among institutionalized patients. Further, memory performance seems to differentiate older patients with schizophrenia from those with Alzheimer's dementia. Older patients with schizophrenia have been shown to be as impaired as those with Alzheimer's dementia regarding learning, but less so on recall [36,39,55,59], suggesting that their memory deficits are driven by an inability to encode information rather than forgetting information. This finding has implications for clinical care as it suggests that simplifying clinical communication to older patients with schizophrenia to optimize encoding is likely to result in compliance with the information being communicated. These findings also support the model that frontal-lobe rather than temporal-lobe dysfunction is behind memory impairments in patients with schizophrenia.

While deficits in working memory, an executive function, have been clearly described in older patients with schizophrenia, studies that separated attention from working memory found variable results with respect to attention. Some studies reported no impairments in attention [35,40,47], while others reported impairments [38,43,52,53,55]. Age at onset was not a factor in determining these deficits [38,43,55].

Cognition and function in older adults with schizophrenia

While it is well known that cognitive impairments are among the strongest predictors of real-world function among adults with schizophrenia [60], much less is known about this relationship among older adults with this illness. Using functional capacity measures as proxy measures for real-world function, the association between cognition and function has been shown to maintain its strength across the adult lifespan, including late in life [9,10]. Thus, this association was not weakened by other aging-related factors that could contribute to functional impairments in later life.

Assessing specific relationships between cognitive domains and function, one study demonstrated that baseline visual memory, information processing speed and executive function predicted functional abilities among mid-life patients with schizophrenia at six months from baseline [61]. A second study found that baseline verbal memory and psychomotor speed predicted function one year later among patients with chronic schizophrenia [62]. A third study found that baseline verbal learning and memory, and sustained attention, predicted functional abilities even at two years of follow-up among patients with chronic schizoaffective disorders [63]. In contrast, among institutionalized patients with schizophrenia, persistent clinical symptoms seem to override the impact of cognition on function [64].

Enhancing cognition and function in older adults with schizophrenia

Few studies have tested pharmacological or non-pharmacological interventions among older patients with schizophrenia specifically to enhance their cognition or daily function.

One study [65–67] randomized 176 patients with schizophrenia aged 60 or older to receive olanzapine or risperidone and assessed change in clinical symptoms and cognition. The two drugs did not differ in their impact on symptoms or cognition and there was improvement in both conditions from baseline in attention and memory.

Another trial [68] randomized 198 patients with schizophrenia (aged 41–75 years) experiencing subsyndromal depression to receive citalopram or placebo. Social functioning improved among those who received citalopram compared to placebo, in addition to their improvement in depressive symptoms.

In an open-label antipsychotic (olanzapine and risperidone) dose-reduction study, 37 chronically stable patients aged 50 or above experienced 40% reduction in the dose of their antipsychotic. The dose reduction resulted in higher dopaminergic receptor availability in the whole striatum. In addition, an association between this availability and overall cognition emerged after the dose reduction, even though there was no improvement in cognition after the dose reduction [69].

Few cognitive remediation studies focused on older patients with schizophrenia, although these may well adhere to this therapy form [70].

Two trials in adult patients with depression, bipolar disorder or schizophrenia assessed the addition of cognitive remediation to vocational rehabilitation. Combining these two studies, 34 patients aged 45 or older were compared to 42 patients aged 44 or younger [71]. The younger group improved on several cognitive measures in response, however there was no improvement in the older group.

A second cognitive remediation study enrolled 55 patients with schizophrenia aged less than 40 and 30 patients aged 40 or above [72]. The younger participants benefited from cognitive remediation with respect to cognitive flexibility, memory and planning. In contrast, older participants improved only in memory.

A third small, randomized controlled trial of patients with schizophrenia aged 60 or above (N = 29) showed that virtual reality cognitive remediation improved overall cognition compared to treatment as usual [73].

A fourth analysis assessed whether patients with schizophrenia aged 40 or above (N = 57) benefited differently from those aged less than 40 (N = 77) in a randomized controlled trial and an observational study of cognitive remediation [74]. In contrast to the younger patients, who experienced improvements in working memory if they received cognitive remediation compared to control condition, older patients did not experience any benefits from cognitive remediation.

Finally, in a pilot study among 22 patients aged 60 or above, cognitive remediation was well tolerated and adhered to. However, patients did not experience improvement in cognition [70].

Few studies aimed at enhancing function among older adults with schizophrenia using psychosocial interventions. Several of these studies are described in detail in Chapter 14. Among these, a manualized weekly group therapy (cognitive behavioral social skills training; CBSST) explicitly includes cognitive functioning as a target, next to behavioral symptoms, communication deficits, and problem solving skills. A 24-week course of CBSST has been shown to improve skills of independent living among a group of 37 patients with schizophrenia aged 42–74 years compared to 39 patients who received treatment as usual [75]. These improvements persisted for one year after the end of the CBSST course [76]. Baseline cognition predicted response to CBSST and treatment as usual [77].

Conclusions

Cognition in older adults with schizophrenia continues to be a critical dimension of the illness in its ability to determine patients' overall level of functioning. Thus, understanding its trajectories is essential to better understand the course of the illness overall and to better develop interventions that could enhance cognition and in turn function in this growing population.

While the current literature suggests different trajectories for different patients, mostly due to their level of cognitive function – and their residential status as a proxy – in late mid-life, larger and longer studies among community-dwelling patients are needed. These patients represent the vast majority of older patients living with schizophrenia. Clinically, their trajectories are not static in late life, with significant fluctuations in symptoms [78]. Thus, larger and longer cognitive studies are needed to have enough power to detect such fluctuations and heterogeneous trajectories with respect to cognition [79]. Such studies will also advance our knowledge of the predictors of these various trajectories and consequently allow intelligent design of interventions that aim at modifying these factors and altering these trajectories.

References

1. Cohen, C.I., Outcome of schizophrenia into later life: an overview. *Gerontologist*, 1990. 30(6): 790–7.

2. Cohen, C.I., Directions for research and policy on schizophrenia and older adults: Summary of the GAP Committee report. *Psychiatric Services*, 2000. 51(3): 299–302.

3. Gurland, B.J. and P.S. Cross, Epidemiology of psycho-pathology in old-age: some implications for clinical services. *Psychiatric Clinics of North America*, 1982. 5(1): 11–82.

4. Palmer, B.W., R.K. Heaton, J.S. Paulsen, et al., Is it possible to be schizophrenic yet neuropsychologically normal? *Neuropsychology*, 1997. 11(3): 437–46.

5. Kahn, R.S. and R.S.E. Keefe, Schizophrenia is a cognitive illness: time for a change in focus. *JAMA Psychiatry*, 2013. 70(10): 1107–12.

6. Cuffel, B.J., D.V. Jeste, M. Halpain, et al., Treatment costs and use of community mental health services for schizophrenia by age cohorts. *American Journal of Psychiatry*, 1996. 153(7): 870–6.

7. Karim, S., R. Overshott, and A. Burns, Older people with chronic schizophrenia. *Aging and Mental Health*, 2005. 9(4): 315–324.

8. Green, M.F. and P.D. Harvey, Neurocognitive deficits and functional outcome in schizophrenia: are we measuring the "right stuff"? *Schizophrenia Bulletin*, 2000. 26(1): 119–36.

9. Kalache, S.M., B.H. Mulsant, S.J.C. Davies, et al., The impact of aging, cognition, and symptoms on functional competence in individuals with schizophrenia across the lifespan. *Schizophrenia Bulletin*, 2015. 41(2): 374–81.

10. Tsoutsoulas, C., B.H. Mulsant, S.M. Kalache, et al., The influence of medical burden severity and cognition on functional competence in older community-dwelling individuals with schizophrenia. *Schizophrenia Research*, 2016. 170(2-3): 330–5.

11. Roth, M., The natural history of mental disorder in old age. *Journal of Mental Science*, 1955. 101(423): 281–301.

12. Holden, N.L., Late paraphrenia or the paraphrenias: a descriptive study with a 10-year follow-up. *British Journal of Psychiatry*, 1987. 150: 635–9.

13. Folstein, M.F., S.E. Folstein, and P.R. McHugh, Mini-Mental State: practical method for grading cognitive state of patients for clinicians. *Journal of Psychiatric Research*, 1975. 12(3): 189–98.

14. Harvey, P.D., L. White, M. Parella, et al., The longitudinal stability of cognitive impairment in schizophrenia: Mini-Mental State scores at one- and two-year follow-ups in geriatric inpatients. *British Journal of Psychiatry*, 1995. 166: 630–3.

15. Harvey, P.D., J. Lombardi, M. Leibman, et al., Cognitive impairment and negative symptoms in geriatric chronic schizophrenic patients: a follow-up study. *Schizophrenia Research*, 1996. 22(3): 223–31.

16. Harvey, P.D., J. Lombardi, M. Leibman, et al., Performance of chronic

schizophrenic patients on cognitive neuropsychological measures sensitive to dementia. *International Journal of Geriatric Psychiatry*, 1996. 11(7): 621–7.

17. Harvey, P.D., J.M. Silverman, R.C. Mohs, et al., Cognitive decline in late-life schizophrenia: a longitudinal study of geriatric chronically hospitalized patients. *Biological Psychiatry*, 1999. 45(1): 32–40.

18. Waddington, J.L. and H.A. Youssef, Cognitive dysfunction in chronic schizophrenia followed prospectively over 10 years and its longitudinal relationship to the emergence of tardive dyskinesia. *Psychological Medicine*, 1996. 26(4): 681–8.

19. McGurk, S.R., P.J. Moriarty, P.D. Harvey, et al., The longitudinal relationship of clinical symptoms, cognitive functioning, and adaptive life in geriatric schizophrenia. *Schizophrenia Research*, 2000. 42(1): 47–55.

20. Friedman, J.I., P.D. Harvey, T. Coleman, et al., Six-year follow-up study of cognitive and functional status across the lifespan in schizophrenia: a comparison with Alzheimer's disease and normal aging. *American Journal of Psychiatry*, 2001. 158(9): 1441–8.

21. McClure, M.M., D.M. Barch, J.D. Flory, et al., Context-procesing deficits in schizotypal personality disorder. *Journal of Abnormal Psychology*, 2004. 113(4): 556–8.

22. Heaton, R.K., J.A. Gladsjo, B.W. Palmer, et al., Stability and course of neuropsychological deficits in schizophrenia. *Archives of General Psychiatry*, 2001. 58(1): 24–32.

23. Savla, G.N., D.J. Moore, S.C. Roesch, et al., An evaluation of longitudinal neurocognitive performance among middle-aged and older schizophrenia patients: use of mixed-model analyses. *Schizophrenia Research*, 2006. 83(2-3): 215–23.

24. Palmer, B.W., M.W. Bondi, E.W. Twamley, et al., Are late-onset schizophrenia spectrum disorders neurodegenerative conditions? Annual rates of change on two dementia measures. *Journal of Neuropsychiatry and Clinical Neurosciences*, 2003. 15(1): 45–52.

25. Laks, J., L.F. Fontenelle, A. Chalita, and M.V. Mendlowicz, Absence of dementia in late-onset schizophrenia: a one year follow-up of a Brazilian case series. *Arquivos de Neuro-Psiquiatria*, 2006. 64(4): 946–9.

26. Brodaty, H., P. Sachdev, A. Koschera, et al., Long-term outcome of late-onset schizophrenia: 5-year follow-up study. *British Journal of Psychiatry*, 2003. 183: 213–19.

27. Loewenstein, D.A., S.J. Czaja, C.R. Bowie, and P.D. Harvey, Age-associated differences in cognitive performance in older patients with schizophrenia: a comparison with healthy older adults. *American Journal of Geriatric Psychiatry*, 2012. 20(1): 29–40.

28. Stern, Y., What is cognitive reserve? Theory and research application of the reserve concept. *Journal of the International Neuropsychological Society*, 2002. 8(3): 448–60.

29. Harvey, P.D., D.A. Loewenstein, and S.J. Czaja, Hospitalization and psychosis: Influences on the course of cognition and everyday functioning in people with schizophrenia. *Neurobiology of Disease*, 2013. 53: 18–25.

30. Thompson, W.K., G.N. Savla, I.V. Vahia, et al., Characterizing trajectories of cognitive functioning in older adults with schizophrenia: does method matter? *Schizophrenia Research*, 2013. 143(1): 90–6.

31. Cohen C.I. and T. Murante, A prospective analysis of the role of cognition in three models of aging and schizophrenia. *Schizophrenia Research*, 2018. 196: 22–8.

32. Ribe, A.R., T.M. Laursen, M. Charles, et al., Long-term risk of dementia in persons with schizophrenia. *JAMA Psychiatry*, 2015. 72(11): 1095–101.

33. Mattis, S., *Dementia Rating Scale*. 1973, Odessa, FL: Psychological Assessment Resources, Inc.

34. Randolph, C., M.C. Tierney, E. Mohr, and T.N. Chase, The repeatable battery for the assessment of neuropsychological status (RBANS): preliminary clinical validity.

Journal of Clinical and Experimental Neuropsychology, 1998. 20(3): 310–19.

35. Almeida, O.P., R.J. Howard, R. Levy, et al., Cognitive features of psychotic states arising in late-life (late paraphrenia). *Psychological Medicine*, 1995. 25(4): 685–98.

36. Davidson, M., P. Harvey, K.A. Welsh, et al., Cognitive functioning in late-life schizophrenia: a comparison of elderly schizophrenic patients and patients with Alzheimer's disease. *American Journal of Psychiatry*, 1996. 153(10): 1274–9.

37. Harvey, P.D., H. Jacobsen, D. Mancini, et al., Clinical, cognitive and functional characteristics of long-stay patients with schizophrenia: a comparison of VA and state hospital patients. *Schizophrenia Research*, 2000. 43(1): 3–9.

38. Jeste, D.V., M.J. Harris, A. Krull, et al., Clinical and neuropsychological characteristics of patients with late-onset schizophrenia. *American Journal of Psychiatry*, 1995. 152(5): 722–30.

39. McBride, T., P.J. Moberg, S.E. Arnold, et al., Neuropsychological functioning in elderly patients with schizophrenia and Alzheimer's disease. *Schizophrenia Research*, 2002. 55(3): 217–27.

40. Miller, B.L., I.M. Lesser, K.B. Boone, et al., Brain-lesions and cognitive function in late-life psychosis. *British Journal of Psychiatry*, 1991. 158: 76–82.

41. Moore, D.J., B.W. Palmer, and D.V. Jeste, Use of the Mini-Mental State Exam in middle-aged and older outpatients with schizophrenia: cognitive impairment and its associations. *American Journal of Geriatric Psychiatry*, 2004. 12(4): 412–19.

42. Patterson, T.L., J.C. Klapow, J.H. Eastham, et al., Correlates of functional status in older patients with schizophrenia. *Psychiatry Research*, 1998. 80(1): 41–52.

43. Sachdev, P., H. Brodaty, N. Rose, and S. Cathcart, Schizophrenia with onset after age 50 years 2: Neurological, neuropsychological and MRI investigation. *British Journal of Psychiatry*, 1999. 175: 416–21.

44. Sachdev, P., H. Brodaty, D. Cheang, and S. Cathcart, Hippocampus and amygdala volumes in elderly schizophrenic patients as assessed by magnetic resonance imaging. *Psychiatry and Clinical Neurosciences*, 2000. 54(1): 105–12.

45. Rajji, T.K., A.N. Voineskos, M.A. Butters, et al., Cognitive performance of individuals with schizophrenia across seven decades: a study using the MATRICS Consensus Cognitive Battery. *American Journal of Geriatric Psychiatry*, 2013. 21(2): 108–18.

46. Bankole, A.O., C.I. Cohen, I. Vahia, et al., Factors affecting quality of life in a multiracial sample of older persons with schizophrenia. *American Journal of Geriatric Psychiatry*, 2007. 15(12): 1015–23.

47. Cohen, C.I., P. Stastny, D. Perlick, I. Samuelly, and L. Horn, Cognitive deficits among aging schizophrenic-patients residing in the community. *Hospital and Community Psychiatry*, 1988. 39(5): 557–9.

48. Evans, J.D., A.E. Negron, B.W. Palmer, et al., Cognitive deficits and psychopathology in institutionalized versus community-dwelling elderly schizophrenia patients. *Journal of Geriatric Psychiatry and Neurology*, 1999. 12(1): 11–15.

49. Palmer, B.W., L.B. Dunn, P.S. Appelbaum, and D.V. Jeste, Correlates of treatment-related decision-making capacity among middle-aged and older patients with schizophrenia. *Archives of General Psychiatry*, 2004. 61(3): 230–6.

50. Zorrilla, L.T.E., R.K. Heaton, L.A. McAdams, et al., Cross-sectional study of older outpatients with schizophrenia and healthy comparison subjects: no differences in age-related cognitive decline. *American Journal of Psychiatry*, 2000. 157(8): 1324–6.

51. Jeste, D.V., B.W. Palmer, P.S. Appelbaum, et al., A new brief instrument for assessing decisional capacity for clinical research. *Archives of General Psychiatry*, 2007. 64(8): 966–74.

52. Evans, J.D., R.K. Heaton, J.S. Paulsen, et al., The relationship of neuropsychological abilities to specific domains of functional capacity in older schizophrenia patients. *Biological Psychiatry*, 2003. 53(5): 422–30.

53. Fucetola, R., L.J. Seidman, W.S. Kremen, et al., Age and neuropsychologic function in schizophrenia: a decline in executive abilities beyond that observed in healthy volunteers. *Biological Psychiatry*, 2000. 48(2): 137–46.

54. Depp, C.A., D.J. Moore, D. Sitzer, et al., Neurocognitive impairment in middle-aged and older adults with bipolar disorder: comparison to schizophrenia and normal comparison subjects. *Journal of Affective Disorders*, 2007. 101(1–3): 201–9.

55. Heaton, R., J.S. Paulsen, L.A. McAdams, et al., Neuropsychological deficits in schizophrenics: relationship to age, chronicity, and dementia. *Archives of General Psychiatry*, 1994. 51(6): 469–76.

56. Kosmidis, M.H., V.P. Bozikas, C.H. Vlahou, et al., Verbal fluency in institutionalized patients with schizophrenia: age-related performance decline. *Psychiatry Research*, 2005. 134(3): 233–40.

57. Moore, R., N. Blackwood, R. Corcoran, et al., Misunderstanding the intentions of others: an exploratory study of the cognitive etiology of persecutory delusions in very late-onset schizophrenia-like psychosis. *American Journal of Geriatric Psychiatry*, 2006. 14(5): 410–18.

58. Dickinson, D., M.E. Ramsey, and J.M. Gold, Overlooking the obvious: a meta-analytic comparison of digit symbol coding tasks and other cognitive measures in schizophrenia. *Archives of General Psychiatry*, 2007. 64(5): 532–42.

59. Ting, C., T.K. Rajji, Z. Ismail, et al., Differentiating the cognitive profile of schizophrenia from that of Alzheimer disease and depression in late life. *PLOS One*, 2010. 5(4): e10151.

60. Green, M.F., What are the functional consequences of neurocognitive deficits in schizophrenia? *American Journal of Psychiatry*, 1996. 153(3): 321–30.

61. Lewandowski, K.E., B.M. Cohen, M.S. Keshavan, S.H. Sperry, and D. Öngür, Neuropsychological functioning predicts community outcomes in affective and non-affective psychoses: a 6-month follow-up. *Schizophrenia Research*, 2013. 148(1–3): 34–7.

62. Tabares-Seisdedos, R., V. Balanzá-Martínez, J. Sánchez-Moreno, et al., Neurocognitive and clinical predictors of functional outcome in patients with schizophrenia and bipolar I disorder at one-year follow-up. *Journal of Affective Disorders*, 2008. 109(3): 286–99.

63. Arts, B., N. Jabben, L. Krabbendam, and J. van Os, A 2-year naturalistic study on cognitive functioning in bipolar disorder. *Acta Psychiatrica Scandinavica*, 2011. 123(3): 190–205.

64. Nemoto, T., H. Niimura, Y. Ryu, K. Sakuma, and M. Mizuno, Long-term course of cognitive function in chronically hospitalized patients with schizophrenia transitioning to community-based living. *Schizophrenia Research*, 2014. 155(1–3): 90–5.

65. Kennedy, J., D. Jeste, C.J. Kaiser, et al., Olanzapine vs haloperidol in geriatric schizophrenia: analysis of data from a double-blind controlled trial. *International Journal of Geriatric Psychiatry*, 2003. 18(11): 1013–20.

66. Harvey, P.D., J.A. Napolitano, L. Mao, and G. Gharabawi, Comparative effects of risperidone and olanzapine on cognition in elderly patients with schizophrenia or schizoaffective disorder. *International Journal of Geriatric Psychiatry*, 2003. 18(9): 820–8.

67. Jeste, D.V., Y. Barak, S. Madhusoodanan, F. Grossman, and G. Gharabawi, International multisite double-blind trial of the atypical antipsychotics risperidone and olanzapine in 175 elderly patients with chronic schizophrenia. *American Journal of Geriatric Psychiatry*, 2003.

11(6): 638–47. [Erratum appears in *American Journal of Geriatric Psychiatry*, 2004. 12(1): 49].

68. Kasckow, J., N. Lanouette, T. Patterson, et al., Treatment of subsyndromal depressive symptoms in middle-aged and older adults with schizophrenia: Effect on functioning. *International Journal of Geriatric Psychiatry*, 2010. 25(2): 183–90.

69. Rajji, T.K., B.H. Mulsant, S. Nakajima, et al., Cognition and dopamine D-2 receptor availability in the striatum in older patients with schizophrenia. *American Journal of Geriatric Psychiatry*, 2017. 25(1): 1–10.

70. Golas, A.C., S.M. Kalache, C. Tsoutsoulas, et al., Cognitive remediation for older community-dwelling individuals with schizophrenia: a pilot and feasibility study. *International Journal of Geriatric Psychiatry*, 2015. 30(11): 1129–34.

71. McGurk, S.R. and K.T. Mueser, Response to cognitive rehabilitation in older versus younger persons with severe mental illness. *American Journal of Psychiatric Rehabilitation*, 2008. 11: 90–105.

72. Wykes, T., C. Reeder, S. Landau, et al., Does age matter? Effects of cognitive rehabilitation across the age span. *Schizophrenia Research*, 2009. 113(2–3): 252–8.

73. Chan, C.L., E.K. Ngai, P.K. Leung, and S. Wong, Effect of the adapted virtual reality cognitive training program among Chinese older adults with chronic schizophrenia: a pilot study. *International Journal of Geriatric Psychiatry*, 2010. 25(6): 643–9.

74. Kontis, D., V. Huddy, C. Reeder, S. Landau, and T. Wykes, Effects of age and cognitive reserve on cognitive remediation therapy outcome in patients with schizophrenia. *American Journal of Geriatric Psychiatry*, 2013. 21(3): 218–30.

75. Granholm, E., J.R. McQuaid, F.S. McClure, et al., A randomized, controlled trial of cognitive behavioral social skills training for middle-aged and older outpatients with chronic schizophrenia. *The American Journal of Psychiatry*, 2005. 162(3):520–9.

76. Granholm, E., J.R. McQuaid, F.S. McClure, et al., Randomized controlled trial of cognitive behavioral social skills training for older people with schizophrenia: 12-month follow-up. *Journal of Clinical Psychiatry*, 2007. 68(5): 730–7.

77. Granholm, E., J.R. McQuaid, P.C. Link, et al., Neuropsychological predictors of functional outcome in cognitive behavioral social skills training for older people with schizophrenia. *Schizophrenia Research*, 2008. 100(1–3): 133–143.

78. Cohen, C.I. and M. Iqbal, Longitudinal study of remission among older adults with schizophrenia spectrum disorder. *American Journal of Geriatric Psychiatry*, 2014. 22(5): 450–8.

79. Shmukler, A.B., I.Y. Gurovich, M. Agius, and Y. Zaytseva, Long-term trajectories of cognitive deficits in schizophrenia: a critical overview. *European Psychiatry*, 2015. 30(8): 1002–10.

Chapter 7

Medical Issues in Older Adults with Schizophrenia

Frank Copeli and Carl I. Cohen, M.D.

This chapter will review recent epidemiological findings concerning medical comorbidity and mortality in older adults with schizophrenia (OAS) and elaborate on several critical elements. First, whether there is an increased or decreased susceptibility to certain medical disorders. In particular, we will assess the OAS population's risk and mortality with regard to cardiovascular, respiratory, metabolic, and malignant neoplastic diseases. Second, to assess whether the services available to this population are comparable with those available to normal community elders, and to determine whether there are any serious impediments to medical treatment. Third, to determine the extent to which existing services are utilized, as well as the level of consumer satisfaction with their health care treatment. Finally, the authors will review some of the recent strategies to improve health care of this population, such as the use of health care managers.

Overall disease prevalence and mortality rates

Several writers have postulated that schizophrenia is considered a state of accelerated aging and there has been an ongoing discussion of the effect of schizophrenia on physical health and mortality [1]. In contrast to younger persons with schizophrenia, few studies have looked into the physical comorbidities of OAS. In 2014, Hendrie et al. [1] reported on a 10-year observational cohort of 31,588 persons without schizophrenia and 1,635 with schizophrenia who were aged 65 and over and living in Indiana. They found that the latter had significantly higher rates of congestive heart failure, chronic obstructive pulmonary disease, dementia, and hypothyroidism, whereas they had lower cancer rates. In contrast, a Danish Registry study reported in 2017 by Brink et al. [2] found no differences between schizophrenia outpatients (N = 667) and the general population (N = 7087) at age 70 with respect to chronic illnesses such as cancer, diabetes, dementia, and cardiovascular, pulmonary, renal, liver, gastrointestinal, and rheumatic diseases. The Danish findings contrast with studies of younger schizophrenia populations and their age peers in which the former typically had higher rates of cardiovascular disease, diabetes, and pulmonary disorders, whereas the cancer rates were more inconsistent [3].

The increased mortality of patients with schizophrenia is widely accepted, with a life expectancy reduced by 15–20 years [4,5]. In 2007, Saha et al. [6], in a meta-analysis of mortality in multiple nations, described a significant disparity between the mortality of people with schizophrenia and the general population, finding a standardized mortality ratio (SMR) of 2.58 compared to the general population and no significant changes after post-hoc analyses and consideration of national economic development. They also noted the SMRs had been increasing in a linear fashion over the preceding three decades.

More recently, Hjorthøj et al. [5] performed a meta-analysis of mortality studies from "all inhabited continents excluding South America." They described an average of "potential life lost" of 14.5 years and a life expectancy of 64.7 years, with a reduced life expectancy for men of 15.9 years, compared to 13.6 years for women. Life expectancy for men in this study was 60 years and 68 for women. Life lost was greatest in Africa and least in Asia, with a life expectancy lowest in the Asian and African continents. The study was not able to assess or isolate patients seeking treatment versus those not seeking treatment because all patients included in the analysis were seeking or had previously sought treatment.

In the past, there has been some difficulty commenting on mortality in OAS patients due to a lack of consensus on the age demarcation for "older adult" [7]; earlier studies have used cut-offs that typically coincide with middle age. However, over the past few years new studies have used more standard definitions of "elderly," e.g., age 60 or 65 and over. Below, we summarize the largest mortality studies of OAS aged 65 and over.

- Talaslahti et al. [3] examined mortality and cause of death in OAS patients aged 65 or older using a sample of 9,461 Finnish patients registered between 1969 and 2008 and followed between 1999 and 2008. They demonstrated an SMR of 2.69 in these OAS patients. For natural causes, an SMR of 2.58 was observed with an SMR of 11.04 for unnatural causes (including accidents and suicides). Of patients who died during follow-up, 31% had at least one psychiatric hospitalization within the five-year period preceding follow-up – their SMR was 3.92, compared to an SMR of 2.37 for patients who were not psychiatrically hospitalized during this period.

- In the previously described study, Hendrie and colleagues [1] found a mortality hazard ratio after controlling for various confounding variables of 1.25 for patients with schizophrenia (p = 0.006). Patients with schizophrenia were more likely to die of pulmonary disease and heart/vascular disease and less likely to die of neurological diseases and cancer.

- An Australian longitudinal study of 37,892 elderly men followed for 14.7 years by Almeida et al. [8] observed an increased age-adjusted mortality hazard of 2.0 for the 444 men with schizophrenia spectrum disorder aged 65–85 compared to older men without severe mental disorder. The authors observed mortality rates that increased with age, even into the 80s. A subset of these patients (N = 12,136) were also assessed with a formal evaluation of "sociodemographic, lifestyle, and clinical variables," but the authors concluded that these variables could not account for increased mortality.

- A five-year prospective study of 157 OAS patients in the Netherlands [9] demonstrated an SMR of 1.89, higher in men than women (2.60 versus 1.78). Higher hazard ratios were associated with increasing age, male gender, and compulsory psychiatric hospitalizations.

- Kredentser's population-based study in Manitoba, Canada [16] described age- and sex-adjusted 10-year mortality rates and noted an increased risk of cancer mortality in middle-aged patients in comparison to younger and older schizophrenia patients. The study also found a relative risk of all-cause mortality of 1.42 in patients older than 60 years, lower than that found in patients aged 10–39 (4.14), 40–59 (2.5), and all ages (1.70). The relative risk of suicide trended downward from the 10–39 to 40–59-year-old age group and was the least frequent cause of death in patients older than 60, so infrequent that a statistically significant SMR could not be established.

- A Danish study [11] of persons with schizophrenia aged 50 and over found suicide rate ratios of 7.0 and 13.7 in 50–69-year-old men and women, respectively, when compared to controls. With patients above the age of 70, the suicide rate ratios dropped to 2.1 and 3.4 in men and women, respectively.
- A cohort study of 150,000 mental health users in South London and Maudsley National Health Services Foundation Trust (NHS SLAM) [12] demonstrated SMRs of 2.25 and 2.52 in patients with schizophrenia and schizoaffective disorders, compared to an SMR of 1.95 in bipolar disorder patients. African and other black patients displayed the highest SMR compared to other ethnicities, and females displayed a decreased SMR compared to men with schizophrenia, but increased mortality in bipolar disorder and schizoaffective disorders compared to men. The study also demonstrated decreasing SMRs of 4.73, 3.44, and 1.63 in schizophrenic patients aged 15–44, 45–64, and 65+, respectively. Schizoaffective patients had decreasing SMRs of 3.96, 2.71, and 2.10 and the SMRs of bipolar disorder patients also decreased to 4.09, 2.58, and 1.51, respective to the above age groups.
- A Danish study by Brink and colleagues of persons aged 70 and over [2] found that while OAS did not differ from their age peers in the prevalence of chronic medical illnesses, they were less likely to receive cardiovascular medications, more likely to be prescribed analgesics, and had fewer encounters as medical outpatients. The authors concluded that the increased mortality commonly found in OAS may be due to underdiagnosis of physical illness or a poor conception of the severity of an established medical diagnosis [13].

In summary, a pattern emerged from these studies that pointed to an increased mortality risk in OAS versus their age peers. On the other hand, OAS consistently experienced reduced all-cause mortality rates compared to younger schizophrenia patients. Moreover, there remains a poor understanding of modifiable risk factors contributing to this mortality. There is a suggestion that the medical illnesses of these patients are likely undertreated or not diagnosed in the primary care or psychiatric setting. The severity of diagnosed physical diseases in these patients may also be underappreciated, requiring an enhanced level of care compared to their age peers with the same diagnosis. Future research should focus more specifically on the etiological factors accounting for the increased mortality versus their age peers.

Common medical disorders

Respiratory disorders

Mortality risk

Over the past decade, there have been advances in our understanding of the association between respiratory disease risk and mortality in schizophrenia patients, including older adults [10,14]. Kredentser et al. [16] observed SMRs rising in a large Canadian population, reaching a value of 59.63 for respiratory diseases above the age of 60, compared to age-matched controls with an SMR of 35.97 and 10.04 for patients in the 40–59 age group. The oldest patient group also had a relative risk of 1.66, dropping from 5.27 in the 40–59 age group. This drop in risk may represent a survival bias. Notably, this age group's mortality risk for respiratory disease was greater than that for lung cancer (SMRs of relative risk of 1.66 and 1.34, respectively). Very-late-onset schizophrenia patients (greater than 60 years old) were shown to have increased SMRs for respiratory diseases compared to earlier-onset patients [17].

Prevalence rates

Hendrie et al. [1] observed an increased risk of chronic obstructive pulmonary disease (COPD) in OAS in Indiana after adjusting for age, sex, and ethnicity, while a nationwide register study in Denmark did not [2]. The latter study's findings may be attributable to differences between the America and Danish health care systems or the possibility that Danish schizophrenia patients were underregistered or undertreated. A population-based study in Taiwan [18] found an increased prevalence of COPD in schizophrenia patients aged 70 years and older.

Several recent mixed-age studies have also yielded interesting findings. A retrospective case–control study of comorbidity in persons with schizophrenia admitted to British hospitals over a 12-year period [19] found an increased odds ratio for COPD in deceased patients with schizophrenia compared to the general population. An increased mortality odds ratio was also found for pneumonia and bronchitis. A population-based study in Spain also found an increased odds ratio for COPD, but not for other respiratory diseases [20]. Increased risk of death was also found in patients with "diseases of the respiratory system." An American study of hospitalizations [21] also found increased risk of chronic hospitalizations for COPD and asthma in schizophrenia patients with a mean age of 49.

Schizophrenia patients in general appear to be more likely to be hospitalized for pneumonia than the general population [22] and this has been associated with worse clinical outcomes [23], including acute respiratory failure, ICU admissions, mechanical ventilation, and mortality [24].

Association with antipsychotic medications

The association of antipsychotic use with respiratory diseases, and community-acquired pneumonia in particular [25–31], has been explored in some detail since the FDA [25] issued a warning about the increased risk of death due to pneumonia in elderly dementia patients taking antipsychotic medications. A review by Trifirò [32] described a general finding in epidemiological investigations of elderly patients being treated with antipsychotics of an apparent dose-dependent relationship in "the early phases of treatment with either typical or atypical antipsychotics." This increased risk may be attributable to increased aspiration risk due to extrapyramidal effects or dopamine receptor blockade resulting in dysfunction of the oropharynx [20]. Similarly, an extensive review by Correll et al. [33] demonstrated a dose-dependent risk for pneumonia of second-generation antipsychotic agents used in mixed-age schizophrenia patients (adjusted risk ratio (ARR) 1.69). These analyses, however, were not focused directly on OAS patients.

Diabetes

Mortality risk

The increased mortality has not been so consistently observed in OAS patients with diabetes. In Hendrie and colleagues' [1] register study in Indiana, diabetes was not identified as a significant cause of death compared to their age peers. An Australian population study [8] similarly found no significant elevation of diabetes mortality in a large population of elderly males with schizophrenia versus their age peers. On the other hand, a population study of American schizophrenia patients did show higher diabetes mortality rates for OAS patients. Patients aged 55–63 had an SMR of 4.1 compared to age peers, the same as the 35–54-year-old schizophrenia patients, but lower than the SMR of 7.3 in the 20–34-year-old schizophrenia group [22].

Prevalence rates

Hendrie's group found OAS patients had a significant, albeit modest (10%), higher prevalence of diabetes comorbidity than their age peers [1]. The Danish study by Brink et al. [2] in a less heterogeneous population and different health care delivery system was unable to demonstrate a statistically significant adjusted odds ratio increase in diabetes mellitus in OAS patients.

Some studies have shown underutilization of diabetic medications in OAS, whereas others have not [34]. Interestingly, a VA study of severe mental illness (SMI) patients [35] (7,529 patients, mean age 54.5 years) found patients with bipolar disorder were 19% more likely to suffer from diabetes than schizophrenic patients. Among 200 individuals with serious mental illness [36], the cohort over the age of 55 averaged a lower HbA1c than their peers under the age of 55; and among the latter, the schizophrenia patients had lower average HbA1c measurements than those with bipolar disorder and major depressive disorder.

Association with antipsychotic medications

It is difficult to separate the metabolic risk profile in OAS patients from the well-described risk [37] inherent in antipsychotic use. The synergistic development of metabolic and cardiovascular diseases along with other environmental behavioral risk factors provides additional challenges. However, it is known that an increased risk for diabetes is present generally in the schizophrenia population [38,39]. Jeste et al. [40] theorized that despite the implication of antipsychotics in metabolic risk, reports of "greater insulin resistance, shorter telomeres, increased oxidative stress markers and mortality" in schizophrenics are not "solely attributable" to these medications and indicate morbidity and mortality are part of the schizophrenia disease state.

Cardiovascular disease

Mortality rates

Cardiovascular disease is one of the most common comorbid disorders in persons with schizophrenia, with increased risk factors and onset at a younger age when compared to patients without schizophrenia, as well as higher mortality rates versus those in the general population [41–45]. Moreover, schizophrenia patients seem to be benefiting less from the drop in cardiovascular disease mortality experienced by the rest of the population [46]. The increased mortality from cardiovascular disease has been attributed to increased rates of smoking, obesity, diabetes, and hyperlipidemia in schizophrenia patients.

In a British retrospective study by Osborn et al. [37], hazard ratios (HRs) for coronary heart disease (CHD) mortality in people with severe mental illness (including schizophrenia, schizoaffective disorder, bipolar disorder, delusional disorder) were 3.22, 1.86, and 1.05 in age groups of 18–49, 50–75, and older than 75, respectively. These ratios were only slightly diminished after further adjustments for smoking status and social deprivation. Patients with schizophrenia and CHD had higher mortality in the 18–49 and 50–75 groups than those with bipolar disorder, but these HRs did not extend into the 75 and older population. Likewise, Kredentser et al. [16], in a Canadian population study, demonstrated an increased mortality relative risk of 1.41 for circulatory disease for patients above the age of 60, and an apparent drop in relative risk compared to younger age groups. The apparent drop in cardiovascular mortality in schizophrenia patients may represent a survival bias.

Prevalence rates

Hendrie et al. [1], in an observational cohort described previously, found an increase in congestive heart failure versus other older adults, but not in other cardiovascular diseases. The Danish register study by Brink and coauthors demonstrated no statistically significant odds ratios for a cardiovascular disease in 70-year-old schizophrenic adults compared to controls [2]. This study also found that these patients were less likely to be prescribed cardiovascular medications, similar to another Danish population study showing underprescription of cardiovascular drugs to schizophrenia patients [41]; an American study of community-dwelling older adults with schizophrenia similarly showed undertreatment of hypertension and heart disease in OAS [34]. Brink et al. [2] also demonstrated a decrease in outpatient utilization of health care amongst these patients, suggesting undertreatment of cardiovascular disease in the primary care setting. A large American study that included schizophrenia patients with a mean age of 62 found that they were significantly less likely than their age peers to receive revascularization [47]. A nationwide cohort of patients with a first diagnosis of myocardial infarction in Sweden, followed over a 12-year period, found schizophrenia patients had a higher 30-day and 1-year mortality than bipolar patients and non-mentally-ill controls [48]. These studies suggest a strong likelihood of undertreatment of cardiovascular disease in this population. It is also possible that the severity of illness is underappreciated in these patients [23], requiring more careful assessment of risk factors in primary care [49] and psychiatric settings [50].

Association with antipsychotic medications

With regard to antipsychotic usage, it is important to recognize that the known metabolic risks associated with these drugs are a likely predisposing factor in the development of cardiovascular disease. A Clinical Antipsychotic Trials of Intervention Effectiveness (CATIE)-based study [51] clarified some of the risks of antipsychotic medications. In a population treated with antipsychotics for a mean of 14 years, the authors found that olanzapine produced the largest elevation of 10-year CHD risk, based on the Framingham scale, with quetiapine having a comparable risk. Risperidone, ziprasidone, and perphenazine were associated with lower overall risk; the largest differences were found in patients with a 10% baseline risk of CHD. A study of a mixed age schizophrenia sample in Sweden revealed a U-shaped pattern in which higher cardiovascular mortality occurred in patients using either high doses or no antipsychotic medications [52]. Osborn et al. [37] showed some increased CHD and stroke mortality in SMI patients older than 75 when on higher prescribed doses of antipsychotics, but cautioned that antipsychotics alone could not explain this increased mortality. The U-shaped mortality curve suggests the need for more research into identifying the optimal antipsychotic dosages for elderly patients.

Cancer

Mortality risk

The increased cancer mortality rate among persons with schizophrenia is well established. A recent meta-analysis by Zhou et al. [53] found a pooled SMR of 1.40 versus the general schizophrenia population. This increased cancer mortality in the general schizophrenia population may extend to OAS, although findings have been inconsistent in older persons. Kredentser's Canadian study [16] of mortality found an increased cancer mortality rate with a relative risk of 2.48 in patients aged 40–59, which subsequently dropped to 0.63 in patients older than 60 years. Lung cancer relative risk in the same study was 1.65 and 1.34 in patients aged 40–59 and 60+, respectively. A study of American schizophrenia patients by Olfson et al. [22] found SMRs for lung cancer of 2.5, 2.4, and 1.5 for 55–64, 35–54, and 20–34 age groups, respectively; 55–64-year-old patients also had elevated SMRs versus other age categories for colon, breast, liver, pancreatic, and "other" cancers. The hematologic cancer SMR was slightly higher for the 55–64-year-old age group compared to 35–54, but the same as the 20–34-year-old group. Talaslahti [54] observed an SMR of 1.9 for "neoplasm" in a Finnish register study of 10,000 OAS patients diagnosed before 59 years of age and an alarming SMR of 5.1 in patients with onset of schizophrenia after the age of 60. On the other hand, a study in Indiana by Hendrie and colleagues [1] showed a decreased identified cause of death from cancer in older schizophrenia patients versus their age peers (14.78% versus 22.63%).

Surprisingly, the high rate of tobacco use in the schizophrenia community did not appear to influence mortality. In a study of the effect of smoking on mortality of schizophrenia patients, 55–69-year-olds who smoked more than one pack per day had an HR of 0.47 for all-cause tobacco-related mortality compared to non-schizophrenia smokers; by contrast, younger schizophrenia smokers (aged 35–54) had an HR of 2.1 compared to non-smokers [55].

There are few data on cancer mortality studies of OAS by ethnicity. In mixed age samples, a longitudinal cohort study in the UK [56] examining mortality in SMI by ethnicity (white British, black Caribbean, black African, South Asian, and Irish) found white British and black African patients had higher SMR for cancer than the other ethnicities in the study. Olfson et al. [22] found the highest SMR in white persons with schizophrenia and lower SMRs for black non-Hispanics and Hispanics.

Incidence rates

With respect to the incidence of cancer, a decreased, similar, or occasionally elevated incidence continues to be observed in multiple studies of mixed-age populations with schizophrenia [57–62]. A Taiwanese study [63] found cancer risk decreases as the duration and age of onset of schizophrenia increase. If schizophrenia is diagnosed before 50, the SMRs for colorectal, breast, cervical, and uterine cancers increased, but if diagnosed after 50, the SMRs for all cancers decreased except for breast cancer. Australian researchers [64] noted that a paradox exists in that cancer incidence among persons with schizophrenia seems to be the same or lower than in their age peers, but their mortality rate is higher. They postulated that this paradox may be due to difficulties in differentiating medically explained and unexplained symptoms, greater case fatality, or inequity in access to specialist procedures.

It may be more profitable to investigate cancer incidence and mortality by specific cancer rather than by this catch-all term that fails to account for the nuanced and wide-ranging pathophysiology and risk factors for each cancer. Brink's Danish register study of 70-year-olds with schizophrenia [2] did not demonstrate significant increased or decreased odds ratios for "malignant neoplasms," "lung cancer," "breast cancer," or "colon cancer." A Taiwanese study [65] found OAS patients had lower risks for pancreatic, prostate, and stomach cancer than age peers, but higher risks of nasopharynx, breast, and uterine cancers.

Bergamo et al. [66], using the Surveillance, Epidemiology, and End Results (SEER) database, linked to Medicare records, examined the diagnosis and treatment of schizophrenia men greater than 66 years old with lung cancer. Although patients with schizophrenia presented with earlier stages of lung cancer, they were less likely than their age peers to undergo diagnostic evaluation or to receive stage-appropriate treatment, resulting in poorer outcomes. The authors called for efforts to increase treatment rates for elderly patients with schizophrenia, which may lead to improved survival in this group. Another SEER retrospective cohort [67] of colon cancer patients 67 years and older found participants with a pre-existing mental illness were less likely to receive no treatment in the form of surgery, chemotherapy, or radiation. Likewise, a London-based study [68] of women aged 50–64 found patients with psychosis were less likely to attend mammogram screening, consistent with other studies finding cancer-screening gaps for schizophrenia patients [69–72]. For women with schizophrenia aged 50 and over, living in a low-income area decreased the likelihood of cancer screening in a population-based study in Manitoba, Canada [73]. Crump et al. [74] found persons with schizophrenia were more likely to die from cancer without being diagnosed.

Association with antipsychotic medications

There is no persuasive evidence that the use of antipsychotics increases risk of cancer in OAS, although data are sparse. Correll et al. [33] reviewed this subject in mixed-age samples and found contradictory studies on breast cancer incidence in women, despite increased prevalence of breast cancer risk factors. Of particular interest is whether prolactin's role in mammary carcinogenesis [75] extends to antipsychotic use. Correll's analysis of first- and second-generation antipsychotic medications predominantly showed no increased risk of breast cancer [33].

Health care utilization

The literature suggests that OAS have appreciable gaps in the adequacy of their primary medical care as compared to age peers, and this appears to cross national borders as well as health care systems. The Indiana study, described previously, by Hendrie and colleagues [1] observed that, compared to their age peers, OAS had more hospital admissions, nursing home days, home health care days, and health care costs billed to Medicare and Medicaid. However, when correcting hospital admissions per year for demographics and comorbidities, there was no significant difference in hospitalizations. Likewise, Brink's [2] study of Danish older patients with schizophrenia found no differences in hospital admissions between OAS and elders in the community, but the former had fewer medical outpatient visits. The study did find OAS patients to be less likely to receive cardiovascular medications despite comparable incidence and more likely to be prescribed analgesics, anxiolytics, and hypnotics. Persons with SMI have been found to more often be placed in a nursing home [76], while preferring to remain in a community setting [77].

Several promising innovative outreach programs have shown success in treating schizophrenia patients, resulting in improved medical outcomes. A VA study of SMI patients [78] successfully reduced mortality through outreach efforts to re-establish care, which included a cohort above the age of 64. Another VA study [79] found success in providing palliative care to elderly schizophrenics with lung cancer. These successes in providing nuanced care requiring interspecialty communication as well as physician–patient partnerships suggest the utility of integrated medical care that leverages the relationships, access, and knowledge of both primary and psychiatric care settings.

In recent years, psychosocial models of integrated care and self-management have been developed with several trials described by Bartels et al. [80] in Chapter 14 of this volume.

Moreover, as described below, several RCTs have examined embedding primary care into the mental health setting, with the intention of leveraging the relationships SMI patients may have with mental health professionals. These have been referred to in the literature as a "reverse-integrated," "colocated," or "reverse-colocated model."

- A VA study [81] of 120 SMI patients (mean age of 45.7 years) embedding primary care into mental health clinics managed to increase primary care utilization and showed improvement in the 36-item Short-Form Health Survey. Other studies have further suggested the utility of this model to increase primary care visits and reduce emergency visits [81–83].

- Primary Care Access, Referral, and Evaluation (PCARE) [84], an RCT of 407 SMI adults with a mean age of 47, showed reduced Framingham Coronary Risk scores, increased primary care utilization, and a non-significant improvement in the SF-36 physical components. At 12 months, adults received 59% of recommended primary prevention compared to 22% in the treatment-as-usual group. They were more likely to receive evidence-based care for cardiometabolic disease and more likely to have a primary care physician.

- Primary and Behavioral Health Care Integration (PBHCI) [85], a study of 447 adults with SMI (mean age of 47 years) showed greater use of preventive services, continuity, and better cardiometabolic care. This study followed important measures of cardiometabolic health such as LDL, Framingham Risk, and HbA1c, but could not demonstrate significant improvements.

- A VA longitudinal cohort study in Providence, Rhode Island of 97 SMI veterans with a mean age of 55 years(age range: 28–86 years) more closely focused on cardiometabolic risks and medical comorbidity in a primary care model colocated in a mental health clinic [86]. After six months, the authors observed statistically significant improvements in attaining target blood pressure, LDL, triglycerides, and BMI goals, but not HDL and HbA1c.

Telehealth and mobile technologies may offer a powerful component in building successful collaborative care models and managing chronic medical conditions. A pilot study of telehealth interventions at Dartmouth Centers for Health and Aging [87], with 70 SMI patients (aged 18 and over), achieved high participation and improvement in self-reported health management, as well as significant decreases in diastolic blood pressure, fasting glucose, and urgent care visits. Another small pilot study (N = 8) of SMI patients over the age of 60 [88] usedeer technology and a smart phone application and also found high participation and improvement in patient self-assessments. SMI patients are engaged with mobile technologies and social media [89–91] and its widespread use across the globe presents promising opportunities to improve utilization of primary care services as well as peer-to-peer support.

Fortuna et al. [92] examined the experience in SMI patients with secondary data from Medical Expenditure Panel Surveys of over 35,000 adults over the age of 50. This study found psychiatric diagnosis to be a predictor of patient satisfaction. Schizophrenia spectrum patients were more likely to report "providers did not explain things in a way that was easily understood" and to find a physician to have "not spent enough time" compared to patients with a mood disorder or older adults without SMI. On the positive side, schizophrenia spectrum patients did not report significant difficulty in shared decision-making processes. Schizophrenia spectrum disorder patients were also not found to report statistically significant difficulty gaining access to care compared to patients without SMI and patients with mood disorders.

For a more extensive discussion of this topic, the reader is referred to an excellent review by De Hert and colleagues [93]. The authors identify 31 barriers to the recognition and management of physical diseases in patients with severe mental illness divided into five categories: patient and illness, treatment, psychiatrist, other physician, and services. The authors propose 17 recommendations at the system and individual levels of action that can address gaps in the assessment and treatment of physical health within this population.

Conclusions

Several key points emerge from this review:

- There are inconsistencies in the prevalence of various medical disorders among OAS, most likely reflecting differences in study methods, age categories, survivor effects, and the ability of health care systems to recognize and treat disorders in this population.
- Recent studies across nations and health care systems have demonstrated about a 2.0 to 2.5 increase in all-cause mortality in OAS compared to age peers. The all-cause mortality risk broadly appears to be improved compared to middle-aged and younger schizophrenics.
- The risk of suicide trends downward in OAS patients after the age of 60, further decreasing past the age of 70. Female OAS patients appear to have a higher suicide risk than males. OAS patients are still at significant risk of suicide compared to their age peers.
- With respect to respiratory disorders, among OAS there is increased mortality for respiratory disease compared to the general population, but reduced compared to younger persons with schizophrenia. Increased prevalence of respiratory diseases in OAS has not been demonstrated consistently. Schizophrenia patients in general are more likely to be hospitalized for pneumonia than the general population and more likely to experience acute respiratory failure, mechanical ventilation, and mortality. OAS patients may have a theoretical increased dose-dependent risk for pneumonia when on antipsychotic medications, but this requires more direct study.
- With respect to diabetes, there has been no demonstrated increase in mortality or prevalence in the OAS population. However, OAS patients may be undertreated and underdiagnosed.

- With respect to cardiovascular disease, OAS patients have a declining mortality from cardiovascular disease as they age compared to their younger counterparts, but still elevated compared to their age peers. A survival bias cannot be ruled out. Prevalence of cardiovascular disease drops with age, but paradoxically, large register studies demonstrate increased mortality, but have not demonstrated increased prevalence versus their age peers. This may reflect a greater likelihood of receiving inadequate treatment. Antipsychotic medication may play a role in increased cardiovascular mortality in OAS patients, e.g., a U-shaped pattern with very high, or very low or none, but more research is needed to optimize dosing in this population.
- With respect to cancer, a wide range of studies have demonstrated increased, decreased, or similar incidence in OAS compared to age peers. Studies by cancer type may provide more clarity. There is a suggestion that a paradox exists in that cancer incidence among all persons with schizophrenia appears to be the same or lower than their age peers, but their mortality rate is higher. This may reflect a variety of patient and systemic factors. Indeed, a screening and treatment gap exists in OAS patients with respect to cancer, which may account for lower incidence rates and higher mortality rates.
- A health care utilization gap for outpatient care exists for OAS patients across nations and health care systems. Integrated health care models show promise in bridging primary and psychiatric care. A variety of self-management, peer support groups, and integrated care models in tandem with advancements in telehealth and mobile technologies offer novel strategies in treating physical disease in OAS patients.

References

1. Hendrie HC, Tu W, Tabbey R, et al. Health outcomes and cost of care among older adults with schizophrenia: a 10-year study using medical records across the continuum of care. *Am J Geriatr Psychiatry* 2014; 22(5):427–36.

2. Brink M, Green A, Bojesen AB, et al. Physical health, medication, and healthcare utilization among 70–year–old people with schizophrenia: a nationwide Danish register study. *Am J Geriatr Psychiatry* 2017; 25:500–9.

3. Talaslahti T, Alanen H-M, Hakko H, et al. Mortality and causes of death in older patients with schizophrenia. *Int J Geriatr Psychiatry* 2012; 27:1131–7.

4. Laursen TM. Life expectancy among persons with schizophrenia or bipolar affective disorder. *Schizophr Res* 2011; 131(1–3):101–4.

5. Hjorthøj C, Stürup AE, Mcgrath JJ, Nordentoft M. Years of potential life lost and life expectancy in schizophrenia: a systematic review and meta-analysis. *Lancet Psychiatry* 2017; 4(4):295–301.

6. Saha S, Chant D, McGrath J. A systematic review of mortality in schizophrenia: is the differential mortality gap worsening over time? *Arch Gen Psychiatry* 2007; 64:1123–31.

7. Cohen CI, Freeman K, Ghoneim D, et al. Advances in the conceptualization and study of schizophrenia in later life. *Psychiatr Clin N Am* 2018; 41:39–53.

8. Almeida OP, Hankey GJ, Yeap BB, et al. Mortality among people with severe mental disorders who reach old age: a longitudinal study of a community-representative sample of 37892 men. *PloS one* 2014; 9(10): e111882.

9. Meesters PD, Comijs HC, Smit JH, et al. Mortality and its determinants in late-life schizophrenia: a 5-year prospective study in a Dutch catchment area. *Am J Geriatr Psychiatry* 2016; 24:272–7.

10. Hoang U, Stewart R, Goldacre, MJ. Mortality after hospital discharge for people with schizophrenia or bipolar disorder: retrospective study of linked English hospital episode statistics, 1999–2006. *BMJ* 2011; 343:d5422.

11. Erlangsen A, Eaton WW, Mortensen PB, Conwell Y. Schizophrenia: a predictor of suicide during the second half of life? *Schizophr Res* 2012; 134(2–3):111–17.

12. Chang CK, Hayes RD, Broadbent M, et al. All-cause mortality among people with serious mental illness (SMI), substance use disorders, and depressive disorders in southeast London: a cohort study. *BMC Psychiatry* 2010; 10:77.

13. Meesters PD. Healthy older schizophrenia patients: exceptions to the rule? *Am J Geriatr Psychiatry* 2017; 25(5):510–11.

14. Crump C, Winkleby MA, Sundquist K, Sundquist J. Comorbidities and mortality in persons with schizophrenia: a Swedish national cohort study. *Am J Psychiatry* 2013; 170(3):324–33.

15. Partti K, Vasankari T, Kanervisto M, et al. Lung function and respiratory diseases in people with psychosis: population-based study. *Br J Psychiatry* 2015; 207(1):37–45.

16. Kredentser MS, Martens PJ, Chochinov HM, Prior HJ. Cause and rate of death in people with schizophrenia across the lifespan: a population-based study in Manitoba, Canada. *J Clin Psychiatry* 2012; 74:154–61.

17. Talaslahti T, Alanen HM, Hakko H, et al. Patients with very-late-onset schizophrenia-like psychosis have higher mortality rates than elderly patients with earlier onset schizophrenia. *Int J Geriatr Psychiatry* 2015; 30(5):453–9.

18. Hsu J-H, Chien IC, Lin CH, Chou YJ, Chou P. Increased risk of chronic obstructive pulmonary disease in patients with schizophrenia: a population-based study. *Psychosomatics* 2013; 54(4):345–51.

19. Schoepf D, Uppal H, Potluri R, Heun R. Physical comorbidity and its relevance on mortality in schizophrenia: a naturalistic 12-year follow-up in general hospital admissions. *Eur Arch Psychiatry Clin Neurosci* 2014; 264(1):3–28.

20. Bouza C, López-Cuadrado T, María Amate J. Physical disease in schizophrenia: a population-based analysis in Spain. *BMC Publ Health* 2010; 10(1):745.

21. Cahoon EK, McGinty EE, Ford DE, Daumit GL. Schizophrenia and potentially preventable hospitalizations in the United States: a retrospective cross-sectional study. *BMC Psychiatry* 2013; 13(1):37.

22. Olfson M, Gerhard T, Huang C, Crystal S, Stroup TS. Premature mortality among adults with schizophrenia in the United States. *JAMA Psychiatry* 2015; 72(12):1172–81.

23. Chen Y-H, Lin H-C, Lin H-C. Poor clinical outcomes among pneumonia patients with schizophrenia. *Schizophr Bull* 2010; 37(5):1088–94.

24. Chou FH-C, Tsai K-Y, Chou Y-M. The incidence and all-cause mortality of pneumonia in patients with schizophrenia: a nine-year follow-up study. *J Psychiatr Res* 2013; 47(4):460–6.

25. U.S. Food and Drug Administration. *Public Health Advisory: Deaths with Antipsychotics in Elderly Patients with Behavioural Disturbances.* Silver Spring, MD: U.S. Food and Drug Administration; 2005.

26. Trifirò G, Gambassi G, Sen EF, et al. Association of community-acquired pneumonia with antipsychotic drug use in elderly patients: a nested case-control study. *Ann Intern Med* 2010; 152:418–25.

27. Knol W, Marum RJ, Jansen PA, et al. Antipsychotic drug use and risk of pneumonia in elderly people. *J Am Geriatr Soc* 2008; 56:661–6.

28. Gau JT, Acharya U, Khan S, et al. Pharmacotherapy and the risk for community-acquired pneumonia. *BMC Geriatr* 2010; 10:45.

29. Star K, Bate A, Meyboom RH, Edwards IR. Pneumonia following antipsychotic prescriptions in electronic health records: a patient safety concern? *Br J Gen Pract* 2010; 60:e385–94.

30. Barnett MJ, Perry PJ, Alexander B, Kaboli PJ. Risk of mortality associated with antipsychotic and other neuropsychiatric drugs in pneumonia patients. *J Clin Psychopharmacol* 2006; 26:182–7.

31. Kuo C-J, Yang S-Y, Liao Y-T, et al. Second-generation antipsychotic medications and risk of pneumonia in schizophrenia. *Schizophr Bull* 2013; 39(3):648–57.

32. Trifirò G. Antipsychotic drug use and community-acquired pneumonia. *Curr Infect Disease Rep* 2011; 13(3): 262–8.

33. Correll CU, Detraux J, De Lepeleire J, De Hert M. Effects of antipsychotics, antidepressants and mood stabilizers on risk for physical diseases in people with schizophrenia, depression and bipolar disorder. *World Psychiatry* 2015; 14(2):119–36.

34. Vahia IV, Diwan S, Bankole AO, et al. Adequacy of medical treatment among older persons with schizophrenia. *Psychiatr Serv* 2008; 59:853–9.

35. Kilbourne AM, Brar JS, Drayer RA, Xu X, Post EP. Cardiovascular disease and metabolic risk factors in male patients with schizophrenia, schizoaffective disorder, and bipolar disorder. *Psychosomatics* 2007; 48(5):412–17.

36. Sajatovic M, Gunzler D, Einstadter D, et al. A preliminary analysis of individuals with serious mental illness and comorbid diabetes. *Arch Psychiatr Nurs* 2016; 30(2):226–9.

37. Osborn DPJ, Levy G, Nazareth I, Petersen I, Islam A, King MB. Relative risk of cardiovascular and cancer mortality in people with severe mental illness from the United Kingdom's General Practice Research Database. *Arch Gen Psychiatry* 2007; 64(2):242–9.

38. Casey DA, Rodriguez M, Northcott C, Vickar G, Shihabuddin L. Schizophrenia: medical illness, mortality, and aging. *Int J Psychiatry Med* 2011; 41(3):245–51.

39. Martens PJ, Chochinov HM, Prior HJ. Where and how people with schizophrenia die: a population-based, matched cohort study in Manitoba, Canada. *J Clin Psychiatry* 2013; 74(6):e551–7.

40. Jeste DV, Wolkowitz OM, Palmer BW. Divergent trajectories of physical, cognitive, and psychosocial aging in schizophrenia. *Schizophr Bull* 2011; 37(3):451–5.

41. Bresee LC, Majumdar SR, Patten SB, et al. Prevalence of cardiovascular risk factors and disease in people with schizophrenia: a population-based study. *Schizophr Res* 2010; 117:75–82.

42. Hahn LA, Mackinnon A, Foley DL, et al. The value of counting WHO-defined cardiovascular risk factors for death and disability in a national sample of adults with psychosis. *Schizophr Res* 2017; 182:13–18.

43. Fors BM, Isacson D, Bingefors K, Widerlov B. Mortality among persons with schizophrenia in Sweden: an epidemiological study. *Nord J Psychiatry* 2007; 61(4):252–9.

44. Goff DC, Cather C, Evins AE, et al. Medical morbidity and mortality in schizophrenia: guidelines for psychiatrists. *J Clin Psychiatry* 2005; 66(2):183–94.

45. Olfson M, Gerhard T, Huang C, Crystal S, Stroup TS. Premature mortality among adults with schizophrenia in the United States. *JAMA Psychiatry* 2015; 72(12):1172–81.

46. Ösby U, Westman J, Hällgren J, Gissler M. Mortality trends in cardiovascular causes in schizophrenia, bipolar and unipolar mood disorder in Sweden 1987–2010. *Eur J Publ Health* 2016; 26(5):867–71.

47. Schulman-Marcus J, Goyal P, Swaminathan RV, et al. Comparison of trends in incidence, revascularization, and in-hospital mortality in ST-elevation myocardial infarction in patients with versus without severe mental illness. *Am J Cardiol* 2016; 117(9):1405–10.

48. Bodén R, Molin E, Jernberg T, et al. Higher mortality after myocardial infarction in patients with severe mental illness: a nationwide cohort study. *J Intern Med* 2015; 277(6):727–36.

49. Viñas CL, Fernández San-Martín MI, Martín López LM. Effectiveness of a joint project between primary care and mental health to improve the recording of cardiovascular risk factors in patients with psychosis. *Aten Primaria* 2012; 45(6):307–14.

50. Rouillon F, Van Ganse E, Vekhoff P, et al. Vigilance level for cardiovascular risk factors in schizophrenic patients. *L'Encephale* 2015; 41(1):70–7.

51. Daumit GL, Goff DC, Meyer JM, et al. Antipsychotic effects on estimated 10-year coronary heart disease risk in the CATIE schizophrenia study. *Schizophr Res* 2008; 105(1–3):174–87.

52. Torniainen M, Mittendorfer-Rutz E, Tanskanen A, et al. Antipsychotic treatment and mortality in schizophrenia. *Schizophr Bull* 2015; 41(3):656–63.

53. Zhou C, Tao R, Jiang R, Lin X, Shao M. Cancer mortality in patients with schizophrenia: systematic review and meta-analysis. *Br J Psychiatry* 2017; 211(1):7–13.

54. Talaslahti T. Finnish older patients with schizophrenia: antipsychotic use, psychiatric admissions, long-term care and mortality. Dissertation, University of Tampere, 2015.

55. Kelly DL, McMahon RP, Wehring HJ, et al. Cigarette smoking and mortality risk in people with schizophrenia. *Schizophr Bull* 2011; 37(4):832–8.

56. Das-Munshi J, Chang CK, Dutta R, et al. Ethnicity and excess mortality in severe mental illness: a cohort study. *Lancet Psychiatry* 2017; 4(5):389–99.

57. Kisely S, Sadek J, Mackenzie A, Lawrence D, Campbell LA. Excess cancer mortality in psychiatric patients. *Can J Psychiatry* 2008; 53:753–61.

58. Kisely S, Crowe E, Lawrence D. Cancer-related mortality in people with mental illness. *JAMA Psychiatry* 2013; 70(2):209–17.

59. Lawrence D, Holman CD, Jablensky AV, Threlfall TJ, Fuller SA. Excess cancer mortality in Western Australian psychiatric patients due to higher case fatality rates. *Acta Psychiatr Scand* 2000; 101(5):382–8.

60. Bushe CJ, Hodgson R. Schizophrenia and cancer: in 2010 do we understand the connection? *Can J Psychiatry* 2010; 55(12):761–7.

61. Goldacre MJ, Kurina LM, Wotton CJ, Yeates D, Seagroat V. Schizophrenia and cancer: an epidemiological study. *Br J Psychiatry* 2005; 187:334–8.

62. Chen LY, Hung YN, Chen YY, et al. Cancer incidence in young and middle-aged people with schizophrenia: nationwide cohort study in Taiwan, 2000–2010. *Epidemiol Psychiatr Sci* 2018; 27(2):146–56.

63. Lin G-M, Chen YJ, Kuo DJ, et al. Cancer incidence in patients with schizophrenia or bipolar disorder: a nationwide population-based study in Taiwan, 1997–2009. *Schizophr Bull* 2013; 39(2):407–16.

64. Kisely S, Forsyth S, Lawrence D. Why do psychiatric patients have higher cancer mortality rates when cancer incidence is the same or lower? *Aus NZ J Psychiatry* 2016; 50(3):254–63.

65. Lin C-Y, Lane HY, Chen TT, et al. Inverse association between cancer risks and age in schizophrenic patients: a 12-year nationwide cohort study. *Cancer Sci* 2013; 104(3):383–90.

66. Bergamo C, Sigel K, Mhango G, Kale M, Wisnivesky JP. Inequalities in lung cancer care of elderly patients with schizophrenia: an observational cohort study. *Psychosom Med* 2014; 76(3):215.

67. Baillargeon J, Kuo YF, Lin YL, et al. Effect of mental disorders on diagnosis, treatment, and survival of older adults with colon cancer. *J Am Geriatr Soc* 2011; 59(7):1268–73.

68. Werneke U, Horn O, Maryon-Davis A, et al. Uptake of screening for breast cancer in patients with mental health problems. *J Epidemiol Community Health* 2006; 60(7):600–5.

69. Irwin KE, Henderson DC, Knight HP, Pirl WF. Cancer care for individuals with schizophrenia. *Cancer* 2014; 120(3):323–34.

70. Aggarwal A, Pandurangi A, Smith W. Disparities in breast and cervical cancer screening in women with mental illness: a systematic literature review. *Am J Prev Med* 2013; 44(4):392–8.

71. Chochinov H, Martena PJ, Prior HJ, Fransoo R, Burland E. Does a diagnosis of schizophrenia reduce rates of mammography screening? A Manitoba population-based study. *Schizophr Res* 2009; 113:95–100.

72. Xiong G, Bermudes R, Torres S, Hales R. Use of cancer screening services among patients with serious mental illness in Sacramento County. *Psychiatr Serv* 2008; 59:929–32.

73. Martens PJ, Chochinov HM, Prior HJ, et al. Are cervical cancer screening rates different for women with schizophrenia? A Manitoba population-based study. *Schizophr Res* 2009; 113(1):101–6.

74. Crump C, Winkleby MA, Sundquist K, Sundquist J. Comorbidities and mortality in persons with schizophrenia: a Swedish national cohort study. *Am J Psychiatry* 2013; 170:324–33.

75. De Hert M, Peuskens J, Sabbe T, et al. Relationship between prolactin, breast cancer risk and antipsychotics in patients with schizophrenia: a critical review. *Acta Psychiatr Scand* 2016; 133(1):5–22.

76. Andrews AO, Bartels SJ, Xie H, et al. Increased risk of nursing home admission among middle aged and older adults with schizophrenia. *Am J Geriatr Psychiatry* 2009; 17(8):697–705.

77. Horan ME, Muller JJ, Winocur S, et al. Quality of life in boarding houses and hostels: a residents' perspective. *Community Ment Health J* 2001; 37(4):323–34.

78. Davis CL, Kilbourne AM, Blow FC, et al. Reduced mortality among Department of Veterans Affairs patients with schizophrenia or bipolar disorder lost to follow-up and engaged in active outreach to return for care. *Am J Publ Health* 2012; 102(Suppl 1):S74–9.

79. Ganzini L, Socherman R, Duckart J, Shores M. End-of-life care for veterans with schizophrenia and cancer. *Psychiatr Serv* 2010; 61:725–8.

80. Bartels SJ, DiMilia PR, Fortuna KL, Naslund JA. Integrated care for older adults with serious mental illness and medical comorbidity: evidence-based models and future research directions. *Psychiatr Clin N Am* 2018; 41(1):153–64.

81. Druss BG, Rohrbaugh RM, Levinson CM, et al. Integrated medical care for patients with serious psychiatric illness: a randomized trial. *Arch Gen Psychiatry* 2001; 58(9):861–8.

82. Saxon AJ, Malte CA, Sloan KL, et al. Randomized trial of onsite versus referral primary medical care for veterans in addictions treatment. *Med Care* 2006; 44(4):334–42.

83. Druss BG. Improving medical care for persons with serious mental illness: challenges and solutions. *J Clin Psychiatry* 2007; 68(Suppl 4):40–4.

84. Druss BG, von Esenwein SA, Compton MT, et al. A randomized trial of medical care management for community mental health settings: the primary care access, referral, and evaluation (PCARE) study. *Am J Psychiatry* 2010; 167(2):151–9.

85. Druss BG, von Esenwein SA, Glick GE, et al. Randomized trial of an integrated behavioral health home: the health outcomes management and evaluation (HOME) study. *Am J Psychiatry* 2017; 174(3):246–55.

86. Pirraglia PA, Rowland E, Wu W-C, et al. Benefits of a primary care clinic co-located and integrated in a mental health setting for veterans with serious mental illness. *Prev Chronic Dis* 2012; 9:E51.

87. Pratt SI, Bartels SJ, Mueser KT, et al. Feasibility and effectiveness of an automated telehealth intervention to improve illness self-management in people with serious psychiatric and medical disorders. *Psychiatr Rehabil J* 2013; 36(4):297–305.

88. Fortuna KL, Dimilia PR, Lohman MC, et al. Feasibility, acceptability, and preliminary effectiveness of a peer-delivered and technology supported

self-management intervention for older adults with serious mental illness. *Psychiatr Q.* 2018; 89(2):293–305.

89. Naslund JA, Aschbrenner KA, Bartels SJ. How people living with serious mental illness use smartphones, mobile apps, and social media. *Psychiatr Rehabil J* 2016; 39(4):364–7.

90. Naslund JA, Aschbrenner KA, Marsch LA, et al. The future of mental health care: peer-to-peer support and social media. *Epidemiol Psychiatr Sci* 2016; 25(2):113–22.

91. Naslund JA, Aschbrenner KA, McHugo GJ, et al. Exploring opportunities to support mental health care using social media: a survey of social media users with mental illness. *Early Interv Psychiatry* 2017:1–9. doi: 10.1111/eip.12496. [Epub ahead of print]

92. Fortuna KL, Lohman MC, Batsis JA, et al. Patient experience with healthcare services among older adults with serious mental illness compared to the general older population. *Int J Psychiatry Med* 2017; 52(4-6):381–98.

93. De Hert M, Cohen D, Bobes J, et al. Physical illness in patients with severe mental disorders. II. Barriers to care, monitoring and treatment guidelines, plus recommendations at the system and individual level. *World Psychiatry* 2011; 10(2):138–51.

Chapter

8

Assessing Outcomes in Schizophrenia in Later Life

Carl I. Cohen, M.D.

It is a daunting task to assess outcome in schizophrenia because it has been influenced by the prevailing views of the disease construct and by what constitutes appropriate parameters of outcome [1]. Based on longitudinal studies of 10 years or less, Hegarty and colleagues [2] found improvement rates in schizophrenia fluctuated historically: ≤1910 (12%), 1920 (10%), 1930 (30%), 1940 (89%), 1950 (25%), 1960 (41%), 1970 (49%), 1980 (38%), and 1990 (20%). They attributed the protean rates of outcome over the twentieth century to the fluctuations in the conceptualization of the disorder, and while treatment may have impacted on outcome, the declines in improvement outcome rates in the 1980s and 1990s were thought to reflect the stricter DSMIII diagnostic criteria. Wing [1] noted that many outcome studies typically combine clinical and social indices, making comparisons even more difficult. Thus, although it may be possible to obtain some consistency between sites with respect to clinical measures, social measures may reflect disadvantages such as poor education, lack of opportunities, intellectual disabilities, low income, and the like, irrespective of the impact of the schizophrenia disorder. Moreover, the clinical disorder itself, its phenomenology and course, may be shaped by cultural (e.g., social stigma) and socioeconomic forces [3].

McGlashan [4] illustrated how the outcomes of three long-term studies reflected differences in geographical settings (urban, suburban, rural), educational levels, socioeconomic status, marital status, premorbid work and social functioning, age of onset, responsiveness to medications, and length of hospitalization. Jääskeläinen and colleagues [5] found that many earlier review studies had been flawed by the failure to include duration of illness criteria and inconsistencies in the definition of recovery so that they might include social recovery, symptomatic recovery, or both. Historically, diagnosis and deteriorating course were intertwined. Several nineteenth-century clinicians (e.g., Morel, Haslam, Burrows, Howels) anticipated Kraepelin's conceptualization of schizophrenia (which he called "dementia praecox") based on a constellation of symptoms and their course [6,7]. This perspective lost favor after Bleuler, who introduced the term "schizophrenia," re-conceptualized its core features, and posited that the disease did not always end with deterioration [8].

By the last quarter of the twentieth century, Kraepelin's formulation regarding the constituents of the core symptoms of schizophrenia as a "weakening" or "defect" of mental processes (i.e., in thinking, volition, or will) along with florid symptoms had been replaced by "negative" and "positive" symptoms along with a recognition that there are typically cognitive deficits in the disorder [8]. Interestingly, late in his career, Kraepelin considered abandoning the categorical disease nosology of schizophrenia/manic-depressive disorders and replacing them with a dimensional model [8]. The latter adumbrated the dimensional model of schizophrenia symptoms described in a special section of the DSM5.

In recent years, outcome studies of older adults with schizophrenia (OAS) have incorporated consumer and gerontological frameworks. The consumer-oriented "recovery" model has had a powerful influence in shaping conceptualizations of outcome. The Substance Abuse and Mental Health Services Administration [9] defines recovery as "A process of change through which individuals improve their health and wellness, live a self-directed life, and strive to reach their full potential." With respect to gerontological theory, recovery in OAS may be conceptualized as a pathway moving from clinical remission to community integration to a positive state of aging ("successful aging") [10]. Other writers have focused on the "paradoxical aging" framework, which refers to the concurrent decline in physical health and cognition with an improvement in subjective quality of life and psychosocial functioning in later life. This is thought to be especially striking in OAS [11].

It is evident that there are many ways to examine outcome in OAS. The literature contains no comprehensive explorations, especially utilizing prospective data; nor is there any consensus as to what constitutes outcome in OAS. Researchers and clinicians have assessed outcome using symptoms or social adaptive functioning, and sometimes both. In addition, it seems reasonable that studies of OAS should incorporate a life course perspective. In this chapter, I will examine outcome from several perspectives (symptomatic, social, aging) and look at the associations between measures and variables that may affect outcome.

Methods

In addition to the references cited from an extensive literature search, primarily derived from younger or mixed-age populations, I have utilized outcome data derived from a community sample of 249 persons aged 55 and over with early-onset (i.e., before age 45) schizophrenia spectrum disorder (e.g., schizophrenia or schizoaffective) living in New York City. Some of these findings are reported elsewhere in greater detail [12], but much of the data in this chapter were derived from analyses conducted specifically for this volume. The sample was generated using a stratified convenience sample of patients living in different community settings: 38% were living independently and 62% were living in various types of supported residence. Persons with moderately severe to severe cognitive impairment, serious medical problems, or a history of serious head trauma or unconsciousness were excluded from the study. The mean age was 61 years; 52% were males; 55% were white, 34% were black, 9% were Latino, and 2% other. A more detailed description and rationale of the sample design are provided in other publications [12,13]. Of the original sample, 88 persons could not be located, primarily because of the closing of several community residences. Of the remaining 161 persons (65%), 40 were deceased, 4 were in nursing homes and too disabled to be interviewed, 14 refused to be interviewed, while 103 participated in the follow-up interview (mean follow-up period was 53 months with a range of 12 to 116 months). A comparison of those with complete data who participated in the follow-up study with those who were not included for any reason indicated that that were no differences at baseline between groups in terms of gender, race, median income, residential status, remission rates, positive or negative symptoms, quality of life indices, anxiety scores, rates of clinical or subclinical depression, number of physical disorders, or cognitive functioning. There was a slight age difference (drop-outs were 1.4 years older), albeit statistically significant. A matched community comparison group for age, race, gender, and income, consisting of 113 persons aged 55 years and older was identified using randomly selected block groups, without replacement, as the primary sampling unit, and is described in detail elsewhere [13].

Can the DSM5 dimensional scale be used to assess outcome?

A promising point of departure for this topic is to consider the utility of the new dimensional framework in a special section of the DSM5 [14]. It offers a potentially novel approach for assessing symptom outcome that is accessible to a wide audience. The DSM5 authors contend that dimensional assessment can assist with "treatment planning, prognostic decision making, and research on pathophysiology (p.742)." Thus, it may have utility for clinicians, but also for investigative studies. To my knowledge, there have been no prior publications that have looked at the DSM5 dimensions in OAS. As can be seen in Table 8.1, which comprises the initial cross-sectional data from our NYC study, depression and cognitive dysfunction were much more common than any of the individual positive symptom domains (delusions, conceptual disorganization, hallucinations, behavioral disorganization) or negative symptom domains (blunted affect, diminished emotional express/avolition). The positive symptom domains had very high inter-correlations (r = 0.37 to r = 0.64) as did the two negative symptom domains (r = 0.67). On the other hand, after the four positive domains were combined into one variable and the two negative domains were also combined into a single variable the correlations between the four symptom domains (cognition, depression, positive and negative symptoms) were fairly modest, ranging from r = 0.03 to 0.27, or 0% to 7% shared variance (r^2). The relative independence of the outcome domains is discussed in the next section. Using the combined positive domain and the combined negative domain, 49%, 13%, 42%, and 53% of persons displayed positive symptoms, negative symptoms, depression, and cognitive symptoms (category $\geq$2; i.e., mild, moderate, or severe symptoms), respectively. Using stricter criteria of category $\geq$3 (moderate or severe symptoms), 33%, 9%, 20%, and 39% of persons displayed positive symptoms,

Table 8.1 Dimensions of psychosis symptom severity using DSM-5 criteria (N = 249)

Domain	Level of Severity (% in each category)				
	0	1	2	3	4
Delusions[a]	53	16	12	11	9
Conceptual disorganization/speech[a]	52	19	14	5	10
Hallucinations[a]	59	13	7	10	10
Behavioral disorganization[a]	71	15	10	4	1
Blunted affect[a]	89	3	2	4	2
Diminished emotional expression/avolition[a]	83	6	6	4	1
Depression[a]	44	14	22	12	8
Impaired cognition[b]	6	41	14	14	25

0 = Not present; 1 = equivocal; 2 = mild; 3 = moderate; 4 = severe.
[a]Derived from PANSS scales; [b]Derived from Dementia Rating Scale
Note: Any positive symptoms domains: 49% ($\geq$2), 33% ($\geq$3). Any negative domains: 13% ($\geq$2), 9% ($\geq$3).

negative symptoms, depression, and cognitive symptoms, respectively. In other words, depending on the cut-off, roughly half to two-thirds of persons were doing *well* on three of the four symptom domains (positive symptoms, depressive symptoms, and cognition) and nearly 90% were doing well on the negative symptom domain. Of note, in our control sample, using the dimensional criteria, only 4% exhibited depression and 14% had cognitive dysfunction that was rated mild or greater. Thus, OAS scored substantially worse than their age peers in the general community on the depression and cognitive domains.

From an epidemiological perspective, subdividing various positive and negative symptoms into individual domains made it difficult to determine the full extent of positive and negative symptomatology, although such subcategories may afford clinically useful information when assessing an individual patient. For example, using only four of seven Positive and Negative Syndrome Scale (PANSS) [15] positive symptom items and two of seven PANSS negative symptom items underestimated the prevalence of positive and negative symptoms. If all items had been used, the percentage of patients having moderate or greater positive or negative symptoms would have been 40% and 41%, respectively. The negative symptoms were especially underestimated. Moreover, as I illustrate below using longitudinal studies, data from a single assessment (i.e., cross-sectional analysis) tend to create an overly optimistic picture of clinical symptoms. It is regrettable that the Global Assessment Scale for functioning was removed from the DSM5, since combining that scale with the various domains might have produced a useful indicator of full recovery (i.e., combined symptom remission and unimpaired social functioning).

In summary, the DSM5 domain framework is a work in progress, and provides clinicians with some benchmarks for measuring outcome. However, the positive and negative symptom items will need to be refined to make it more useful as a research tool.

To what extent are various symptoms domains unique, i.e., independent from each other?

The authors of the DSM5 domains drew from schizophrenia literature that had identified four symptom domains: positive symptoms, negative symptoms, cognitive functioning, and depressive symptoms. However, it is reasonable to ask whether we need four outcome domains or do they all measure essentially the same thing? Would one global scale suffice? As shown in Table 8.2, the correlations between PANSS positive symptoms, PANSS negative symptoms, depressive symptoms using the Center for Epidemiologic Studies Depression Scale (CES-D) [16], and cognitive functioning as measured by the Dementia Rating Scale (DRS) [17] ranged from 0.03 to 0.56, with a median correlation of 0.23. Correlations (r values) of 0.1, 0.3, and 0.5 are considered small, medium, and large, respectively. Although four of six correlations were statistically significant, only two of the correlations might be considered large and the shared variances (r^2) across the analyses were fairly modest, ranging from 0% to 31% with a median value of 5%. Negative symptoms seemed to be the least independent outcome measure, exhibiting high associations with positive symptoms and cognition. These findings suggest clinical strategies targeted at the latter two variables might have effects on negative symptoms, or conversely, strategies aimed at negative symptoms might have an impact on positive symptoms or cognition. Below, I will use longitudinal data to explore this possibility. The important take-home message is that for OAS these outcome categories are sufficiently independent to warrant their separate consideration.

Table 8.2 Correlations among symptom categories (N = 249)

Domain	PANSS negative symptoms	CES-D (depressive symptoms)	DRS (cognitive functioning)
PANSS positive symptoms	0.56*	0.23*	−0.31*
DRS (cognitive functioning)	−0.47*	0.03	
CES-D (depressive symptoms)	0.06		

*p < 0.001

What are the prospects for "recovering" and "recovery"?

Liberman and Kopelowicz [18] have contended that the consumer definition of recovery as a process is more akin to "recovering" as opposed to empirical measures of "clinical recovery," which should include clinical remission and unimpaired psychosocial functioning. The final goal of this process might be "positive" mental health, i.e., mental and social well-being and not solely the absence of disease or disability. To assess these outcome indicators within a gerontological perspective, our group has operationalized four measures: clinical remission, community integration, clinical recovery, and successful aging.

Our group [12] utilized an adaptation of the original criteria established by the Remission in Schizophrenia Working Group [19] to assess remission rate, both at baseline and in the follow-up study. In order to meet the criteria of remission, subjects had to score 3 or below on each of the eight symptom domains derived from PANSS and were required to have no history of hospitalization within the previous year. The latter is a modification of the working group criteria that symptoms had to be stable for six months. Remission correlated highly with PANSS positive (r = −0.62) and negative (r = −0.53) scales.

The literature contains a variety of strategies for assessing social functioning. Indeed, for many years, the GAS-F component of the DSM was a popular and quick method to capture this domain. However, because our group was focused on community-dwelling elders, we wished to use a broader and more detailed evaluation of community integration. We developed an instrument based on the work of Wong and Solomon [20] who proposed using Moos' Ecosystem Model [21] to explore factors associated with community integration. The model theorizes that community integration is affected by personal determinants such as sociodemographics, psychiatric symptoms, and health and functioning, as well as by environmental determinants, especially various features of the consumer's treatment and housing programs. We used a modified version of this model with a focus on the personal components, and when data were available, we included some environmental factors [22]. Our 12-item Community Integration Scale consisted of four components derived from the literature: *independence* (goes places, shopping); *psychological integration* ("moderate/very satisfied" on neighborhood satisfaction, house/apartment/residence satisfaction, emotional support from non-family, emotional support from family); *physical integration* (joins activities, does not avoid others, favorable self-esteem score), and *social integration* (≥3 reliable kin members, ≥3 formal network ties, attends church, senior center, or recreational programs).

Using an adaptation of the operational criteria suggested by Strawbridge et al. [23] from the framework of Rowe and Kahn [24], our group [25] created the Successful Aging Scale, comprising the summed score (range: 0–6) of three domains: *Avoiding disease and disability*: (a) absence of cancer heart, lung, diabetic disease, symptoms of stroke, no smoking, body mass index ≤30, and no untreated hypertension and (b) no disabilities in Basic Activities of Daily Living; *High cognitive and physical function*: (a) Dementia Rating Scale: 130 (maximum 144) and (b) Instrumental Activities of Daily Living: 25 of maximum score of 28; *Engagement with life*: (a) ≥3 confidants and (b) ≥3 instrumental (i.e., helps or gives advice to others) linkages and/or working and/or does heavy and light housework.

To attain "clinical recovery," a person had to meet the aforementioned criteria for clinical remission as well as for community integration. The latter was defined as scoring 9 or more on the Community Integration Scale, which was the median value for the community comparison group.

As can be seen in Figure 8.1, cross-sectional data showed that nearly half of patients attained clinical remission, about two-fifths attained community integration, one-fifth attained "clinical recovery," and only 2% attained successful aging.

The prevalence rate of clinical remission (46%) in the NYC sample was similar to that found in a San Diego community sample of older and middle-aged adults with schizophrenia [26], but was greater than the 29% found in a Dutch sample that included some institutionalized patients and late-onset cases [27]. The San Diego and our NYC samples showed higher rates of clinical remission than in most younger samples in which the prevalence of clinical remission using Remission in Schizophrenia Working Group criteria varied widely across reported studies (17% to 88%); however, for most samples in cross-sectional studies in naturalistic settings, approximately one-third of individuals had symptomatic remission [28].

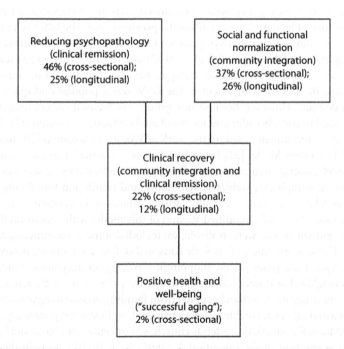

Figure 8.1 Cross-sectional and longitudinal outcome of recovery process (N: cross-sectional = 249; longitudinal = 104)

Social recovery in OAS (37%) was lower than the rates reported in World Health Organization (WHO) and catamnestic studies from various global sites, which reported rates ranging from nearly half to three-quarters of middle-aged and older subjects [29,30]. The latter studies used global measures of social outcome and there were differences from our group in the criteria for determining social recovery. In younger samples, Warner [31] reported social recovery rates ranging from 22% to 53%.

The cross-sectional level of clinical recovery (22%) in our sample was higher than the rates of 10% to 14% in younger samples [32] and the 12% and 8% reported in older persons by Ciompi [33] and Auslander and Jeste [34]. The meta-analysis by Jääskeläinen and coauthors found recovery rates of 13.5% among younger persons who met persistence of recovery criteria for two years or more [5]. Notably, our longitudinal recovery rate of 12% was similar to the latter studies.

Finally, with respect to successful aging, only 2% of the sample met the criteria. Of our community comparison group, 19% met criteria for successful aging, which was similar to the rate found in other elderly samples [35]. Thus, successful aging is difficult to attain in normal community elders, and highly unlikely among OAS. Interestingly, persons in both the normal and schizophrenia samples perceived themselves to be higher in successful aging using self-rated scales [36], although the OAS remained substantially lower than their healthy age peers: 13% of the schizophrenia sample and 27% of the community comparison group perceived themselves as aging successfully.

In summary, based on limited data in OAS that may be confounded by differences in study sites and assessment criteria, a point prevalence snapshot suggests that OAS do somewhat better than their younger counterparts with respect to clinical remission and clinical recovery, and about the same with respect to social recovery. However, as I will discuss in the next section, longitudinal data paint a more nuanced picture of these findings.

What are the outcome trajectories and associated risk factors?

There have been remarkably little longitudinal data available on changes in various outcome domains in OAS. Several writers have characterized later life as a period of "quiescence" [37], a stable phase" [38], or an "end state" [33]. However, research at our center on 104 OAS who were re-interviewed at a mean of 52 months found considerable fluidity in various outcome measures. As shown in Table 8.3, between one-quarter and two-fifths of the sample changed outcome statuses between baseline and follow-up (going in either direction). This fluctuation in various clinical and psychosocial indicators suggests that there may be opportunities for further recovery in later life. Conversely, there is also the potential for decline.

There have been several longitudinal studies of clinical remission and associated predictors in younger persons with schizophrenia that may be instructive with respect to long-term predictors of remission in older adults (Table 8.4). Among the former, the rates of clinical remission following an initial clinical episode ranged from 17% to 88% [39,40]. On follow-up, the percentage of patients maintaining remission ranged from 50% to 89% [41,42], with remission occurring in some of the originally non-remitted patients over time. For example, in one study, 57% of relapsed patients flipped back to remission on follow-up [43].

In our group's sample of OAS [12], there was a non-significant decline in the cross-sectional prevalence attaining clinical remission (49% baseline; 40% follow-up); however,

Table 8.3 Longitudinal assessments for various outcome domains (mean: 52 months follow-up)

Outcome domains	Never	Time 1 (yes); Time 2 (no)	Time 1 (no); Time 2 (yes)	Always
Remission (%)	35	25	16	25
High community integration (%)	39	16	19	26
Recovery: remission and high community integration (%)	18	31[a]	3[a]	12
Normal cognition: DRS ≥130 (%)	25	18	14	43
Not depressed: CES-D <8 (%)	44	10	16	30

[a]70% were various combinations of remission and high community integration
Note: N = 103; DRS = Dementia Rating Scale; CES-D = Center for Epidemiologic Studies–Depression Scale

25% were in remission at both assessments, 35% were not in remission at either assessment, 25% went from remission to non-remission, and 16% went from non-remission to remission. Thus, while the point prevalence for remission rates was found to be approximately half in several recent studies as well as in most of the catamnestic studies, our longitudinal data indicate that only a quarter of the sample remained in persistent remission.

In younger samples, numerous variables predicted remission on follow-up: female gender, younger age, later age of onset, taking antipsychotic medication, rapid onset, duration of untreated psychosis, baseline social functioning, better cognitive functioning, less severe negative symptoms, employment status, premorbid adjustment, and a diagnosis of schizoaffective disorder; conversely, baseline remission has been found to predict better life quality, more social contacts, and higher psychosocial functioning (see [12] for specific citations and Table 8.4 for summary of findings). Because different remission criteria were used, there have been many inconsistencies in these findings. Surprisingly, in our study of OAS [12], there were only four significant baseline predictors of remission at follow-up: higher community integration, greater number of entitlements, fewer psychotropic medications, and lower frequency of psychiatric services. Baseline remission status predicted having more total contacts at follow-up.

In looking at depression, findings from the few longitudinal investigations of younger and mixed-age populations with schizophrenia are informative. These studies found 25% to 40% of persons remained depressed clinically at baseline and follow-up, 35% to 45% were non-depressed at both baseline and follow-up, 10% to 17% became depressed over time, and 13% to 19% transitioned to non-depression over time [44–46]. These studies suggested that there is a core group of depressed (roughly one-third) and non-depressed (one-third to two-fifths) individuals, and the remainder fluctuate between these two states. Our group examined whether this pattern persists into later life. As shown in Table 8.3, we found that 44% had persistent syndromal or subsyndromal depression, 30% were never depressed, and the remainder (26%) fluctuated between the two states [47]. Thus, the pattern of depression resembled that of younger people.

In younger and mixed-age populations, several baseline factors were associated with the presence of depression on follow-up: higher levels of relapse-related mental health services, including hospitalization, suicidal ideation, and substance-related problems; conversely, depression was associated with lower levels of social and family relationships,

Table 8.4 Longitudinal studies: predictors and trajectories

	Younger and mixed-aged samples	Older adults with schizophrenia
Remission	**Predictors:** fewer negative symptoms, higher cognitive functioning, higher education, better social and vocational functioning, fewer hospitalizations, better premorbid functioning, higher Strauss–Carpenter Scale **Remission rates:** 7% to 52% References: [12,39–42]	**Predictors:** baseline higher community integration, greater number of entitlements, fewer psychotropic medications, and lower frequency of psychiatric services **Remission rates:** 25% persistent; 35% never; 16% absent to present; 25% present to never Reference: [12]
Social functioning	**Predictors:** older age of onset, better baseline social functioning, fewer negative symptoms, less severe positive symptoms, better cognitive functioning, negative family history of non-affective psychosis **Social functioning outcome rates:** GAF-D >60, 51% to 60% (WHO); 1st episode functional recovery: 42%; GAF criteria 55%; 22% to 53% social recovery References: [29,31,54–57]	**Predictors of better community integration:** lower depression, higher cognitive functioning, fewer mental health services **Community integration outcome rates:** 26% persistent; 39% never; 19% absent to present; 16% present to absent Social recovery (catamnestic studies) = 47% to 77% References: [30,58]
Depression	**Predictors:** baseline depressive symptoms, higher number of psychotropic medications, age of onset of psychotic symptoms **Depression outcome:** 25% to 40% persistent depression; 35 to 45% persistent non-depression; 13% to 19% depressed to non-depressed; 10% to17% non-depressed to depressed References: [44,47]	**Predictors of depression on follow-up:** baseline depression; greater number of psychotropic medications **Outcome:** 44% persistent depression; 30% persistent non-depression; 16% depressed to non-depressed; 10% non-depressed to depressed Reference: [47]
Cognition	**Predictors of poorer cognition:** unemployed, lower education, age of onset (not clear if early or late), male gender, negative symptoms, poor premorbid adjustment, more severe psychiatric symptoms, substance abuse **Cognitive outcome:** stable: short-term studies (mean: 12 months); stable in study over 10 years References: [11,50]	**Predictors of poorer cognition on follow-up:** lower baseline cognition, residential status (institutionalized), lower education, older age, female, Caucasian, shorter duration of illness, later age of onset. positive symptoms, negative symptoms. **Outcome:** 10% to 19% rapid decliners (>2.1/y on DRS); 25 to 40% modest decliners (0.21–2.1/y); stable 11%; 26% modest improvers (0.21–2.1/y); 19% rapid improvers (>2.1/y). References: [51,52]

quality of life, global level of functioning, mental and physical health, medication adherence, life satisfaction (see [47] for specific citations and Table 8.4 for summary of findings). Like remission, our study of OAS found few predictors of depression. There were only two significant baseline predictors of depression at follow-up: depression and greater number of psychotropic medications. Depression at baseline predicted having higher anxiety scores at follow-up [47].

A majority of broad-age-range studies suggest that schizophrenia is associated with mild premorbid cognitive deficits that are approximately one-third to two-thirds of a standard deviation below age-matched controls [11]. A recent study of persons aged 50 and over found that schizophrenia is associated with cognitive deficits that are nearly two standard deviations below control participants [48], which may represent an aging effect or capture an accelerated decline seen in persons after age 65, especially among persons with long institutional histories. Follow-up studies in younger persons have generally found stable cognitive function as long as 10 years post-baseline [49,50]. In older adults, a study in San Diego of middle-aged and older persons with schizophrenia [51] and our follow-up data of OAS in NYC [52] identified a variety of trajectories: Rapid decliners (>2.1/year on DRS), 10% (San Diego), 19% (NYC); modest decliners (0.21–2.1/year), 40% (San Diego), 25% (NYC); stable, 11% (NYC); modest improvers (0.21–2.1/year), 26% (NYC); rapid improvers (>2.1/year), 19% (NYC). The San Diego study lumped the last three categories into a single "stable" category comprising 50% of the sample. Another illustration of the fluctuation in cognition in our NYC sample using the DRS cut-off for probable dementia is shown in Table 8.3: about two-fifths are persistently cognitively intact, one-quarter are persistently impaired, and about one-third fluctuate between these states.

In younger samples, predictors of poorer cognition have included unemployment, lower education, age of onset (either early or late), male gender, negative symptoms, poor premorbid adjustment, more severe psychiatric symptoms, and substance abuse (see [52] for specific citations and Table 8.4 for summary of findings). In middle-aged and OAS, predictors of poorer cognition at follow-up have included lower baseline cognition, residential status (living in institutions), older age, female sex, race (white), shorter duration of illness, later age of onset, positive symptoms, and negative symptoms; baseline cognitive functioning has been a strong predictor of subsequent adaptive functioning [52,53]. For many of the studies of older adults, the time interval between follow-up observations was short, e.g., median 16.5 months (range: 1 to 18 years). Moreover, 11 of the 13 longitudinal studies with mean age over 54 have been with chronically institutionalized patients or mixed-setting patients, although 85% of OAS now reside in community settings [52]. In our study of OAS, we found only three predictors of higher cognition on follow-up: baseline cognition, decline in anxiety score, and race (white). Higher baseline cognitive functioning predicted clinical remission at follow-up (Table 8.4).

With respect to community functioning over time, various international studies and literature reviews of younger samples have found favorable outcome ranging from 22% to 60%, depending on the location, historical period, and criteria for social functioning [29,31,54–57] (Table 8.4). Typically rates have been around 50%. In our longitudinal study of OAS, we found that community integration criteria were met persistently in 26% of persons, never present in 39%, and fluctuated between the two states in 35% of persons [58].

In younger adults with schizophrenia, predictors of subsequent social recovery included older age of onset, better baseline social functioning, fewer negative symptoms, less severe positive symptoms, better cognitive functioning, and negative family history of non-affective psychosis [54–56] (Table 8.4). Among OAS, our group found that lower depression, higher cognitive functioning, and fewer mental health services predicted subsequent community integration. Conversely, baseline community integration predicted remission, fewer positive symptoms, and less general psychopathology at follow-up [58].

Finally, "clinical recovery," based on whether a person attained clinical remission and community integration, was found to be persistent in only 12% of persons in our NYC sample. This rate was similar to longitudinal rates found in younger samples [5]. Conversely, 18% of individuals were unable to attain remission or community integration at any point in time. The rest of the people (70%) showed some combination of these outcome measures over time. At the more extreme ends within these combinations, 5% of patients had persistent clinical remission, but never attained community integration; obversely, 6% of individuals showed persistent community integration but never attained remission.

Several important conclusions emerged from the longitudinal studies of OAS: (1) Cross-sectional data give an overly optimistic perspective of outcome, and the prospective data suggest as many as two-fifths of persons may fluctuate between favorable and unfavorable outcome categories. (2) Heterogeneity in course persists into later life so that outcome for many persons still remains uncertain; consequently, proactive care must continue into later life. (3) It is unclear whether the relatively few predictor variables found in our studies reflect differences in methods or vicissitudes that accompany older age; moreover, the fact that there were few predictor variables makes it more difficult to predict outcome or identify points for intervention. (4) For most of the outcome variables, baseline status was the strongest predictor of subsequent outcome ("time 1 predicts time 2") although it was not an overwhelming determinant, and for remission, it did not obtain. Nevertheless, the limited number of predictor variables suggests that focusing interventions on enhancing baseline levels of the outcome variables may yield the biggest payoff with respect to subsequent outcome. This is addressed a bit more in the next section.

To what extent do the outcome indicators affect each other over time?

As seen in Table 8.5, in cross-sectional and longitudinal analyses the broad outcome indicators (depression, cognition, community integration, remission) are modestly correlated with each other, although none of the associations account for more than 19% $((r = 0.44)^2)$ of shared variance. For this reason, these outcome variables will need to be addressed largely by separate treatment strategies. Other chapters in this volume propose strategies for intervention. On the other hand, it is useful to explore some of the potential casual relationships among these indicators since interventions with one outcome variable might have impact, albeit moderate, on other outcome variables. As shown in Figure 8.2, after controlling for time since baseline, race (white), education, gender, age, residential status, and baseline value of the dependent variable, longitudinal data analyses indicated that: (1) lower depressive symptoms ($\beta = -0.18$) had a significant, albeit small, association with subsequent community integration;

Table 8.5 Correlations among the four broad outcome indicators at baseline (T1) and follow-up (T2) (N = 103)

	Remission T1	Remission T2	DRS T1	DRS T2	CES-D T1	CES-D T2
Community Integration T1	0.24[a]	0.32[b]	0.12	0.00	−0.44[b]	−0.34[b]
Community Integration T2	0.22[a*]	0.23[a]	0.18	0.27[a]	−0.36[b]	−0.47[b]
CES-D T1	−0.16	−0.04	0.05	−0.04		
CES-D T2	0.04	−0.24[a]	0.06	−0.10		
DRS T1	0.40[b]	0.20[a]				
DRS T2	0.22[a]	0.18				

[a]p < .05; [b]p < .01

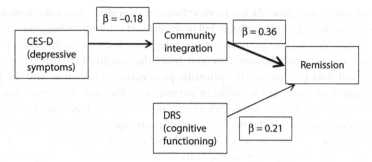

Figure 8.2 Possible pathways linking various outcome indicators (N = 103)
Note: Controlling for time since baseline, race (white), education, gender, age, residential status, and baseline value of the dependent variable

(2) community integration had a moderately strong association ($\beta = 0.36$) with subsequent clinical remission; there was a modest trend (that did not quite attain statistical significance) suggesting that improved cognition is associated with subsequent remission ($\beta = 0.21$). Of course, these are temporal relationships so causality cannot be certain. Nevertheless, the findings indicate that remission may result in part from improvements in other clinical and social measures, and conversely, clinical remission has no appreciable effect on the other clinical and social outcome measures. This does not mean that clinical remission might not have an effect on other clinical and social variables at other points across the lifespan; rather, among OAS, such effects seem to be attenuated.

Does the paradoxical aging model apply to outcome in later life?

"Paradoxical aging" refers to the concurrent decline in physical health and cognition with an improvement in subjective quality of life and psychosocial functioning [11]. This paradox is thought to be even more pronounced in OAS, in which there are higher rates of mortality and physical disease in tandem with a trend towards fewer relapses, higher rates of clinical remission, and better self-management. When looked at longitudinally, the evidence for paradoxical aging in OAS suggests a more nuanced picture. First, data comparing younger samples with our data indicate few appreciable differences in the outcome measures, although data vary because of variations in samples and follow-up periods (Table 8.4). Second, as seen in Table 8.6, for three of the outcome measures – remission, community integration, and depression – between half and three-fifths of persons either persistently *did not* attain positive cut-off values or dropped below these values over time. On the other hand, for the cognitive and health outcome variables, roughly three-fifths attained positive cut-off values or improved over time. As can be seen in Figure 8.3, there is a wide variability in favorable outcomes with 9% showing no favorable outcomes (i.e., unfavorable in all categories) to 6% showing favorable outcome in all categories; 28% showed favorable outcomes in four or five categories. Thus, the paradoxical aging pattern seems to be true for some people, but there is a mosaic of outcomes across domains.

Does heterogeneity in course remain fluid into later life?

"Heterogeneity of course" refers to the multitude of trajectories and outcomes found in schizophrenia [59]. Several investigators have suggested that in later life, persons with

Table 8.6 Components of paradoxical aging: 52-month follow-up status (N = 103)

	Persistently unfavorable or worse over time (%)	Persistently favorable or better over time (%)
Remission	59	41
Community integration	55	45
Depression	54	46
Cognitive functioning	43	57
Self-health (excellent/good)	36	64

Note: Self-health was used a proxy measure of health. At baseline, correlations of self-health with number of physical disorders and the activities of daily living total score were r = −0.29 (p = 0.003) and r = 0.32 (p = 0.001), respectively.

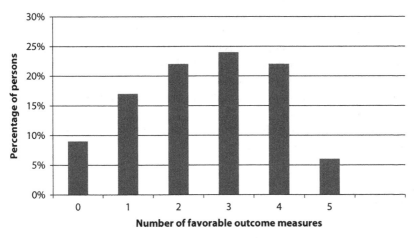

Figure 8.3 Number of favorable outcome measures (maximum = 5)

schizophrenia reached a stable end-state [33,37,38]. This was based primarily on clinical observations of institutionalized patients and has not taken into account the stultifying impact of long-term hospitalization and lack of data about outcome in OAS in the post-deinstitutionalization era. However, as I described above, our longitudinal analyses indicated that even in later life there is a substantial minority of persons (one-quarter to two-fifths) who continue to alter their status on various outcome indices (Table 8.3). Moreover, with more complex outcome measures such as recovery, there are even more transitions between various statuses.

Summary

1. The definition of outcome is an unsettled area of debate in psychiatry that has varied historically and across investigative sites. It has included symptom as well as social indices. As most people with OAS now live in the community, it is imperative to incorporate the recovery model into an outcome framework, which is an integral component of community psychiatry. Moreover, the inclusion of a life-span perspective is essential when investigating older adults.

2. At this historical moment, clinical outcome measures such as cognition, clinical remission, and depressive symptoms, along with social indices such as community integration and quality of life are the most commonly used for OAS.

3. Contrary to earlier reports of a quiescent end stage in later life, heterogeneity in course persists into later life. Prospective data suggest as many as two-fifths of persons may fluctuate between favorable and unfavorable outcome categories. Consequently, outcome for many remains uncertain, and for most OAS, active clinical engagement must continue into later life. Because of the fluidity in the various combinations of favorable outcome categories, "recovering" remains a viable conceptual framework in later life.

4. Although the outcome indices are largely independent of each other, provisional data suggest that over time, alleviation of depressive symptoms is associated with improved community integration, which in turn is associated with higher rates of remission; improved cognitive function may also augment clinical remission.

5. There were few predictors of the various outcome indices, suggesting that clinical strategies need to target the specific clinical or social domain.

6. The novel DSM5 domain approach is best used to assess outcome in individual patients. For research purposes, more comprehensive positive and negative symptom scales need to be considered.

7. Paradoxical aging is valid for some OAS, but most show a variegated pattern of outcomes across domains.

8. Because of the various combinations of outcome and the relative independence among outcome dimensions, optimal care can best be achieved through an individualized care approach.

References

1. J. Wing, Long-term outcome in schizophrenia, *Schizophrenia Bulletin*, 14, 669–73, 1988.

2. J.D. Hegarty, R.J. Baldessarini, M. Tohen, et al., One-hundred years of schizophrenia: a meta-analysis of the outcome literature, *American Journal of Psychiatry*, 151, 1409–16, 1994.

3. C. Cohen, Poverty and the course of schizophrenia: Implications for research and policy, *Hospital and Community Psychiatry*, 22, 951–8, 1993.

4. T. McGlashan, A selective review of recent North American long-term followup studies of schizophrenia, *Schizophrenia Bulletin*, 14, 515–42, 1988.

5. E. Jääskeläinen, J. Paulina, N. Hirvonen, et al., A systematic review and meta-analysis of recovery in schizophrenia, *Schizophrenia Bulletin*, 39, 1296–306, 2013.

6. Adityanjee, Y.A. Aderibigbe, D. Theodoridis, and W. V. Vieweg, Dementia praecox to schizophrenia: the first 100 years, *Psychiatry and Clinical Neurosciences*, 53, 437–48, 1999.

7. A. Ebert and K.-J. Bar, Emil Kraepelin: a pioneer of scientific understanding of psychiatry and psychopharmacology, *Indian Journal of Psychiatry*, 52, 191–2, 2010.

8. A. Jablensky, The diagnostic concept of schizophrenia: its history, evolution, and future prospects, *Dialogues in Clinical Neuroscience*, 12, 271–87, 2010.

9. SAMHSA, *SAMHSA's Working Definition of Recovery*, Rockville, MD: SAMHSA, 2012.

10. C. Cohen, K. Freeman, D. Ghoneim, et al., Advances in the conceptualization and study of schizophrenia in later life, *Psychiatric Clinics of North America*, 41, 39–53, 2018.

11. D.V. Jeste, O.M. Wolkowitz, and B.W. Palmer, Divergent trajectories of physical, cognitive, and psychosocial aging in schizophrenia, *Schizophrenia Bulletin*, 37, 451–5, 2011.

12. C.I. Cohen and M. Iqbal, A longitudinal study of remission among older adults with schizophrenia spectrum disorder, *American Journal of Geriatric Psychiatry*, 22, 450–8, 2014.

13. S. Diwan, C.I. Cohen, A. Bankole, et al., Depression in older adults with schizophrenia spectrum disorders: prevalence and associated factors, *American Journal of Geriatric Psychiatry*, 12, 991–8, 2007.

14. American Psychiatric Association, *Diagnostic and Statistical Manual of Mental Disorders*, 5th edn., Arlington, VA: American Psychiatric Publishing, 2013.

15. S. Kay, L. Opler, and A. Fiszbein, *Positive and Negative Syndrome Scale User's Manual*, North Tonawanda, NY: Multi-Health Systems, 1992.

16. J.S. Radloff, The CES-D scale: a self-report depression scale for research in the general population, *Journal of Applied Psychological Measurement*, 1, 385–401, 1977.

17. J.M. Coblentz, S. Mattis, L.H. Zingesser, et al., Presenile dementia: clinical aspects and evaluation of cerebrospinal fluid dynamics, *Archives of Neurology*, 29, 299–308, 1973.

18. R.P. Liberman, Recovery from schizophrenia: a concept in search of research, *Pychiatric Services*, 56, 735–42, 2005.

19. N.C. Andreasen, W.T. Carpenter, J.M. Kane, et al., Remission in schizophrenia: proposed criteria and rationale for consensus, *American Journal of Psychiatry*, 162, 441–9, 2005.

20. Y.I. Wong and P.L. Soloman, Community integration of persons with psychiatric disabilities in supportive independent housing: a conceptual model and methological considerations, *Mental Health Services Research*, 4, 13–28, 2002.

21. R.H. Moos, *Evaluating Treatment Environments: The Quality of Psychiatric and Substance Abuse Programs*, 2nd edn., New Brunswick, NJ: Transaction, 1997.

22. C. Abdallah, C.I. Cohen, M. Sanchez-Almira, et al., Community integration and associated factors among older adults with schizophrenia, *Psychiatric Services*, 12, 1642–8, 2009.

23. W.J. Strawbridge, M.I. Wallhagen, and R.D. Cohen, Successful aging and well being: self-rated compared with Rowe and Kahn, *Gerontologist*, 42, 727–33, 2002.

24. J.W. Roew and R.L. Kahn, Human aging: usual and successful, *Science*, 237, 143–9, 1987.

25. F. Ibrahim, C.I. Cohen, and P.M. Ramirez, Successful aging in older adults with schizophrenia: prevalence and associated factors, *American Journal of Geriatric Psychiatry*, 18, 879–86, 2010.

26. W.W. Leung, C.R. Bowie, and P.D. Harvey, Functional implications of neuropsychological normality and symptom remission in older outpatients diagnosed with schziophrenia: a cross-sectional study, *Journal of the International Neuropsycholical Society*, 14, 479–88, 2008.

27. P.D. Meesters, H.C. Comijs, L. de Haan, et al., Symptomatic remission and associated factors in a catchment area based population of older patients with schizophrenia, *Schizophrenia Research*, 126, 237–44, 2011.

28. S.N. Mosolov, A.A. Potapov, and U.V. Ushakov, Remission in schizophrenia: results of cross-sectional with 6 month follow-up period and 1-year observational therapeutic studies in an outpatient popuation, *Annals of General Psychiatry*, 11, 1–10, 2012.

29. G. Harrison, K. Hopper, T. Craig, et al., Recovery from psychotic illness: a 15- and 25-year international follow-up study, *British Journal of Psychiatry*, 178, 506–17, 2001.

30. C. Harding, Changes in schizophrenia across time: paradoxes, patterns, and predictors, in *Schizophrenia Into Later*

Life, Arlington, VA: American Psychiatric Publishing, 2003, 19–41.

31. R. Warner, Recovery from schizophrnenia, in *Psychiatry and Political Economy*, 3rd edn., Hove, East Sussex: Bruner-Routledge, 2004.

32. D.G. Robinson, M.G. Woerner, M. McMeniman, et al., Symptomatic and functional recovery from a first episode of schizophrenia of schizoaffective disorder, *American Journal of Psychiatry*, 161, 473–479, 2004.

33. L. Ciompi, Catamnestic long-term study on the course of life and aging of schizophrenics, *Schizophrenia Bulletin*, 6, 606–18, 1980.

34. L.A. Auslander and D.V. Jeste, Sustained remission of schizophrenia among community-dwelling older outpatients, *American Journal of Psychiatry*, 161, 1490–3, 2004.

35. C.A. Depp and D.V. Jeste, Definitions and predictors of successful aging: a comprehensive review of larger quantitative studies, *American Journal of Geriatric Psychiatry*, 14, 6–20, 2006.

36. C.I. Cohen, I. Vahia, P. Reyes, et al., Schizophrenia in later life: clinical symptoms and well-being, *Psychiatric Services*, 59, 232–4, 2008.

37. R. Belitsky and T.H. McGlashan, The manifestations of schizophrenia in late life: a dearth of data, *Schizophrenia Bulletin*, 19, 683–5, 1993.

38. R. Tandon, H.A. Nasrallah, and M.S. Keshavan, Schizophrenia, "just the facts." 4. Clinical features and conceptualization, *Schizophrenia Research*, 110, 1–23, 2009.

39. R. Emsley, B. Chiliza, L. Asmal, et al., The concepts of remission and recovery in schziophrenia, *Current Opinion in Psychiatry*, 114, e121, 2011.

40. F.U. Lang, M. Kosters, S. Lang, et al., Psychopathological long-term outcome of schizophrenia: a review, *Acta Psychiatrica Scandinavica*, 127, 173–82, 2013.

41. I. Gasquet, J.M. Haro, S. Tcherny-Lessenot, et al., Remission in the outpatient care of schizophrenia: 3-year results from the Schizophrenia Outpatient Health Outcomes (SOHO) study in France, *European Psychiatry*, 23, 491–6, 2008.

42. J. Bobes, A. Ciudad, E. Alvarez, et al, Recovery from schizophrenia: results from a 1-year follow-up observational study of patients in symptomatic remission, *Schziophrenia Research*, 115, 58–66, 2009.

43. A. Ucok, S. Serbest, and P. E. Kandemir, Remission after first-episode schizophrenia: results of a long-term follow-up study, *Psychiatry Research*, 189, 33–7, 2011.

44. R.R. Conley, H. Ascher-Svanum, B. Zhu, et al., The burden of depressive symptoms in the long-term treatment of patients with schizophrenia, *Schizophrenia Research*, 90, 186–97, 2007.

45. I.M. Lako, K. Taxis, R. Bruggerman, et al., The course of depressive symptoms and prescribing patterns of antidepressants in schizophrenia in a one year follow-up study, *European Psychiatry*, 27, 240–4, 2012.

46. J.R. Sands and M. Harrow, Depression during the longitudinal course of schizophrenia, *Schizophrenia Bulletin*, 25, 157–71, 1999.

47. C.I. Cohen and H.H. Ryu, A longitudinal study of the outcome and associated factors of subsyndromal and syndromal depression in community-dwelling older adults with schizophrenia spectrum disorder, *American Journal of Geriatric Psychiatry*, 23, 925–33, 2015.

48. C. Tsoutsoulas, B.H. Mulsant, S.M. Kalache, et al., The influence of medical burden severity and cognition on functional competence in older community-dwelling individuals with schizophrenia, *Schizophrenia Research*, 170, 330–5, 2016.

49. A. Szoke, A. Trandafir, M.-E. Dupont, et al., A systematic review of longitudinal outcome studies of first-episode psychosis, *British Journal of Psychiatry*, 192, 248–57, 2008.

50. R.S. Keefe, A longitudinal course of cognitive impairment in schizophrenia: an examination of data from premorbid

through posttreatment phases of illness, *Journal of Clinical Psychiatry*, 75, Suppl 2, 8–13, 2014.

51. W.K. Thompson, G.N. Savla, I.V. Vahia, et al., Characterizing trajectories of cognitive functioning in older adults with schizophrenia: does method matter? *Schizophrenia Research*, 143, 90–6, 2013.

52. C.I. Cohen and T. Murante, A prospective analysis of the role of cognition in three models of aging and schizophrenia, *Schizophrenia Research*, 196, 22–8, 2018.

53. S. Bergh, C. Hjorthoj, H. J. Sorensen, et al., Predictors and longitudinal course of cognitive functioning in schizophrenia spectrum disorder, 10 years after baseline: the OPUS study, *Schizophrenia Research*, 175, 57–63, 2016.

54. M.F. Green, R.S. Kern, and R.K. Heaton, Longitudinal studies of cognition and functional outcome in schizophrenia: implications for MATRICS, *Schizophrenia Research*, 72, 41–51, 2004.

55. E. Velthorst, A.J. Fett, A. Reichenberg, et al., The 20-year longitudinal trajectories of social functioning in individuals with psychotic disorders, *American Journal of Psychiatry*, 174, 1075–85, 2017.

56. C.M. Diaz-Caneja, L. Pina-Camacho, A. Rodriguez-Quiroga, et al., Predictors of outcome in early-onset psychosis: a systematic review, *NPJ Schizophrenia*, 1, 14005, 2015.

57. N.M. Menezes, T. Arenovich, and R.B. Zipursky, A systematic review of longitudinal outcome studies, *Psychological Medicine*, 36, 1349–62, 2006.

58. C. Jimenez, H.H. Ryu, E. Garcia-Aracena, and C.I. Cohen, Predictors of community integration in older adults with schizophrenia, in *American Psychiatric Association Annual Meeting, Philadelphia, PA., 2012*, Washington, D.C.: American Psychiatric Association, 2012.

59. A.B. Shmuckler, I.Y. Gurovich, M. Agius, and Y. Zaytseva, Long-term trajectories of cognitive deficits in schizophrenia: a critical overview, *European Psychiatry*, 30, 1002–10, 2015.

Positive Psychiatry for Schizophrenia and Other Psychotic Disorders

Graham Eglit, Ph.D., Barton W. Palmer, Ph.D., and Dilip V. Jeste, M.D.

Defining positive psychiatry

Psychiatry has traditionally focused on reducing the symptoms caused by mental and behavioral disorders. This approach has led to important advances in the characterization and assessment of psychopathology and treatment of psychiatric symptoms. However, traditional psychiatry has often overlooked broader aspects of well-being among individuals with psychiatric disorders. Positive psychiatry is an approach to mental health that attempts to expand the scope of psychiatry to the promotion of well-being in the population at large. Positive psychiatry may be defined as the "science and practice of psychiatry that seeks to understand and promote well-being through assessments and interventions aimed at enhancing positive psychosocial factors among people who have or are at high risk for developing mental and physical illnesses" ([1], p. 2–3). Relevant positive psychosocial factors in positive psychiatry include resilience, optimism, social engagement, wisdom, post-traumatic growth, hope, and personal mastery, among others. As a branch of medicine, positive psychiatry is focused on discerning the biological substrates of these traits, including their neurocircuitry, neurochemistry, and genetic basis, as well as developing biomarkers of these positive factors [2,3]. Importantly, positive psychiatry is not intended to replace traditional psychiatry but rather to complement it. This is accomplished by shifting the focus from treating pathology to maintaining health and from treating symptoms to enhancing well-being.

Historical background

While a relatively new subfield, positive psychiatry can be traced back to some of the earliest researchers in psychology. As early as 1906, William James argued for a new approach to research and clinical practice that was guided by the healing power of positive emotions and beliefs – the so-called "mind cure" [4]. The importance of positive psychological capacities was further emphasized in the mid-twentieth century through the development of humanistic psychology by Abraham Maslow and colleagues. Probably the most important and immediate precursor to positive psychiatry, however, was the positive psychology movement of the late 1990s, pioneered by Martin Seligman. This movement was focused on elucidating factors that foster positive human functioning and flourishing [5]. Positive psychiatry built upon this knowledge and expanded the focus to studies of biology of positive traits and outcomes, as well as promotion of well-being among people with or at risk for mental or physical illnesses. The first ever book on positive psychiatry was published in 2015 [1].

The importance of positive psychiatry to schizophrenia was underappreciated until recently due to long-standing notions about the course of this illness. Traditionally, schizophrenia was assumed to be an intractable illness with an inevitably poor prognosis. Research during the latter part of the twentieth century, however, began to call these pessimistic assumptions into question. Starting with Manfred Bleuler, studies in this era documented a wide range of positive outcomes several decades after initial hospitalization among many individuals with schizophrenia [6].

Positive mental health outcomes in schizophrenia

Research has shown that there is a divergence of trajectories of physical, cognitive, and psychosocial functioning with aging in persons with schizophrenia [7]. Thus, physical health declines faster in these patients than in the general population, cognitive functioning is impaired, but the age-related rate of decline is similar to that in people without schizophrenia, and psychosocial functioning tends to improve with aging. Older adults with schizophrenia living in the community generally exhibit improved mental-health-related quality of life [8,9], greater acceptance and self-management abilities with respect to their symptoms, improved medication adherence, a reduction in positive symptoms, and a decreased rate of psychotic relapse and hospitalization [10,11]. A possible explanation for the better functioning in older persons with schizophrenia is "survivor bias" – i.e., the sickest individuals die young (from suicide or physical illnesses) and only the healthiest survive into old age. However, several longitudinal follow-up studies have shown progressive improvement in functioning among adults with schizophrenia. Indeed, a small percentage of patients (approximately 10%) exhibit sustained functional recovery in late life [12]. The 2001 movie "A Beautiful Mind," which won the Academy Award for the Best Picture, told the true story of John Nash, a Nobel Laureate, who had suffered from schizophrenia since his youth, but began functioning better in later life and went back to productive research and teaching after nearly three decades of severe psychosocial disability.

These heterogeneous and sometimes remitting courses raised the question of what factors promote positive outcomes in schizophrenia. A number of studies have begun to address this question. Contrary to traditional pessimistic views, studies in first-episode schizophrenia have found comparable levels of happiness and satisfaction with life among first-episode schizophrenia patients and non-psychiatric controls, despite significant functional impairments in the former group [13]. In general, individuals with schizophrenia report lower levels of happiness and satisfaction with life than non-psychiatric comparison subjects, suggesting a possible decline in subjective well-being shortly after the first episode. Nonetheless, there is substantial heterogeneity in happiness among these patients, with a sizable minority of the patients with schizophrenia reporting levels similar to those of non-psychiatric individuals [14,15]. Happiness and satisfaction with life are associated with lower levels of depressive symptoms and higher levels of motivation [15,16].

Positive psychosocial factors in schizophrenia

Edmonds et al. [17] further explored levels of resilience and optimism, in addition to happiness and perceived stress, among individuals with schizophrenia. Similar to the aforementioned studies, while individuals with schizophrenia reported lower mean levels of these positive psychosocial factors relative to an age-comparable non-psychiatric group, they exhibited considerable variation, with over one-third of schizophrenia participants reporting values similar to those of their non-psychiatric counterparts. Of particular importance, these positive psychosocial factors were also associated with lower levels of biomarkers of inflammation and insulin resistance, especially among individuals with schizophrenia. Taken together, this research suggests that positive psychosocial factors, generally lower in schizophrenia, may be viable treatment targets and have the potential to improve these individuals' well-being and even physical/biological health. The role of family and social support in improving the likelihood of positive outcomes in schizophrenia has been well established [6].

A recently published study involved qualitative interviews of 20 high functioning individuals with schizophrenia who had reached a level of recovery defined by their occupational status [18]. Eight categories of coping strategies were identified: avoidance behavior, utilizing supportive others, taking medications, enacting cognitive strategies, controlling the environment, engaging spirituality, focusing on well-being, and being employed or continuing their education. These strategies were used flexibly in a preventive fashion, and in varied combinations, depending on the context. They seemed to support these high-functioning individuals in achieving their occupational goals.

Positive psychiatry interventions in schizophrenia

Several recent positive psychotherapeutic interventions have directly targeted quality of life and functional improvement in schizophrenia – instead of just symptom relief – with promising results. Cognitive behavioral social skills training (CBSST) involves challenging thoughts and misinterpretations of experiences, as well as developing social skills in order to pursue meaningful goals identified by the patient. This intervention has been shown to improve cognitive insight and mastery of core cognitive-behavioral and social skills among adults with schizophrenia. More importantly, individuals with schizophrenia who participated in CBSST reported improvements in self-esteem and life satisfaction, as well as a reduction of amotivation, a core feature of schizophrenia, especially among persons with defeatist or pessimistic attitudes at baseline [19].

Individual Placement and Support (IPS) is a manualized supported employment intervention that emphasizes competitive work, integrated mental health, and supported employment services. Relative to a conventional vocational rehabilitation program, individuals who participated in IPS exhibited higher rates of gainful employment, weeks worked, and wages earned [20].

Treatment of persons with schizophrenia must involve promotion of a healthy lifestyle – i.e., regular physical exercise, cognitive activity, appropriate socialization, healthy diet, a focus on stress reduction, sleep hygiene, avoidance (or at least, reduction) of smoking, abstinence from substances of abuse, and a positive attitude.

Conclusion

Positive psychiatry has a great potential to improve the lives of individuals with schizophrenia and other psychotic disorders. Current research in this area is at an early stage. Further investigations are needed to develop and validate measures of positive psychosocial factors with adequate psychometric properties, to explore the biological and cognitive underpinnings of these factors, and to elucidate their longitudinal course and impact on physical, mental, and cognitive health outcomes. A positive, albeit realistic, attitude toward schizophrenia and other serious mental illnesses is essential among treating clinicians. Only then can we encourage our patients and their caregivers to adopt an optimistic perspective that there can be a light at the end of even a very long tunnel.

Acknowledgment

This work was supported, in part, by NIH grants 5R01MH094151-04 and 5T32 MH019934-21 (Jeste), and UC San Diego Stein Institute for Research on Aging.

References

1. Jeste, D.V., and Palmer, B.W. (2015). Introduction: What is positive psychiatry? In. D.V. Jeste and B.W. Palmer (Eds.), *Positive Psychiatry (1–16)*. Washington, D.C.: American Psychiatric Association.

2. Jeste, D.V., Palmer, B.W., Rettew, D.C., and Boardman, S. (2015). Positive psychiatry: its time has come. *Journal of Clinical Psychiatry*, 76(6), 675–83.

3. Jeste, D.V., Palmer, B.W., and Saks, E.R. (2017). Why we need positive psychiatry for schizophrenia and other psychotic disorders. *Schizophrenia Bulletin*, 43(2), 227–9.

4. Froh, J.J. (2004). The history of positive psychology: truth be told. *The Psychologist*, 16(3), 18–20.

5. Seligman, M.E.P. and Csikszentmihalyi, M. (2000). Positive psychology: an introduction. *American Psychologist*, 55(1), 5–14.

6. Harding, C.M. and Zahniser, J.H. (1994). Empirical correction of seven myths about schizophrenia with implications for treatment. *Acta Psychiatrica Scandinivica Supplement*, 384, 140–6.

7. Jeste, D.V., Wolkowitz, O.M., and Palmer, B.W. (2011). Divergent trajectories of physical, cognitive, and psychosocial aging in schizophrenia. *Schizophrenia Bulletin*, 37, 451–5.

8. Reine, G., Simeoni, M.C., Auquier, P., et al. (2005). Assessing health-related quality of life in patients suffering from schizophrenia: a comparison of instruments. *European Psychiatry*, 20(7), 510–19.

9. Folsom, D.P., Depp, C., Palmer, B., et al. (2009). Physical and mental health-related quality of life among older people with schizophrenia. *Schizophrenia Research*, 108(1–3), 207–13.

10. Post, F. (1971). Schizo-affective symptomatology in late life. *British Journal of Psychiatry*, 118(545), 437–45.

11. Shepherd, S., Depp, C.A., Harris, G., et al. (2012). Perspectives on schizophrenia over the lifespan: a qualitative study. *Schizophrenia Bulletin*, 38(2), 295–303.

12. Auslander, L.A. and Jeste, D.V. (2004). Sustained remission of schizophrenia among comunity-dwelling older outpatients. *American Journal of Psychiatry*, 161, 1490–3.

13. Agid, O., McDonald, K., Siu, C., et al. (2012). Happiness in first-episode schizophrenia. *Schizophrenia Research*, 141(1), 98–103.

14. Palmer, B.W., Martin, A.S., Depp, C.A., Glorioso, D.K., and Jeste, D.V. (2014). Wellness within illness: happiness in schizophrenia. *Schizophrenia Research*, 159, 151–6.

15. Fervaha, G., Agid, O., Takeuchi, H., Foussias, G., and Remington, G. (2016). Life satisfaction and happiness among young adults with schizophrenia. *Psychiatry Research*, 242, 174–9.

16. Mankiewicz, P.D., Gresswell, D.M., and Turner, C. (2013). Subjective wellbeing in psychosis: mediating effects of psychological distress on happiness levels amongst individuals diagnosed with

paranoid schizophrenia. *International Journal of Wellbeing*, 3(1), 35–59.

17. Edmonds, E.C., Martin, A.S., Palmer, B.W., et al. (2018). Positive mental health in schizophrenia and healthy comparison groups: relationships with overall health and biomarkers. *Aging and Mental Health*, 22(3), 354–62.

18. Cohen, A.N., Hamilton, A.B., Saks, E.R., et al. (2017). How occupationally high-achieving individuals with a diagnosis of schizophrenia manage their symptoms. *Psychiatric Services*, 68, 324–9.

19. Granholm, E., Holden, J., Link, P.C., McQuaid, J.R., and Jeste, D. V. (2013). Randomized controlled trial of cognitive behavioral social skills training for older consumers with schizophrenia: defeatist performance attitudes and functional outcome. *American Journal of Geriatric Psychiatry*, 21(3), 251–62.

20. Twamley, E.W., Vella, L., Burton, C.Z., et al. (2012). The efficacy of supported employment for middle-aged and older people with schizophrenia. *Schizophrenia Research*, 135(1), 100–4.

Chapter

10

Social Functioning among Older Community-Dwelling Persons with Schizophrenia

Paul D. Meesters, M.D.

Introduction

Social functioning is a key concept when evaluating the impact of a disorder as severe as schizophrenia. First, this concerns the individual patient whose opportunities to lead a socially satisfactory life often are significantly constrained by the disorder. Likewise, family and significant others have to deal with the individual's difficulties in relating socially in an adequate way. Next, the societal consequences of schizophrenia may range from the provision of social services to the imposing of legal restraints when the disorder brings along socially unacceptable behaviour. Nowadays, improving social functioning is seen as a crucial treatment goal, with a relevance over and above that of freedom from troubling psychotic symptoms and relapses [1].

No consensus definition of social functioning is available, and a range of related concepts is intertwined, such as community integration and social adaptation. Concepts were often introduced by their intuitive appeal rather than by underlying theoretical models [2]. Mueser and Tarrier [3] elegantly combined objective and subjective aspects of social functioning, defining it as 'the ability of individuals to meet societally defined roles and their satisfaction with their ability to meet these roles'. A DSM5 diagnosis of schizophrenia requires that for a significant portion of the time since the onset of the disturbance, level of functioning in one or more major areas, such as work, interpersonal relations or self-care, is markedly below the level achieved prior to the onset.

The aim of this chapter is to examine the conceptualization and measurement of social functioning as it applies to older persons with schizophrenia and to review relevant studies regarding the level of social functioning and associated factors in this population.

Measuring social functioning

In the light of this complexity, measuring social functioning poses serious challenges. A large number of scales can be found in the literature, often with overlapping scopes. Initiatives have been taken to bring unity to the field [3]. Self-reports, ratings by clinicians, informant reports and behavioural observation all combine advantages with limitations. Principally, assessment of social functioning is strongly influenced by the perspective of evaluation. Significant discordances have been reported between self-reports and observer-based ratings [4]. This is not unique to schizophrenia, but has been reported in many areas of social research. Today, the relevance of including the appraisal by schizophrenia patients themselves is undisputed. Apart from valuing patient perceptions, it also pinpoints blind spots in others who lack the actual experience of living with a disorder as severe as schizophrenia. However, one must keep in mind that poor insight and cognitive limitations may colour appraisals and limit the reliability and the validity of self-reports. Furthermore, self-reports of objective facts (e.g., number of friends) call upon different mental faculties than self-reports of the valence of factual states (e.g., the importance of friendships).

Clinician ratings also have their shortcomings, as these are subject to interrater variability and assume that the clinician disposes of sufficient and relevant information about the patient. Ratings of social skills in simulated situations (for instance, meeting someone or making a phone call) have the advantage of standardized conditions. Still, assessments of competence are at best proxies for real-world activities, where the actual occurrence of behaviour may depend on factors like motivation or the availability of social support. Only a limited part of the variance in real-world social functioning is explained by social skills competence in simulated settings. All in all, when measuring social functioning it is preferable to combine self-reports with observer-based ratings. If research yields incongruities between subjective appraisals and evaluations by others, these should not be merely seen as obstacles to progress, but may be appreciated as eye-openers that elucidate the relevance of the adopted perspective when evaluating such an intricate phenomenon as social functioning.

Obviously, social functioning is a multifaceted phenomenon that is affected by a wide variety of factors. Individual characteristics, like gender and coping style, interact with contextual variables, such as social network and socioeconomic parameters. Ageing-associated changes may negatively impact on the level of social functioning. Examples of these are deteriorating mobility, sensory deprivation or a declining social network. Then again, positive factors like extravert coping styles or the availability of social support services may partially compensate for losses. While some factors will directly impact on social functioning, others may exert their influence through mediators. For example, the consequences of cognitive dysfunction may partly be mediated through functional impairments (e.g., not knowing how to use a hearing aid). The complex interaction of all contributing factors explains the considerable heterogeneity of social functioning in later life.

Quantitative research on social functioning

In younger schizophrenia patients, social impairments have been well documented. In contrast, less is known about the social adaptation of their older counterparts. The shortage in research on this topic is worrisome, as a large majority of older schizophrenia patients are community-based. In the United States about 85% of older persons with schizophrenia live in the community [5]. In a study in the Netherlands, 75% of a catchment-area-based sample (mean age, 67 years) resided in the community [6]. Aiming to synthesize the available scientific evidence, we reviewed the literature on social functioning in community-dwelling schizophrenia patients over 55 years [7]. Of the 36 publications included, 81% originated from the United States and 17% from Europe, while one study was performed in rural China [8]. For a list of all included studies, we refer to our original publication [7]. Due to methodological heterogeneity, data proved unfit for a quantitative review. Here we summarize the main findings, adding some relevant studies that have been published since our review.

Four older follow-up (catamnestic) studies of hospitalized patients, beginning in the 1930s and 1940s, were designed to observe the course of schizophrenia, but also provided information on social functioning. Although important developments during the second half of the last century (e.g., introduction of neuroleptics, deinstitutionalization) and methodological diversities limit extension of the findings to present-day populations, a number of consistent findings from these laborious investigations still bear relevance. Common to all studies was a heterogeneous disease course. Moderate to good general outcomes, suggestive of symptomatic remission according to present-day criteria, were reported for a substantial number of surviving patients. Improvement or even recovery in later phases was not exceptional. Nonetheless, another key finding was that recovery on a symptomatic level was not synonymous with social recovery. A Switzerland-based study, for example, found 49% of the participants to be either recovered or in a 'mild end state' [9]. Nevertheless, 72% of the subjects were 'definitely poor in social relations'. This shows that the significant social shortcomings that patients develop in early, more active phases of their disease cannot be fully compensated for in later stages, although these may be milder from a symptomatic point of view. This is also suggested by another long-term study with an intervention design [10]. In this North American study, chronically disabled back-ward patients were deinstitutionalized in the late 1950s to participate in an intensive psychosocial rehabilitation programme. At follow-up, general outcomes were noticeably positive, with 68% of the subjects without any positive or negative symptoms and around 50% not using psychotropic medication. Nevertheless, social outcomes (with the exception of employment) were not significantly different from a matched comparison group that received traditional custodial care.

In the literature available from 1995 onwards, our review focused on social roles, social support and social skills as critical areas of social functioning. With respect to social roles, older schizophrenia patients in comparison to their healthy peers have been married less often, have fewer social contacts, live independently less often and have lower occupational achievements. A similar pattern emerges in comparison to older individuals with mood disorders. Schizophrenia patients living in supported residences are even more disadvantaged with respect to marital status and social contacts. In a recent Dutch study designed to evaluate depressive symptoms [11], older schizophrenia patients (mean age, 67 years) scored unfavourably on all social indicators, relative to an age- and gender-matched comparison group from the general population. Only 25% of the patients lived in residential settings. Of all patients, 18% had a partner and 50% had children, compared to 66% with a partner and 80% with children in the comparisons. One in every four patients had either a very small or no social network outside of their household, compared to one in every fifty comparisons. Likewise, 41% of the patients could not name a confidant, in contrast to only 5% of the comparisons.

No publications principally evaluated social support in older schizophrenia patients, but a number of studies with a broader perspective reported on social network variables (size, density, role of network members). Most of these relate to the New York City cohort, a large convenience sample of outpatients with early onset schizophrenia (mean age, 62 years [5]). Participants reported smaller network sizes and lower proportions of sustaining and reliable network members, compared to healthy age-peers. Findings supported the notion that network aspects are relevant for clinical functioning (depression, symptomatic remission) and for well-being and quality of life. The complex interpretation of network factors is illustrated by the finding that both smaller network size and higher proportion of intimate network members were predictive of symptomatic remission [12]. The association with smaller network size was related to having disproportionately fewer non-kin members.

All publications evaluating social skills were North American and reported on relatively young urban patients (mean age, 56 to 59 years), with males overrepresented. The New York State group [13] used objective measures to evaluate social skills competence and real-world performance. These studies stand out because of the sophisticated measures applied, in combination with large sample sizes. While cognitive abilities contributed strongly to social skills competence, their contribution to real-world performance was largely mediated by functional skills competence [13]. Clinical symptoms contributed independently to real-world performance [14]. A range of studies by the San Diego group [15] evaluated social skills from the perspective of the patient. In one study patients judged themselves less capable than controls in some, but not all, social roles [16]. Positive, negative and depressive symptoms explained 45% of the variance in their perceived social functioning. In another study evaluating interpersonal competence, patients judged themselves less capable than controls in a number of interpersonal situations, though again not in all. Emotional support from others was a positive predictor of interpersonal competence [17]. In a more recent study comparing social skills in older schizophrenia and mood disorder outpatients [18], individuals with schizophrenia (mean age, 61 years) had worse social skills than those with bipolar disorder or major depression, with individuals with schizoaffective disorder positioned in between. Older age was associated with worse social skills in all groups. Higher levels of social contact and cognitive functioning (especially executive functions and verbal fluency) strongly predicted social skills in people with schizophrenia and schizoaffective disorder, but not in those with mood disorder. Apart from a blunted affect, symptoms were not predictive of social skills in both groups. No association of gender with social skills was found.

Finally, three studies contrasted objective and subjective evaluations of social skills. Results showed wide discrepancies in the appraisal of social functioning by patients and other observers. In one of these studies, patients who underestimated their real-world performance had better cognitive skills and higher self-rated depression than those who overestimated [4]. Accurate raters demonstrated greater social skills than both overestimators and underestimators, while overestimators were most cognitively impaired.

A more granular picture has emerged from this review. Clearly, most older people with schizophrenia are well behind their healthy age-peers with respect to social achievements. At the same time, there is no stereotype of the older patient with schizophrenia, as several studies make a case for heterogeneity as a crucial characteristic of social functioning in later life. The social spectrum ranges from socially isolated and severely incapacitated patients to socially integrated near-normal functioning individuals. The multidimensionality of this spectrum should be acknowledged, as patients may perform relatively well in one realm of social functioning, but relatively poorly in another.

Furthermore, with time patients may move within this spectrum. With positive symptoms attenuating and coping skills maturing, a substantial number of patients may become better socially integrated as they age. On the other hand, ageing patients also run the risk of decline in social functioning, when unfavourable factors (e.g., physical illness, bereavement) dominate the picture. These processes have still received little attention. One study by the New York City group sought to quantify these processes, employing the connected concept of community integration [19]. Community integration relates to the extent to which people live, participate and socialize in the community. Physical, social and psychological integration constitute the three major contributing dimensions. Of all participants, 23% scored above the cut-off for high community integration, versus 41% of a community comparison group. Community integration was, among other variables, positively associated with lower levels of positive, negative and depressive symptoms. At four-year follow-up, 34% of the participants that could be traced fluctuated between high and low community integration [20]. Fewer depressive symptoms, higher cognitive functioning and greater financial well-being at baseline predicted higher community integration at follow-up. Next, higher community integration at baseline predicted symptomatic remission at follow-up [21]. Extending this type of longitudinal research is essential to detect key factors for social functioning that are amenable to intervention.

Determinants of social functioning

Among the clinical variables that are associated with social functioning, cognitive abilities appear to be predominant, outweighing psychotic symptoms. This finding aligns with research in younger patients. A recent study that used a life-span approach to examine functional competence in a simulated setting (with participants aged between 19 and 79 years) found that a comprehensive measure of cognition accounted for 31% of the variance in communication skills, regardless of age [22]. Certain cognitive domains bear more relevance regarding the social realm than others. For example, one of the above cited New York State studies [14] demonstrated a central role for processing speed, attention and working memory, and executive functioning, with differences in the contribution of each function to specific social abilities.

While available research is mainly dedicated to neurocognition, social cognition is another topic awaiting further exploration. One study, with participants ranging in age from 18 to 65 years, reported that older age was related to poorer emotion recognition in both patients and controls, but older patients showed better abilities to decipher hints than younger ones [23]. Another small study found lower performances on a hinting task in older early-onset schizophrenia patients (mean age, 66 years), but not in patients with late-onset schizophrenia (mean age, 67 years), in comparison to healthy age-peers [24].

When evaluating the relative importance of clinical symptoms for social functioning, it is suggested that negative and depressive symptoms have more impact than positive symptoms. However, the lack of a strong association between positive symptoms and social functioning may also reflect the relative ineffectiveness of available treatments to address negative and cognitive deficits, rather than a lack of deleterious social impact of positive symptoms when present. A study examining anxiety symptoms found these to have a greater impact on social functioning than depressive symptoms [25].

Still, the combined effects of cognitive and clinical variables only explain a modest part of the total variance in social functioning. The search for other relevant factors is still underway. As stated above, the availability and quality of social support is underexplored in older patients with schizophrenia. Studies in younger patients with schizophrenia (and in other mental disorders) have highlighted the importance of social support. In the general population, stronger social relationships are associated with a lower mortality risk [26]. Also, in schizophrenia, a relation between the amount of social support and longevity has been suggested [27]. How social networks may change with age was demonstrated in inner-city outpatients in New York City (age range 18–78 years) [28]. While network size diminished with age, dependence on remaining network members did not increase and patients reported more satisfactory relationships with them. This aligns with a study of symptom management strategies by the same author, in which social diversion (increasing social contact by calling friends or talking to someone) was associated with increased age in schizophrenia outpatients (age range 19–69 years) [29].

Two other, partly intertwined, factors with social relevance are gender and age at onset of disease. Gender has been shown to be of major significance for social outcome in schizophrenia, but few studies have specifically addressed this issue. In patients with an early age at onset, women start off with an advantage over their male counterparts that relates to higher premorbid psychosocial functioning and a later mean onset of illness [30], although this advantage may be diluted in the long run. Patients with late-onset schizophrenia differ in their clinical picture from patients with an early onset of disease [31]. Relevant differences relate to female preponderance, fewer negative symptoms and milder cognitive deficits among late-onset patients. Combined with higher premorbid functioning, these features lead to better social integration compared with their early-onset counterparts. Many other underexplored factors possibly impacting on social functioning in later life await future research. Examples are socioeconomic characteristics (e.g., education, urbanicity, financial means), physical health status, coping styles and the impact of stigmatization. When designing new studies, the complex interplay between relevant variables must be kept in mind. For example, a study into the interaction of psychiatric symptoms and psychosocial variables in relation to social functioning and well-being found, contrary to the general idea of psychosocial stressors evoking psychiatric symptoms, that psychiatric symptoms at least partly preceded psychosocial disturbances (e.g., increase in life events, decrease of social support) [16].

Qualitative research on social functioning

In addition to the quantitative data reviewed above, qualitative study methods provide a valuable approach to examine more in-depth subjective perceptions of social functioning by individuals actually living with schizophrenia. Qualitative methods can make a complementary contribution, shedding light on topics that quantitative approaches may overlook. Although numerous qualitative studies have been performed in gerontology there is a striking paucity in relation to older patients with schizophrenia. This most likely relates to concerns about poor insight and cognitive impairment in patients. However, the few existing studies demonstrate that interviewees can provide meaningful information to open-ended queries (e.g., [32]).

In a recent North American qualitative study, 32 older persons with schizophrenia (mean age, 56 years; mean duration of illness, 35 years) were asked how they perceived their functioning over their lifespan [33]. The sample was evenly distributed between individuals living independently versus residing in board and care homes. Median income fell below the poverty line. While most participants described social isolation during the earlier course of their illness, many had made adaptations to their social networks, with peers and facility staff replacing family relationships in some. Nearly all reported improvement in the personal impact of symptoms of schizophrenia in later life, after having experienced the greatest degree of disruption in the early years of the illness. Despite these consistencies, participants strongly differed in their outlook toward the future. Three subgroups of participants were discerned. Some participants chiefly expressed despair over lost opportunities and failure to achieve the goals they had once set for themselves. Others appeared to have accepted their situation, and no longer compared themselves to their peers in the community, but rather with those who were doing worse. Financial limitations were mentioned as one of the greatest barriers to making changes in their lives. The third subgroup of participants were hopeful about the future, attaining functional milestones (e.g., keeping a job) for the first time in their lives and taking pride in their ability to participate in normal activities.

Quality of life

Quality of life is a comprehensive construct that seeks to integrate elements of social functioning and well-being [34]. There now is broad consensus within medicine that self-appraisals are the gold standard of quality of life and that objective assessments should be complementary to self-appraisals. Thus, subjective quality of life (SQOL) is now an established outcome measure in the care of persons with schizophrenia [35]. It has been demonstrated that schizophrenia patients can report SQOL with a high degree of reliability and concurrent validity [36]. In younger patients, relatively high SQOL levels have been documented [34]. Favourable social factors (e.g., independent living, more social support) contribute to a higher SQOL [37], while in the long term, improvement in psychosocial factors [38] as well as meeting unmet needs for care [39] appear to increase SQOL. In addition, patients with schizophrenia generally rate their SQOL as more favourable than those with mood and neurotic disorders, while in all three disorders a positive association between age and SQOL has been demonstrated [40].

In older schizophrenia patients, a smaller number of studies have evaluated quality of life. A cross-sectional study [41] of middle-aged and older community-dwelling patients with schizophrenia found older age to be associated with greater mental-health quality of life, suggesting that quality of life may actually improve with aging. Using a generic concept, Bankole et al. [42] found a lower SQOL in elderly schizophrenia patients in the New York City sample, compared to age-matched peers. However, the mean SQOL in the schizophrenia group was well above the threshold for a positive level of satisfaction and the absolute differences between the two groups were only modest. Six variables predicted a higher SQOL: fewer depressive symptoms, more cognitive deficits, fewer acute life stressors, fewer medication side effects, lower financial strain and better self-rated health. Overall, the model explained 55% of variance in SQOL. A longitudinal study of the same sample [43] found no significant group differences in SQOL between baseline and follow-up (range 12–116 months). However, at an individual level, 57% experienced sizeable changes (either increases or decreases) in their SQOL. Among the baseline predictors of higher SQOL at follow-up were having fewer depressive symptoms and higher religiousness. Having a higher SQOL at baseline predicted fewer anxiety, depressive and positive symptoms at follow-up.

In addition to these North American findings, in our catchment-area sample of older Dutch schizophrenia patients [44] almost half of all participants (48%) reported a global favourable SQOL. Fewer self-reported depressive symptoms, worse global neurocognition, and higher observer-rated social functioning predicted a higher SQOL, explaining 53% of the total variance. Notably, depressive symptoms are suggested to be a more important source of distress than psychotic symptoms, on which treatment traditionally tends to focus. The association between self-reported depressive symptoms and SQOL needs cautious evaluation. SQOL and self-reported depressive symptoms may partially reflect the same underlying affective state [40]. Next, while depressive mood may lead to a lower SQOL, experiencing a lower SQOL may in turn have negative affective consequences. This was suggested by the findings of the longitudinal New York City sample described above.

SQOL relates to the gap between the aspirations of an individual and perceived reality. Comparisons with original ambitions, as well as comparisons with the life situation and achievements of others, influence appraisal of SQOL. Internal standards of comparison may change over time, as patients adjust to their disorder [45]. As a result, while living in conditions that may seem adversarial and unpleasant to others, patients can nevertheless be relatively satisfied with their life. This is reflected in the low correlations between SQOL and objective indicators of quality of life in schizophrenia [40]. In elderly populations, a survivor bias should also be acknowledged, as higher-functioning patients may stand a better chance of surviving into old age. Other factors that intuitively might relate to SQOL are still underresearched in older schizophrenia populations. Physical health, personal coping styles and stigmatization are examples of potentially relevant variables that may be amenable to intervention.

Conclusion

Without any doubt, most elderly people with schizophrenia are well behind their healthy age-peers in their social achievements, such as marital relations, friendships and independent residence. Schizophrenia patients also appear to be socially disadvantaged in comparison to elderly patients with other mental illnesses, although to a lesser extent. Next, there is a marked heterogeneity in the level of social functioning. In a wide spectrum of social functioning, severely incapacitated, socially isolated patients occupy the negative extreme. When the content of their psychosis withholds them from accepting help, they may lead a sorrowful life, largely out of sight of society. At the positive extreme, patients are found in whom the negative impact of their disorder has been limited, and who have shown resilience both emotionally and socially. If they enjoy good physical health, they could even come close to full recovery or to successful ageing [46]. Still, successful ageing remains elusive for most patients with schizophrenia [47].

If recovery is considered as an all-or-nothing goal, these findings are clearly discouraging. However, such a dichotomous approach does not do justice to the versatile reality of coping with everyday life for most older schizophrenia patients, who can be identified at some point in between these extremes. With time they may move in one direction or the other, in line with present knowledge that schizophrenia in later life is not a stable end state but one of fluctuation, in both symptomatology and functioning. Many patients show significant improvements in social functioning and subjective quality of life as they age. Interestingly, this parallels the finding in successful ageing research that positive self-appraisal increases with age, even in the midst of physical and cognitive decline [48].

In adult schizophrenia care, the diversity of treatments has greatly expanded in recent decades, but still few of these gains have seeped through to old age mental health services. Nevertheless, some excellent North American studies have been conducted in the field of psychological and social interventions that fit older patients with severe mental illness [49]. These are extensively reviewed in Chapter 14. However, the majority of older patients receive few if any of the available effective interventions. Lack of adequate funding is one reason for this science-to-service gap, but ageism on the side of professionals also may come into play. This defeatism about the ability of elderly schizophrenia patients to profit from psychosocial interventions needs to be overcome.

Next, the supply of day care facilities that offer participants a hospitable and non-demanding social environment should be encouraged. These may serve various purposes at the same time, such as overcoming social deprivation, improving cognitive functioning and promoting a healthy lifestyle. Input of participants when developing this type of facilities ought to be encouraged. Finally, there is a need for residential and nursing homes to expand specific facilities for elderly patients with severe mental illnesses, given the rapid growth in their numbers. In the development of such services, the specific vulnerabilities of this patient group should be taken into account, as they may run a higher risk of social isolation in these living arrangements [50].

References

1. Harvey, P.D. and Bellack, A. S. (2009). Toward a terminology for functional recovery in schizophrenia: Is functional remission a viable concept? *Schizophrenia Bulletin*, 35(2), 300–6.

2. Priebe, S. (2007). Social outcomes in schizophrenia. *British Journal of Psychiatry*, 191 (Suppl. 50), s15–20.

3. Mueser, K.T. and Tarrier, N. (eds) *Handbook of Social Functioning in Schizophrenia*. Boston, MA: Allyn and Bacon, 1998, XI.

4. Bowie, C.R., Twamley, E.W., Anderson, H., et al. (2007). Self-assessment of functional status in schizophrenia. *Journal of Psychiatric Research*, 41(12), 1012–18.

5. Cohen, C.I., Vahia, I., Reyes, P., et al. (2008). Schizophrenia in later life: clinical symptoms and social well-being. *Psychiatric Services*, 59(3), 232–4.

6. Meesters, P.D., de Haan, L., Comijs, H.C., et al. (2012). Schizophrenia spectrum disorders in later life: prevalence and distribution of age at onset and sex in a dutch catchment area. *American Journal of Geriatric Psychiatry*, 20(1), 18–28.

7. Meesters, P.D., Stek, M.L., Comijs, H.C., et al. (2010). Social functioning among older community-dwelling patients with schizophrenia: a review. *American Journal of Geriatric Psychiatry*, 18(10), 862–78.

8. Ran, M.S., Xiang, M.Z., Conwell, Y., et al. (2004). Comparison of characteristics between geriatric and younger subjects with schizophrenia in community. *Journal of Psychiatric Research*, 38(4), 417–24.

9. Ciompi, L. (1980). Catamnestic long-term study on the course of life and aging of schizophrenics. *Schizophrenia Bulletin*, 6(4), 606–18.

10. Harding, C.M., Brooks, G.W., Ashikaga, T., Strauss, J.S. and Breier, A. (1987). The Vermont longitudinal study of persons with severe mental illness. II: Long-term outcome of subjects who retrospectively met DSM-III criteria for schizophrenia. *American Journal of Psychiatry*, 144(6), 727–35.

11. Meesters, P.D., Comijs, H.C., Sonnenberg, C.M., et al. (2014). Prevalence and correlates of depressive symptoms in a catchment-area based cohort of older community-living schizophrenia patients. *Schizophrenia Research*, 157(1–3), 285–91.

12. Bankole, A., Cohen, C.I., Vahia, I., et al. (2008). Symptomatic remission in a multiracial urban population of older adults with schizophrenia. *American Journal of Geriatric Psychiatry*, 16(12), 966–73.

13. Bowie, C.R., Reichenberg, A., Patterson, T., et al. (2006). Determinants of real-world functional performance in schizophrenia. *American Journal of Psychiatry*, 163(3), 418.

14. Bowie, C.R., Leung, W.W., Reichenberg, A., et al. (2008). Predicting schizophrenia patients' real-world behavior with specific neuropsychological and functional capacity measures. *Biological Psychiatry*, 63(5), 505–11.

15. Jeste, D.V., Twamley, E.W., Eyler Zorrilla, L.T., et al. (2003). Aging and outcome in schizophrenia. *Acta Psychiatrica Scandinavica*, 107(5), 336–43.

16. Patterson, T.L., Semple, S.J., Shaw, W.S., et al. (1997). Self-reported social functioning among older patients with schizophrenia. *Schizophrenia Research*, 27(2–3), 199–210.

17. Semple, S.J., Patterson, T.L., Shaw, W.S., et al. (1999). Self-perceived interpersonal competence in older schizophrenia patients: the role of patient characteristics and psychosocial factors. *Acta Psychiatrica Scandinavica*, 100(2), 126–35.

18. Mueser, K.T., Pratt, S.I., Bartels, S.J., et al. (2010). Neurocognition and social skill in older persons with schizophrenia and major mood disorders: an analysis of gender and diagnosis effects. *Journal of Neurolinguistics*, 23(3), 297–317.

19. Abdallah, C., Cohen, C.I., Sanchez-Almira, M., Reyes P. and Ramirez, P. (2009). Community integration and associated factors among older adults with schizophrenia. *Psychiatric Services*, 60(12), 1642–8.

20. Jimenez Madiedo, C., Garcia-Aracena, E.F., Ryu, H.H. and Cohen, C.I. (2012). Community integration in older adults with schizophrenia on 4-year follow-up. *American Journal of Geriatric Psychiatry*, 20, S91.

21. Cohen, C.I. and Iqbal, M. (2014). Longitudinal study of remission among older adults with schizophrenia spectrum disorder. *American Journal of Geriatric Psychiatry*, 22(5), 450–8.

22. Kalache, S.M., Mulsant, B.H., Davies, S.J., et al. (2015). The impact of aging, cognition, and symptoms on functional competence in individuals with schizophrenia across the lifespan. *Schizophrenia Bulletin*, 41(2), 374–81.

23. Pinkham, A.E., Kelsven, S., Kouros, C., Harvey, P.D. and Penn, D.L. (2017). The effect of age, race, and sex on social cognitive performance in individuals with schizophrenia. *Journal of Nervous and Mental Disease*, 205(5), 346–52.

24. Smeets-Janssen, M.M.J., Meesters, P.D., Comijs, H.C., et al. (2013). Theory of mind differences in older patients with early-onset and late-onset paranoid schizophrenia. *International Journal of Geriatric Psychiatry*, 28(11), 1141–6.

25. Wetherell, J.L., Palmer, B.W., Thorp, S.R., et al. (2003). Anxiety symptoms and quality of life in middle-aged and older outpatients with schizophrenia and schizoaffective disorder. *Journal of Clinical Psychiatry*, 64(12), 1476–82.

26. Holt-Lunstad, J., Smith, T.B. and Layton, J.B. (2010). Social relationships and mortality risk: a meta-analytic review. *PLoS Medicine*, 7(7), e1000316.

27. Christensen, A.J., Dornink, R., Ehlers, S.L. and Schultz, S.K. (1999). Social environment and longevity in schizophrenia. *Psychosomatic Medicine*, 61(2), 141–5.

28. Cohen, C.I. and Kochanowicz, N. (1989). Schizophrenia and social network patterns: a survey of black inner-city outpatients. *Community Mental Health Journal*, 25(3), 197–207.

29. Cohen, C. (1993). Age-related correlations in patient symptom management strategies in schizophrenia: an exploratory study. *International Journal of Geriatric Psychiatry*, 8, 211–13.

30. Leung, A. and Chue, P. (2000). Sex differences in schizophrenia, a review of the literature. *Acta Psychiatrica Scandinavica*, 101, 3–38.

31. Vahia, I.V., Palmer, B.W., Depp, C., et al. (2010). Is late-onset schizophrenia a subtype of schizophrenia? *Acta Psychiatrica Scandinavica*, 122(5), 414–26.

32. Palinkas, L.A, Criado, V., Fuentes, D., et al. (2007). Unmet needs for services for older adults with mental illness: comparison of views of different stakeholder groups. *American Journal of Geriatric Psychiatry*, 15, 530–40.

33. Shepherd, S., Depp, C.A., Harris, G., et al. (2012). Perspectives on schizophrenia over the lifespan: a qualitative study. *Schizophrenia Bulletin*, 38(2), 295–303.

34. Katschnig, H. (2000). Schizophrenia and quality of life. *Acta Psychiatrica Scandinavica Supplementum*, 102, 33–7.

35. Awad, A.G. and Voruganti, L.N. (2012). Measuring quality of life in patients with schizophrenia: an update. *Pharmacoeconomics*, 30(3), 183–95.

36. Voruganti, L., Heslegrave, R., Awad, A.G. and Seeman, M.V. (1998). Quality of life measurement in schizophrenia: reconciling the quest for subjectivity with the question of reliability. *Psychological Medicine*, 28, 165–72.

37. Yanos, P.T. and Moos, R.H. (2007). Determinants of functioning and well-being among individuals with schizophrenia: an integrated model. *Clinical Psychology Review*, 27, 58–77.

38. Ritsner, M.S., Lisker, A. and Arbitman, M. (2012). Ten-year quality of life outcomes among patients with schizophrenia and schizoaffective disorders: I. Predictive value of disorder-related factors. *Quality of Life Research*, 21(5), 837–47.

39. Slade, M., Leese, M., Cahill, S., Thornicroft, G. and Kuipers, E. (2005). Patient-rated mental health needs and quality of life improvement. *British Journal of Psychiatry*, 187, 256–61.

40. Priebe, S., Reininghaus, U., McCabe, R., et al. (2010). Factors influencing subjective quality of life in patients with schizophrenia and other mental disorders: a pooled analysis. *Schizophrenia Research*, 121(1–3), 251–8.

41. Folsom, D.P., Depp, C., Palmer, B.W., et al. (2009). Physical and mental health-related quality of life among older people with schizophrenia. *Schizophrenia Research*, 108(1–3), 207–13.

42. Bankole, A.O., Cohen, C.I., Vahia, I., et al. (2007). Factors affecting quality of life in a multiracial sample of older persons with schizophrenia. *American Journal of Geriatric Psychiatry*, 15, 1015–23.

43. Cohen, C.I., Vengassery, A. and Garcia Aracena, E.F. (2017). A longitudinal analysis of quality of life and associated factors in older adults with schizophrenia spectrum disorder. *American Journal of Geriatric Psychiatry*, 25(7), 755–65.

44. Meesters, P.D., Comijs, H.C., de Haan, L., et al. (2013). Subjective quality of life and its determinants in a catchment area based population of elderly schizophrenia patients. *Schizophrenia Research*, 147(2–3), 275–80.

45. Franz, M., Meyer, T., Reber, T. and Gallhofer, B. (2000). The importance of social comparisons for high levels of subjective quality of life in chronic schizophrenic patients. *Quality of Life Research* 9, 481–9.

46. Reichstadt, J., Sengupta, G., Depp, C.A., Palinkas, L.A and Jeste, D.V. (2010). Older adults' perspectives on successful aging: qualitative interviews. *American Journal of Geriatric Psychiatry*, 18(7), 567–75.

47. Ibrahim, F., Cohen, C.I. and Ramirez, P.M. (2010). Successful aging in older adults with schizophrenia: prevalence and associated factors. *American Journal of Geriatric Psychiatry*, 18(10), 879–86.

48. Jeste, D.V., Savla, G.N., Thompson, W.K., et al. (2013). Association between older age and more successful aging: critical role of resilience and depression. *American Journal of Psychiatry*, 170, 188–96.

49. Bartels, S.J. and Pratt, S.I. (2009). Psychosocial rehabilitation and quality of life for older adults with serious mental illness: recent findings and future research directions. *Current Opinion in Psychiatry*, 22(4), 381–5.

50. Depla, M.F.I., de Graaf, R., van Weeghel, J. and Heeren, T.J. (2005). The role of stigma in the quality of life of older adults with severe mental illness. *International Journal of Geriatric Psychiatry*, 20, 146–53.

Depression in Older Adults with Schizophrenia

11

Aninditha Vengassery, M.D. and John Kasckow, M.D.

Depression is a common cause of comorbidity in older persons with schizophrenia. The 0.5% prevalence of schizophrenia in older adults underscores the importance of studying depressive symptoms in this population [1,2]. In middle-aged and older adults over 45 the prevalence of depression ranges from 44 to 75% [1]. The increase in the number of older adults worldwide and the negative impact of depression, along with debilitating symptoms of schizophrenia highlight the strong significance of studying depressive symptoms in patients with schizophrenia [2]. Depression is one of the common comorbidities in patients with schizophrenia in conjunction with other outcomes, such as higher risk for suicide. People with schizophrenia have an 8.5-fold greater risk of suicide than those in the general population [3]. Depression in schizophrenia is linked with poor outcomes, such as functional impairment and poor interpersonal skills [4]. Comorbid depression impacts negatively on quality of life, functioning, and overall psychopathology and comorbid medical conditions. Older patients with schizophrenia often have cognitive deficits along with multiple comorbidities, which make the diagnosis of depression more difficult [5]. Detection and management of depressive symptoms in patients with schizophrenia has an important role in the management of this population.

The goal of this chapter is to review the impact of depression in patients with schizophrenia and the available treatment modalities, updating the reviews by Kasckow et al. in 2008 [5] and Felmet et al. in 2011 [6]. We will focus on the various forms of depression that clinicians can encounter in older patients with schizophrenia.

Overview of depressive symptoms in schizophrenia

In older patients with schizophrenia, depressive symptoms have been reported to be more severe compared to geriatric patients without schizophrenia [2]. A study by Zisook et al. [7] on 60 outpatients with schizophrenia between the ages of 45 and 79 years vs. 60 normal comparison subjects without major neuropsychiatric disorders showed that depression is more frequent and severe in schizophrenia patients compared to controls. Several research studies have shown that depressive symptoms are associated with disability, recurrence of illness, demoralization and poor motivation, and risk of suicide [8–11].

The following studies have helped us better understand the nature of depressive symptoms in older patients with schizophrenia. Diwan et al. [12] examined 198 patients aged 55 and older with schizophrenia living in an urban population. The schizophrenia group had 32% individuals with clinical depression compared to 11% in the control group. In logistic regression analysis, six variables linked to the presence of depression were physical illness, quality of life, presence of positive symptoms, proportion of confidants, coping by using medications, and coping with conflicts by keeping calm. A longitudinal study by Ryu et al. [13] in the same cohort reported persistent depression in 44% of patients; 30% remained persistently non-depressed and 26% fluctuated between depression and non-depression. Another study [14] examining comorbidity in schizophrenia in a mixed-age sample of 1446 adults with schizophrenia determined that 27.7% were found to have comorbid major depression and a total of 56.0% had at least one comorbid mental health disorder such as obsessive compulsive disorder, substance use, or anxiety.

Meesters et al. [2] examined self-reported depressive symptoms in a sample of 99 community-living older Dutch adults with schizophrenia (mean age 67 years). In the schizophrenia group, 47.5% reported depressive symptoms at a level indicating clinically relevant depression, in contrast to 12.1% in their age peers. Factors associated with depression were functional limitations, chronic physical disorders, and poor social support. A study by Van Liempt et al. [15] in the same cohort found that lower social functioning was associated with both negative symptoms and depressive symptoms.

In the above-cited study [4] on depression and cognition in 71 patients with schizophrenia over 50 years of age, depression severity predicted patient's performance on memory and attention tasks. However, it did not influence the global functional ability of the patients. The study signaled that patients with intact cognition who were living in nursing homes or adult homes experienced more depression due to their needs not being met.

Research has indicated that subsyndromal depression symptoms are more prevalent than major depressive episodes in patients with schizophrenia, with projected rates ranging over 80% in all age groups [16,17]. In DSM V [18] subsyndromal depression can be coded as "other specified depressive disorder." This diagnosis is applied when depressive symptoms cause significant impairments in social and/or occupational areas of functioning, but do not sufficiently meet criteria for a depressive disorder. Zisook et al. in the study cited above [7] found that around two-thirds of patients with schizophrenia without a major depressive episode had at least mild depressive symptoms (Hamilton Depression Rating Scale score ≥ 7), and over 30% of patients reported depressed mood, feelings of guilt, and feelings of hopelessness. Another study by the same research group [19] demonstrated that subsyndromal depression was associated with worse overall psychopathology, positive and negative symptoms, severity of medical conditions, physical and mental functioning, anxiety, and suicidality.

Finally, a British study by Graham et al. [20] in patients with schizophrenia aged over 65, living in the community, found that 40% had a Geriatric Depression Score (GDS) score of >4 indicating "comorbid diagnosis of probable depression."

Suicidality

Suicide is considered the 17th leading cause of death in adults 65 years and older [21]. Palmer et al. performed a meta-analysis on life-time suicide risk in patients with schizophrenia (age 18 and older) and determined an estimated risk of 4.5% [22]. Suicide also is a leading cause of premature death in patients with schizophrenia and depression [23]. In a psychological autopsy case series on 92 patients diagnosed with schizophrenia, one-third of the patients were above the age of 40; 64% of these were diagnosed with depression [24].

Cohen et al. [25] reported a higher prevalence of current and lifetime suicidality among those with schizophrenia compared to individuals in the community (current: 10% vs.

0.6%; lifetime: 56% vs. 7%), as well as a higher number of past suicidal attempts (30% vs. 4%). The variables associated with suicide were subsyndromal depression and trauma in earlier life. Kasckow et al. [26] studied a sample of middle-aged and older patients (mean age 52.5 years) with schizophrenia and subthreshold depressive symptoms. Their study concluded that suicidal ideation was positively correlated with depressive symptoms, but there was no association with age. Another study by Kasckow et al. [27] examined suicidal behavior in 146 patients 40 and older with schizophrenia and depression. Logistic regression analysis indicated that lower quality of life scores predicted suicidality, whereas age, medication management, and everyday functioning were not predictive.

A cohort study in Denmark by Erlangsen et al. [28] examined suicide risk in adults 50 years and older with schizophrenia. They found an increased risk of suicide in older adults diagnosed with schizophrenia compared to those without schizophrenia. An older study [29] examined 243 patients with a family history of suicide and compared them with 5602 patients with no family history of suicide. A family history of suicide significantly increased the risk for a suicide attempt in patients with a wide variety of diagnoses: schizophrenia, unipolar and bipolar affective disorders, depressive neurosis, and personality disorders.

Depression in schizophrenia and its impact on functioning and quality of life and daily functioning

Many studies have shown a connection between depression and quality of life in schizophrenia patients. Recently, Cohen et al. [30] longitudinally examined quality of life in patients with schizophrenia aged 55 or older. The study determined that quality of life was not static in later life and found depression to be a predictor of quality of life at follow-up. Bowie et al. [31] studied the course of neuropsychological performance, symptom severity, and functional capacity in older adults with schizophrenia (50–85 years). They found that interpersonal and work skills were negatively influenced by depression. Roseman et al. [32] found in middle-aged to older adults with schizophrenia and subsyndromal depression that poor insight interacted with negative symptoms to diminish quality of life.

Pharmacotherapy

The treatment of schizophrenia involves pharmacotherapy in combination with psychosocial interventions. A comprehensive discussion of the pharmacological treatment of older adults with schizophrenia in general is found in Chapter 13 and a discussion of psychosocial interventions is provided in Chapters 14 and 18. Evidence-based studies examining the treatment of depression in patients with schizophrenia are very limited. We will discuss below what knowledge base is available. In 2001, Siris et al. [33] conducted an international survey among psychiatrists regarding the treatment of comorbid depression in patients with schizophrenia. The study concluded that most US clinicians prefer to treat depression in schizophrenia patients with both second-generation antipsychotics and an SSRI. However, the same study also indicated that almost one-quarter of clinicians never prescribed or rarely prescribed antidepressants (28% of US psychiatrists, compared with 33% of psychiatrists world-wide).

A systematic review [34] of 3608 mixed-age study participants from 82 trials showed that adding an antidepressant to antipsychotics was effective for treating negative and depressive symptoms in patients with schizophrenia. The 1999 Expert Treatment Guidelines [35] for patients with schizophrenia and major depression recommended treating patients initially with optimal dosages of second-generation antipsychotics. If depression persists it was recommended that an SSRI is added to the regimen. If depressive symptoms still continued, venlafaxine would be the next option, followed by buprorion [36]. Given that these guidelines are now nearly 20 years old, newer ones need to be formulated and they must include some consideration of the appropriate strategies for older adults with schizophrenia.

There are few studies examining antidepressant augmentation in older patients with schizophrenia. Two out of three initial placebo-controlled studies on patients with schizophrenia (mean 42.2 years) with depressive symptoms suggested that fluoxetine may not be beneficial over placebo [37–39]. Kasckow et al. in 2001 [40] performed an open-label study of citalopram in chronically hospitalized patients aged greater than 55 years with schizophrenia and depressive symptoms. In this study, 19 patients were already on antipsychotic medication and 9 of them were augmented with antidepressant citalopram. The citalopram group demonstrated significant improvement in Hamilton Depression scale (HAMD) scores.

Zisook et al. in 2009 [41] conducted a double-blind, randomized, placebo-controlled, two-site study of 198 participants with schizophrenia, aged 40 to 75 years, to examine the effectiveness and safety of citalopram for 12 weeks. In this study, subsyndromal depression was defined as having two to four of the nine DSM-IV symptoms for major depression present for the majority of a two-week period. Almost 90% of participants were on antipsychotics. They were randomly assigned to a "flexible dose treatment" plan with citalopram, or the placebo group. Citalopram-treated participants showed an improvement in their depressive and negative symptoms – validated by HAMD and Calgary depression rating scale (CDRS) scores – vs. the placebo. Kasckow et al. [42] then showed in the same group that citalopram augmentation of antipsychotic medication led to improvements in social functioning and quality of life. However, no improvements were noted for physical functioning or medication management. A study of persons with schizophrenia aged 40 and over by Vahia et al. in 2013 [43] found that augmentation with citalopram improved negative symptoms, depressive symptoms, quality of life, and some motor retardation. They hypothesized that improvements in negative symptoms probably arise secondary to the improvement of depression.

A recent study in the general population has suggested clozapine has higher antidepressant effects relative to quetiapine and equivalent effects relative to olanzapine and risperidone in chronic schizophrenia [44]. Clozapine has also been shown to have a substantial positive effect on reducing suicidal behaviors in patients with schizophrenia. In 2002, the FDA Psychopharmacologic Drugs Advisory Committee approved the use of clozapine for the treatment of suicidal behavior in patients with schizophrenia or schizoaffective disorder. However, studies with older adults still need to be conducted [45].

Psychosocial treatment

Psychosocial therapy in tandem with pharmacotherapy is essential in older adults with schizophrenia [46]. Medication improves the acute symptoms. Psychotherapy in conjunction with other psychosocial treatments presumably improves the residual symptoms, social functioning, and overall quality of life. Interventions such as cognitive behavioral therapy, assertive community treatment, cognitive remediation, family psychoeducation, illness self-management training, supported employment, and social skills training have been found to be successful in improving overall functioning in middle-aged and older adults with schizophrenia. These programs are described in Chapter 14. However, there is a paucity of research data on psychosocial treatments aimed specifically towards treating depression in older adults with schizophrenia.

Summary

1. Prevalence rates in middle age and older adults with schizophrenia range from 44 to 75%, with a majority of persons exhibiting subsyndromal depression. About one-quarter of persons fluctuate between depression and non-depression over time.
2. Depression has its greatest impact on quality of life and daily functioning.
3. Suicide risk is higher in older adults with schizophrenia than their age peers. Depression is the strongest predictor of suicidality.
4. Treatment is understudied in older persons. Adding an antidepressant to an antipsychotic agent may diminish depressive symptoms. Little is known with respect to psychosocial treatment for depression in this population.

References

1. Cohen CI, Meesters PD, Zhao J. New perspectives on schizophrenia in later life: implications for treatment, policy and research, *Lancet Psychiatry* 2015;2:340–50.

2. Meesters PD, Comijs HC, Sonnenberg CM, et al. Prevalence and correlates of depressive symptoms in a catchment-area based cohort of older community-living schizophrenia patients, *Schizophr Res* 2014;157:285–91.

3. Harris EC, Barraclough B. Suicide as an outcome for mental disorders: a meta-analysis, *Br J Psychiatry* 1997;170:205–28.

4. Antonio ED, Serper MP. Depression and cognitive deficits in geriatric schizophrenia, *Schizophr Res* 2012;134:65–9.

5. Kasckow JW, Zisook S. Co-occurring depressive symptoms in the older patient with schizophrenia, *Drugs Aging* 2008;25:631–47.

6. Felmet K, Zisook S, Kasckow JW. Elderly patients with schizophrenia and depression: diagnosis and treatment, *Clin Schizophr Relat Psychoses* 2011;4:239–50.

7. Zisook S, McAdams LA, Kuck J, et al. Depressive symptoms in schizophrenia, *Am J Psychiatry* 1999;156:1736–43.

8. Kessler RC, McGonagle KA, Zhao S, et al. Lifetime and 12-month prevalence of DSM-III-R psychiatric disorders in the United States, *Arch Gen Psychiatry* 1994;51:8–19.

9. American Psychiatric Association. *Diagnostic and Statistical Manual of Mental Disorders, Text Revision.* 3. Washington, DC: American Psychiatric Association; 2000.

10. Roy A. Suicide in chronic schizophrenia, *Br J Psychiatry* 1982;141:171–7.

11. Johnson DA. Studies of depressive symptoms in schizophrenia, *Br J Psychiatry* 1981;139:89–101.

12. Diwan S, Cohen CI, Bankole AO, et al. Depression in older adults with schizophrenia spectrum disorders: prevalence and associated factors, *Am J Geriatr Psychiatry* 2007;15(12):991–8.

13. Ryu HH, Cohen CI. A longitudinal study of the outcome and associated factors of subsyndromal and syndromal depression in community-dwelling older adults with schizophrenia spectrum disorder, *Am J Geriatr Psychiatry* 2015;23:925–33.

14. Jack T, Robert RA. Psychiatry comorbidity among adults with schizophrenia: a

latent class analysis, *Psychiatry Res* 2013;210:16–20.

15. Van Liempt S, Dols A, Schouws S, Stek ML, Meesters PD. Comparison of social functioning in community-living older individuals with schizophrenia and bipolar disorder: a catchment area-based study, *Int J Geriatr Psychiatry* 2017;32:532–8.

16. Bartels SJ, Drake RE. Depressive symptoms in schizophrenia: comprehensive differential diagnosis. *Compr Psychiatry* 1988;29(5):467–83.

17. Leff, J. Depressive symptoms in the course of schizophrenia. In *Depression in Schizophrenia*, ed. LE DeLisi, Washington, DC: American Psychiatric Press; 1990. 3–23.

18. American Psychiatric Association. *Diagnostic and Statistical Manual of Mental Disorders, DSM-V.* Washington, DC: American Psychiatric Association; 2013.

19. Zisook S, Montross L, Kasckow J, et al. Subsyndromal depressive symptoms in middle-aged and older persons with schizophrenia, *Am J Geriatr Psychiatry* 2007;15(12):1005–14.

20. Graham C, Arthus A, Howard R. The social functioning of older adults with schizophrenia, *Aging Ment Health* 2002;6:149–53.

21. Centers for Disease Control and Prevention (CDC). Suicide facts at a glance 2015; stacks.cdc.gov/view/cdc/21865/cdc_21865_DS1.pdf (accessed October 2018).

22. Palmer BA, Pankratz VS, Bostwick JM. The lifetime risk of suicide in schizophrenia: a reexamination, *Arch Gen Psychiatry* 2005;62:247–53.

23. Kaskow JW, Golshan S, Zisook S. Does age moderate the relationship between depressive symptoms and suicidal ideation in middle aged and older patients with schizophrenia and subthreshold depression? *Am J Geriatr Psychiatry* 2014;22(5):437–41.

24. Heilä H, Isometsä ET, Henriksson MM, et al. Suicide and schizophrenia: a nationwide psychological autopsy study on age- and sex-specific clinical characteristics of 92 suicide victims with schizophrenia, *Am J Psychiatry* 1997;154:1235–42.

25. Cohen CI, Abdallah GC, Diwan S. Suicide attempts and associated factors in older adults with schizophrenia, *Schizophr Res* 2010;119:253–7.

26. Kasckow J, Golshan S, Zisook S. Does age moderate the relationship between depressive symptoms and suicidal ideation in middle aged and older patients with schizophrenia and subthreshold depression? *Am J Geriatr Psychiatry* 2014;22(5): 437–41.

27. Kasckow J, Montross L, Golshan S, et al. Suicidality in middle aged and older patients with schizophrenia and depressive symptoms: relationship to functioning and quality of life, *Int J Geriatr Psychiatry* 2007;22:1223–8.

28. Erlangsen A, Eaton WW, Mortensen PB, Conwell Y. Schizophrenia: a predictor of suicide during the second half of life, *Schizophr Res* 2012;134(2–3):111–17.

29. Roy A. Family history of suicide, *Arch Gen Psychiatry* 1983;40:971–4.

30. Cohen CI, Vengassery A, Aracena EF. A longitudinal analysis of quality of life and associated factors in older adults with schizophrenia spectrum disorder, *Am J Geriatr Psychiatry* 2017;25(7):755–65.

31. Bowie CR, Reichenberg A, Patterson TL, Heaton RK, Harvey PD. Determinants of real-world functional performance in schizophrenia subjects: correlations with cognition, functional capacity, and symptoms, *Am J Psychiatry* 2006;163(3):418–25.

32. Roseman AS, Kasckow J, Fellows I, et al. Insight, quality of life, and functional capacity in middle-aged and older adults with schizophrenia, *Int J Geriatr Psychiatry* 2008;23(7):760–5.

33. Siris SG, Addington D, Azorin J, Calinescu E. Depression in schizophrenia: recognition and management in the USA, *Schizophr Res* 2001;47:185–97.

34. Helfer B, Samara TM, Huhn M, et al. Efficacy and safety of antidepressants added to antipsychotics for schizophrenia: a systematic review and meta-analysis, *Am J Psychiatry* 2016;173(9):876–86.

35. McEvoy JP, Scheifler PL, Frances A. The Expert Consensus Guidelines Series: treatment of schizophrenia, *J Clin Psychiatry* 1999;60(Suppl 11): 1–80.

36. Alexopoulos GS, Streim J, Carpenter D, Docherty JP; Expert Consensus Panel for Using Antipsychotic Drugs in Older Patients. Using antipsychotic agents in older patients, *J Clin Psychiatry* 2004;65(Suppl 2):5–99.

37. Micallef J, Fakra E, Blin O. Use of antidepressant drugs in schizophrenic patients with depression, *Encephale* 2006;32:263–9.

38. Eiber R, Even C. Actual approaches to post-psychotic depression, *Encephale* 2001;27(4):301–7.

39. Hausmann A, Fleischhacker WW. Depression in patients with schizophrenia, *CNS Drugs* 2000;14(4):289–99.

40. Kasckow JW, Mohamed S, Thallasinos A, et al. Citalopram augmentation of antipsychotic treatment in older schizophrenia patients, *Int J Geriatr Psychiatry* 2001;16(12):1163–7.

41. Zisook S, Kasckow JW, Golshan S, et al. Citalopram augmentation for subsyndromal symptoms of depression in middle-aged and older outpatients with schizophrenia and schizoaffective disorder: a randomized controlled trial, *J Clin Psychiatry*. 2009;70(4):562–571.

42. Kasckow J, Lanouette N, Patterson T, et al. Treatment of subsyndromal depressive symptoms in middle-aged and older adults with schizophrenia: effect on functioning, *Int J Geriatr Psychiatry* 2010;25(2):183–90.

43. Vahia IV, Lanouette NM, Golshan S, et al. Adding antidepressants to antipsychotics for treatment of subsyndromal depressive symptoms in schizophrenia: impact on positive and negative symptoms, *Indian J Psychiatry* 2013;55:144–8.

44. Nakajima S, Takeuchi H, Fervaha G, et al. Comparative efficacy between clozapine and other atypical antipsychotics on depressive symptoms in patients with schizophrenia: analysis of the CATIE Phase 2E data, *Schizophr Res* 2015;161:429–33.

45. Gareri P, De Fazio P, Russo E, et al. The safety of clozapine in the elderly, *Expert Opin Drug Saf* 2008;7(5):525–38.

46. Mueser KT, Deavers F, Penn DL, Cassisi JE. Psychosocial treatments for schizophrenia, *Annu Rev Clin Psychol* 2013;9:465–97.

Chapter

12

Community Treatment Needs

Paul D. Meesters, M.D.

This chapter will explore objective and subjective environmental, physical, psychological, and social needs of older persons with schizophrenia, and examine the individual and socio-political factors that are associated with these needs. In contrast to the past, the large majority of older patients nowadays reside in the community. This specifically shapes the character of their needs, with major implications for the services required to meet these needs.

Case Study 12.1

Mr C, a 73-year-old man, was raised by his grandparents. After leaving school he had several jobs. At 21, he joined the army to pursue a military career. Early on in his training, he got confused. He talked incessantly about religious issues and was found walking around naked on the army base. Persuaded to do so, he reported to a mental institution, where medication was started. He was diagnosed with schizophrenia. After leaving the hospital prematurely, he set out to sea. In the following years, return of his florid delusions frequently caused social turmoil, leading to new hospitalizations. He repeatedly stopped taking his medication and disengaged with outpatient mental health services some time later. In the meantime, he got married and had two daughters, but his wife left him after another readmission. After residing in a facility for the homeless for several years, he was able to acquire a house of his own. As an outgoing person, he met with several people on a daily basis, but was never visited by them at his place. At age 66, after throwing household goods from his window, he was readmitted involuntarily, showing agitation, paranoia, and visual hallucinations. His gait was unsteady and he had suffered some falls. Eventually he accepted antipsychotic medication. He was diagnosed with diabetes and chronic obstructive pulmonary disease, and now needed a walker. In addition to schizophrenia-related neurocognitive deficits, mild memory impairments were documented that were possibly linked to former periods of alcohol abuse. After stabilization, he accepted a move into a residential home with specific accommodation for older individuals with mental illnesses. Here, he integrated fairly easily. Brought up in a religious family, he has restarted attending church and is frequently visited by one of its volunteers. His brightly decorated room is filled with electrical equipment, which he collects and repairs. Asked where his two daughters reside nowadays, he says he does not know or care.

Introduction

For the delivery of appropriate and comprehensive services to persons suffering from schizophrenia, understanding their specific needs for care is a prerequisite. At an individual level it helps clinicians to provide individually tailored high-quality care. At a group level it informs service providers and policy makers to attune mental health and social welfare services to this population. Individuals with schizophrenia often have complex needs. Some needs will have a universal character (e.g., housing), but many relate to the specific condition of living with a mental disorder as severe and disruptive as schizophrenia. In mental health care, focus has traditionally been on clinically orientated needs (e.g., treatment of psychotic symptoms). Recent years have seen a shift to a wider scope that acknowledges needs with a more subjective or existential character (e.g., finding meaning in life). This more inclusive view does justice to the complex interrelatedness of needs. For example, a person who experiences purpose in his life will be more motivated to take medication or to adopt a healthier lifestyle. A primordial prerequisite in this approach of needs is the inclusion of the patient's own perspective. This may highlight needs that go undetected or underestimated by staff. In addition, valuing the patient's opinions improves collaboration and negotiation with professional caregivers. Differences between patients and significant others in prioritization of needs also have relevance. Nowadays, the importance of putting emphasis on patient preferences when developing services in schizophrenia care is undisputed [1].

Research among younger schizophrenia patients has demonstrated that their needs for care are prevalent and heterogeneous [2]. The prevalence of unmet needs relates to both patient characteristics (e.g., severity of symptoms) and external factors (e.g., service provision). Patients tend to report psychosocial needs as being the most frequently unmet, including daily activities, company, and intimate relationships [3]. Various studies have documented that higher rates of patient-rated unmet needs are strongly associated with a lower subjective quality of life [4,5]. In addition, there is longitudinal evidence that meeting unmet needs can improve subjective quality of life [6], although this relationship should be interpreted with some caution as various items assessing perceived quality of life relate to need areas. Changes associated with aging (e.g., physical illness, social losses) may generate new care needs or modify existing ones. In spite of the substantial numbers of older schizophrenia patients, their specific needs are still poorly understood.

Assessment of needs

The validity of the need concept has been criticized for being over-simplified and not doing justice to the versatile and highly individual character of care [7]. Keeping in mind its possible shortcomings, needs assessment nevertheless is a sensible starting point in everyday clinical practice. It helps patients, as well as staff and families, to determine which issues bear relevance and which treatment goals should be given priority. Thus, it may inspire a well-negotiated treatment plan that can be evaluated and adjusted periodically depending on its effectiveness.

In a common definition, a need for care refers to an illness or impairment for which there is an effective and acceptable method of intervention [8]. This definition avoids inclusion of needs that are principally or practically unfulfillable (e.g., wanting a partner). While some needs have a more neutral (e.g., housing) and others a more subjective character (e.g., company), assessment of a need inevitably involves a value judgment. Therefore, needs preferably should be evaluated from a multiple perspective, including at least that of the patient and preferably of the (in)formal carer. A met need refers to a situation in which the individual has had difficulties in a particular area that now are being adequately taken care of. An unmet need exists when the individual is believed not to receive the appropriate care or the adequate level of care.

A number of instruments have been developed to evaluate care needs in a comprehensive way. The Camberwell Assessment of Need for the Elderly (CANE) [9] was introduced in 2000 and at present is the most well-researched instrument to assess needs in older persons. The CANE, derived from the Camberwell Assessment of Need (CAN) [10], is a semi-structured interview that covers 24 areas of environmental, physical, psychological, and social needs. For each area, needs are rated as either non-existent, existing but met, or existing and unmet. Interviews with the patient, a staff member and – if available – an informal carer each yield specific need profiles that can be compared with each other.

Studies of needs in older individuals with schizophrenia

Only a few studies have specifically investigated the care needs of older schizophrenia patients. McNulty and colleagues studied 58 patients (mean age, 75 years) in a catchment area in Scotland (UK), with 64% of the participants living in the community [11]. Needs were evaluated with the Cardinal Needs Schedule, which applied a somewhat different assessment from the subsequently introduced CANE. The reported high levels of unmet needs in many patients raised concerns about the standards of care for this group. However, the study was performed in a notably underserviced and socioeconomically deprived area, questioning the generalizability of findings. A North American study by Auslander and Jeste used a consumer-based questionnaire, examining the priority assigned to various needs in a convenience sample of 72 stable outpatients (mean age, 55 years) with schizophrenia and related disorders [12]. Participants assigned the highest priority to improvement of physical health and memory, while several needs related to social functioning were also highly valued. Whether needs were met or unmet was not assessed. An Australian study of a convenience sample of 97 patients (mean age, 66 years; 62% diagnosed with schizophrenia), reported that, in contrast to other needs, the majority of social needs (measured with the CANE) were unmet [13]. Key unmet social needs were company, daily activities, and having a close confidant.

Our group documented the needs of 114 older schizophrenia patients in a well-serviced psychiatric catchment area in Amsterdam, the Netherlands [14], applying the CANE. On average, patients (mean age, 69 years) reported a total of 7.6 needs, slightly lower than the 8.6 needs reported by their staff members. Both patients and staff rated approximately one in five needs as unmet. Patients and staff showed consensus on the presence of most needs, although some discrepancies existed in individual need areas. Needs within the psychological and social domains were unmet notably more often than environmental and physical needs, according to both the patients and the staff. The total number of unmet needs correlated with several patient variables, with the strongest association found for self-reported quality of life, accounting for 36% of the variance in unmet needs.

Clearly, it is impossible to draw firm conclusions from the limited evidence on care needs in older schizophrenia patients. Nevertheless, a pattern emerges that resembles the more extensive findings in younger populations, in which – provided that socioeconomic conditions guarantee that needs in more basic areas (e.g., accommodation, income) are satisfied – the most relevant unmet needs are to be found in social and psychological domains. In younger populations it has been demonstrated that needs in these domains show a tendency to persist over time, more than other needs [15].

One can question to what extent these findings on unmet needs are unique for schizophrenia. For example, in a study of elderly Dutch depressed outpatients, psychological distress, daytime activities, and company were among the most frequently reported unmet needs [16]. Psychological and social unmet needs have also been reported with considerable frequency among community-dwelling older individuals with dementia [17], older patients in primary care [18] and older people living in sheltered housing [19]. All in all, older people with schizophrenia may not be that exceptional in their frequent reports of unmet psychological and social needs. Most likely, these needs are also connected with aging in general and with the limited formal support provided for these types of need.

Need domains

Delineating a specific area of need inevitably is an artificial and arbitrary process. The same holds true for categorizing the various needs areas into readily distinguishable domains. For example, the need for accommodation covers both basic requirements (having a roof above one's head) as well as social prerequisites (being able to easily encounter other people). Next, needs do not stand alone but interact with each other. Lack of income may impede access to transportation facilities, which hinders meeting others, and so forth. Keeping in mind this interrelatedness, it is still helpful to discern domains of needs that share a similar character.

Environmental needs

This refers to basic needs such as income, food and housing. Clearly, in countries with low socioeconomic standards of living these needs will be unmet more often and will be more difficult to fulfill. In addition, this may also apply to countries with more unequal distribution of wealth. In younger schizophrenia patients, a large European study found more unmet needs in large urban areas, where poverty, unemployment, and related problems were more severe [20]. As many individuals with severe mental illnesses due to limited financial resources depend on social security systems, lack or incomplete coverage of these systems may put them in jeopardy. Next, even when support systems are available, schizophrenia patients may experience difficulty in accessing them. Lack of information, fear of contact in general, or paranoia against institutions are amongst the many reasons that may affect their entitlement to these services.

Appropriate housing and accommodation is often challenging to obtain for older persons with schizophrenia. In contrast to earlier times, nowadays a large majority lives in the community (see Chapter 2). While this in itself may be seen as a positive development, it is important to realize that adequate support to continue living independently in later life is often needed. Just like older people in general, patients with schizophrenia often require support with tasks related to physical care, household, or management of their finances. Apart from obstacles to accessing the appropriate facilities, staff providing for these type of needs can experience difficulty in relating to the specific habits or peculiarities that patients sometimes show. Consultation and advice provided by mental health services is often facilitating in this respect. The same holds true once again for patients living in residential or nursing homes.

Physical needs

With aging, physical needs become more prominent in the care of patients with schizophrenia. The accelerated aging process that takes place in schizophrenia implies that the biological age of many patients is largely ahead of their actual age. Genetic, disease-specific, lifestyle, and treatment-related factors account for this phenomenon (see

Chapters 7 and 9). Other potentially contributing factors are chronic elevation of stress levels, limitations in access to general health care, or inadequate coordination of care. The most common cause of death in patients with schizophrenia is cardiovascular disease. Guidelines have been developed to implement screening, monitoring, and prevention of cardiometabolic risk factors [21]. However, guidelines are often not or only partially followed in clinical practice. In addition to major medical disorders, sensory deficits, reduced mobility, and urinary incontinence are other examples of conditions with relevance for a patient's well-being and ability to function independently.

Older adults with schizophrenia are at risk for undetected or inadequately treated medical disorders. Both individual and systemic factors are responsible for this. Symptoms of the disorder can contribute to diminished access to health care. For example, one study showed that higher rates of positive symptoms were associated with inadequate treatment of four common medical disorders [22]. Next, there are also strong indications that schizophrenia patients often do not receive the amount of care that corresponds to their clinical need. For example, a large register-based Finnish study [23] that documented morbidity, mortality, and quality of medical care over three decades, found that patients with schizophrenia had an increased risk of hospitalization for and markedly increased mortality from coronary heart disease. However, patients with schizophrenia received less lipid-lowering and blood pressure medication compared to their age-peers. These associations were not age-specific, implying that both younger and older patients were exposed to these risks. This study was not able to clarify underlying factors for these disparities, but it is conceivable that negative countertransference in treating staff may partially explain this under-treatment.

Psychological needs

In spite of the tendency of positive psychotic symptoms to attenuate somewhat with aging, at least half of all older individuals with schizophrenia do not reach persistent symptomatic remission [24,25] and continue to live with the burden of – for example – intrusive voices or frightening delusions. Nevertheless, in the course of their disease process many patients find ways to cope with their symptoms [26]. At the same time, one should realize that the present generation of older patients has not had the opportunity to profit from skill training (e.g., [27]) that nowadays is available to younger persons who develop schizophrenia. The same holds true for information about their disorder. Informing people about their diagnosis and its consequences was an exception to the rule at the time that most now older individuals with schizophrenia fell ill. Interestingly, in our study on needs, 11% of the participants reported an unmet need concerning information on their illness, while none of the staff members did so [14].

As psychotic symptoms by their nature are not easily overlooked, this doesn't hold true for a range of psychiatric comorbidities that co-occur frequently with schizophrenia. Depressive disorders, anxiety disorders, posttraumatic stress disorders, and substance abuse rank high in this respect. Many older patients tend not to draw attention to lowered mood, while staff or family too often interpret mood-related symptoms as a natural phenomenon of old age. In the same realm, anxiety- or phobia-related symptoms in patients that live socially withdrawn or actively avoid social contact may too readily be understood as being primarily psychosis-related. Furthermore, it is now recognized that many schizophrenia patients have gone through traumatic experiences, in their youth as well as in the course of their disease [28]. No specific studies on the prevalence of posttraumatic stress disorders in older schizophrenia patients have been published. In younger individuals, offering specific therapeutic interventions for posttraumatic symptoms is rapidly becoming part of the therapeutic armory [29]. Once again, very few older patients profit from this recognition, either through the lack of specialized psychotherapists or the stigmatizing idea that in late life such interventions are not worth the effort. Finally, the general finding that substance abuse often goes undetected or underestimated in old age also applies to older schizophrenia patients. This problem will be even greater in individuals reluctant to accept help, or out of sight of mental health services.

Social needs

As reviewed extensively in Chapter 10, the social achievements of older individuals with schizophrenia remain largely below those of older people in general. Essentially, this relates to the social scars that patients bear dating back to earlier stages of their disorder. At crucial stages, many have missed educational and occupational opportunities, as well as chances for intimate relationships and friendships. Their smaller networks and social isolation are sustained by enduring impairments in social skills. As the network size of older schizophrenia patients is smaller compared to that of their healthy age-peers [30], greater strain is put on formal carers to provide support for needs (see Chapter 17). At the same time, levels of social functioning vary markedly from one individual to another. Most importantly, with aging a substantial number of individuals can improve significantly in social functioning and may show more openness to social opportunities than earlier on in their disease course.

Social needs outnumber other types of need in many studies of younger individuals with schizophrenia [3]. A similar finding has been reported in the more limited number of studies in older age. In our study [14], the two most prevalent unmet needs according to patients were company (24%) and daytime activities (16%). Staff rated even higher percentages, both for company (29%) and daytime activities (28%).

Meeting needs

Which type of intervention is required to meet a specific need and by whom this intervention preferably should be delivered obviously varies with the type of need involved. Several chapters in this book deal with interventions directed at specific need areas (e.g., see Chapter 14 on social skills training and cognitive behavioral strategies, and model programs that integrate social integration and health care). Underlying the actual arrangements for meeting needs lies the more fundamental question of if and when meeting needs goes beyond what mental health services can reasonably be expected to provide through their resources alone. This certainly holds true for several basic needs (e.g., providing financial support or appropriate accommodation). But it also pertains to support for more sophisticated needs such as meeting other people and leading a fulfilling life, which directly relate to a justified longing for social inclusion and societal integration. Not only do mental health services run short of adequate means to supply enough help in this respect, but, more importantly, meeting these needs ought to be seen as a task for which society as a whole should take responsibility. Leaving this task exclusively to mental health services is one more example of the stigmatization that is attached to having a severe mental illness.

The clubhouse model of psychosocial rehabilitation started in 1948 at the Fountain House in New York City [31] and is now a well-established facility that is being offered in many Western countries. Funding sources for clubhouses vary along with country and local situation, with contributions from government, mental health, and social services, as well as private funding. The goal of clubhouses is to help members lead vocationally productive and socially satisfying lives. Participants contribute to the operation of the clubhouse by working side-by-side with staff in a rehabilitative environment that is meant to be a catalyst for recovery. Positive effects on quality of life and social relationships have been reported [32]. With its focus on education and work placement as means of societal reintegration, clubhouses are mainly attended by younger adults and older participants are a small minority. Similar facilities for older people with severe mental illnesses are still very scarce.

In contrast to younger adults, recovery in older age is predominantly focused on the here and now. To illustrate what role mental health services can play in the fulfillment of psychological and social needs of older persons with schizophrenia and how they can cooperate with allied social facilities and the local government, we here describe the case of The New Club, a novel Dutch facility that provides a welcome and non-demanding social environment to older individuals with severe mental illnesses (mostly schizophrenia; Box 12.1).

A qualitative study illustrated how the New Club contributes at various levels to the psychological and social needs of its participants [33]. At the individual level, participants may profit from very basic achievements. This is well illustrated by the observation that for some, attending the facility is a positive accomplishment of its own. Next, the feeling expressed by participants that at the facility they can be who they are emerged as a crucial aspect. Related to the exceptional nature of their experiences, many older persons with schizophrenia share the experience of being looked at as odd, laughable, or even threatening. The facility counteracts this stigmatization [34], which often has been internalized by patients. At the social level, the opportunity to engage with others in a welcoming environment emerges as a major benefit. For some participants just being among people suffices, while others develop reciprocal friendships and eventually meet

---

Box 12.1 The New Club

The New Club, founded in 2011, offers activities with the aim to promote self-reliance and social participation, and to contribute to the resilience of its participants. It is situated in a community center in an old and lively neighborhood in Amsterdam (the Netherlands), facilitating exchange with other age groups that take part in activities at the center. The New Club is a collaboration of the local mental health organization (GGZ inGeest) and a welfare service (Combiwel), while the local council supplies funding. A relatively stable pool of around 20 participants attend the New Club, most of whom live independently, although some reside in a sheltered home. When necessary, participants are offered travel arrangements to attend the meetings. The age of participants varies between 60 and 80 years, with a mean around 70 years. Men are slightly overrepresented in comparison to women. The three main components of the New Club are: (1) weekly daytime activities (e.g., fitness, painting, games) combined with lunch; (2) weekly dinner, including cooking and singing; (3) weekly outings (e.g., cinema, hikes, museums). The activities are coordinated and supervised by well-trained activity coordinators who are joined by a number of volunteers. Whenever possible, participants are given the lead in the choice and design of the employed activities. The mental health organization provides an experienced psychiatric nurse who coaches the staff at the facility.

up outside of the facility. Participants may learn from social skills demonstrated by one another, acknowledging that some peers are more skilled or experienced than others. The social interconnectedness of participants is reflected in the sense of community and the self-correcting mechanisms that are visible within the group. The community-based location, avoiding the connection to a mental health institution, once more strengthens the non-stigmatizing character of the facility and lowers the threshold to participation.

Another age-specific characteristic of facilities like the New Club is that for many participants the club is an endpoint instead of a stepping stone to wider societal opportunities. For many participants meeting others at the New Club constitutes their main source of social contact. At the same time, the example of the New Club demonstrates that participants may enlarge their social scope and engage in more societal activities than they did before joining.

Programs such as the New Club can be implemented successfully if a number of organizational requirements are fulfilled. Adequate funding is a *sine qua non*. Funding agencies tend to underestimate the number and quality of staff necessary to ensure a minimum quality of the facility. Appropriate selection and training of staff that familiarizes them with the values and the basic recovery components of the facility are key elements to its success. Next, ongoing consultation by a skilled psychiatric health worker needs to be ensured. Provided these minimum requirements are fulfilled, one should realize that facilities such as the New Club with relatively limited means are able to make a difference for this fragile and under-served group of patients.

A UK-based pilot study [35] offering 16 weekly sessions to older schizophrenia patients (mean age, 63 years) reported similar encouraging results in the social realm. At a group level, participants made improvements in self-esteem and negative symptoms. Feedback interviews suggested that participants valued the social contact provided by the group and made actual changes in their day-to-day lives as a result of attending. Various North American studies reported on psychotherapeutic group interventions in severe mental illnesses in later life [36–38]. Chapters 15 and 16 discuss these studies, among others, extensively. It is very likely that in addition to the specific therapeutic effects of these relatively high-structured interventions, the implicit opportunities for social contact have also added positive value for participants. Of note, the mean age of participants in these studies (55 to 60 years) was significantly lower than that of the population of the New Club. Inspired by the same objectives as these more specialized interventions, facilities such as the New Club can offer a feasible alternative tailored for patients who lack either the mental or physical capacity, or the motivation to engage in more demanding psychotherapeutic interventions.

Individuals unengaged with mental health services

Nearly all scientific information available on needs in schizophrenia relates to patient populations in contact with mental health services. This points to the pitfall of "the clinician's illusion." North American research suggests that possibly 40% or more of all individuals with schizophrenia are not connected to mental health care, although this figure may be more favorable in later life [39,40]. Little is known about the pattern and level of needs in the hidden population of persons who decline help or are overlooked by services.

A Dutch study [41] carried out in patients who were treated by an Assertive Community Treatment (ACT) team that specifically targeted 70 older patients with severe mental illnesses who were difficult to engage with treatment (mean age, 72 years;

53% schizophrenia) found that those who were less motivated for psychiatric treatment had greater unmet care needs than those who were more motivated, and had more problems in social functioning. Less motivated patients had greater unmet care needs with regard to daytime activities, psychotic symptoms, behavioral problems, and addiction. With ACT involvement, the number of patients who were not motivated for treatment decreased sharply over time (71% at baseline vs. 31% at 18 months) [42]. A decrease in unmet needs was associated with improvement in motivation, suggesting that it may be possible to increase motivation for treatment by addressing unmet needs.

Conclusion

In schizophrenia care, the merits of the traditional medical model are many. However, its scope inevitably is restricted due to its focus on disorders, symptoms, and limitations. Mental health services too often have been restricted to routine prescriptions of medication and infrequent follow-up visits, the more so in older age. Recent years have seen a widening of the scope to prioritize the specific wants and desires of each individual living with schizophrenia. A needs-directed approach that prioritizes patient preferences may enrich the orientation of mental health services. Psychological and social needs have emerged as highly prevalent and frequently being unmet. Mental health services clearly have a role in meeting these needs. Interventions with different scopes and intensities are certainly available. However, the wide science-to-service gap implicates that at present many patients are not being offered this type of help. This holds even more true for older persons with schizophrenia. Next, one should also be aware of the limited extent to which mental health services on their own can contribute in meeting these needs. This implies that in this realm a broader effort is needed on a political and societal level.

References

1. Rosenheck, R., Stroup, S., Keefe, R.S.E., et al. (2005). Measuring outcome priorities and preferences in people with schizophrenia. *British Journal of Psychiatry*, 187, 529–34.

2. Wiersma, D. (2006). Needs of people with severe mental illness. *Acta Psychiatrica Scandinavica Supplementa*, 429, 115–19.

3. Torres-Gonzalez, F., Ibanez-Casas, I., Saldivia, S., et al. (2014). Unmet needs in the management of schizophrenia. *Neuropsychiatric Disease and Treatment*, 10, 97–110.

4. Hansson, L., Sandlund, M., Bengtsson-Tops, A., et al. (2003). The relationship of needs and quality of life in persons with schizophrenia living in the community: a Nordic multi-center study. *Nordic Journal of Psychiatry*, 57, 5–11.

5. Slade, M., Leese, M., Taylor, R., Thornicroft, G. (1999). The association between needs and quality of life in an epidemiologically representative sample of people with psychosis. *Acta Psychiatrica Scandanivica*, 100(2), 149–57.

6. Slade, M., Leese, M., Cahill, S., Thornicroft, G., Kuipers, E. (2005). Patient-rated mental health needs and quality of life improvement. *British Journal of Psychiatry*, 187, 256–61.

7. Priebe, S., Huxley, P., Burns, T. (1999). Who needs needs? *European Psychiatry*, 14, 186–8.

8. Wing, J.K. (1990). Meeting the needs of people with psychiatric disorders. *Social Psychiatry and Psychiatric Epidemiology*, 25(1), 2–8.

9. Reynolds, T., Thornicroft, G., Abas, M., et al. (2000). Camberwell Assessment of Need for the Elderly (CANE): development, validity and reliability. *British Journal of Psychiatry*, 176, 444–52.

10. Phelan, M., Slade, M., Thornicroft, G., et al. (1995). The Camberwell Assessment of Need: the validity and reliability of an instrument to assess the needs of people with severe mental illness. *British Journal of Psychiatry*, 167(5), 589–95.

11. McNulty, S.V., Duncan, L., Semple, M., Jackson, G.A., Pelosi, A.J. (2003). Care needs of elderly people with schizophrenia: assessment of an epidemiologically defined cohort in Scotland. *British Journal of Psychiatry*, 182, 241–7.

12. Auslander, L.A., Jeste, D.V. (2002). Perceptions of problems and needs for service among middle-aged and elderly outpatients with schizophrenia and related psychotic disorders. *Community Mental Health Journal*, 38(5), 391–402.

13. Futeran, S., Draper, B.M. (2012). An examination of the needs of older patients with chronic mental illness in public mental health services. *Aging and Mental Health*, 16(3), 327–34.

14. Meesters, P.D., Comijs, H.C., Dröes, R.-M., et al. (2013). The care needs of elderly patients with schizophrenia spectrum disorders. *American Journal of Geriatric Psychiatry*, 21(2), 129–37.

15. Wiersma, D., van den Brink, R., Wolters, K., et al. (2009). Individual unmet needs for care: are they sensitive as outcome criterion for the effectiveness of mental health services interventions? *Social Psychiatry and Psychiatric Epidemiology*, 44, 317–24.

16. Houtjes, W., van Meijel, B., Deeg, D.J.H., Beekman, A.T.F. (2010). Major depressive disorder in late life: a multifocus perspective on care needs. *Aging and Mental Health*, 14(7), 874–80.

17. van der Roest, H.G., Meiland, F.J., Comijs, H.C., et al. (2009). What do community-dwelling people with dementia need? A survey of those who are known to care and welfare services. *International Psychogeriatrics*, 21(5), 949–65.

18. Walters, K., Iliffe, S., Tai, S.S., Orrell, M. (2000). Assessing needs from patient, carer and professional perspectives: the Camberwell assessment of need for elderly people in primary care. *Age and Ageing*, 29, 505–10.

19. Field, E., Walker, M., Orrell, M. (2004). The needs of older people living in sheltered housing. In *CANE: Camberwell Assessment of Need for the Elderly; A Needs Assessment for Older Mental Health Service Users*, ed. Orrell, M., Hancock, G. London, UK: Gaskell, 35–44.

20. McCrone, P., Leese, M., Thornicroft, G., et al. (2001). A comparison of needs of patients with schizophrenia in five European countries: the EPSILON Study. *Acta Psychiatrica Scandinavica*, 103, 370–9.

21. De Hert, M., Cohen, D., Bobes, J., et al. (2011). Physical illness in patients with severe mental disorders. II. Barriers to care, monitoring and treatment guidelines, plus recommendations at the system and individual level. *World Psychiatry*, 10(2), 138–51.

22. Vahia, I.V., Diwan, S., Bankole, A.O., et al. (2008). Adequacy of medical treatment among older persons with schizophrenia. *Psychiatric Services*, 59(8), 853–9.

23. Lahti, M., Tiihonen, J., Wildgust, H., et al. (2012). Cardiovascular morbidity, mortality and pharmacotherapy in patients with schizophrenia. *Psychological Medicine*, 42(11), 2275–85.

24. Meesters, P.D., Comijs, H.C., de Haan, L., et al. (2011). Symptomatic remission and associated factors in a catchment area based population of older patients with schizophrenia. *Schizophrenia Research*, 126(1–3), 237–44.

25. Cohen, C. I., Iqbal, M. (2014). Longitudinal study of remission among older adults with schizophrenia spectrum disorder. *American Journal of Geriatric Psychiatry*, 22(5), 450–8.

26. Cohen, C.I., Hassamal, S.K., Begum, N. (2011). General coping strategies and their impact on quality of life in older adults with schizophrenia. *Schizophrenia Research*, 127(1–3), 223–8.

27. Liberman, R.P., Wallace, C.J., Blackwell, G., et al. (1998). Skills training versus psychosocial occupational therapy for

persons with persistent schizophrenia. *American Journal of Psychiatry*, 155, 1087–91.

28. Achim, A.M., Maziade, M., Raymond, É., et al. (2011). How prevalent are anxiety disorders in schizophrenia? A meta-analysis and critical review on a significant association. *Schizophrenia Bulletin*, 37(4), 811–21.

29. van den Berg, D. (2015). Prolonged exposure vs eye movement desensitization and reprocessing vs waiting list for posttraumatic stress disorder in patients with a psychotic disorder: a randomized clinical trial. *JAMA Psychiatry*, 72, 259–67.

30. Meesters, P.D., Stek, M.L., Comijs, H.C., et al. (2010). Social functioning among older community-dwelling patients with schizophrenia: a review. *American Journal of Geriatric Psychiatry*, 18(10), 862–78.

31. Beard, J., Propst, R., Mulamud, T. (1982). The Fountain House model of psychiatric rehabilitation. *Psychosocial Rehabilitation Journal*, 5(1), 47–53.

32. Warner, R., Huxley, P., Berg, T. (1999). An evaluation of the impact of clubhouse membership on quality of life and treatment utilization. *International Journal of Social Psychiatry*, 45(4), 310–20.

33. Meesters, P.D., van der Ham, L., Dominicus, M., Stek, M.L., Abma, T. (2018). Promoting personal and social recovery in older persons with schizophrenia: the case of the New Club, a novel Dutch facility offering social contact and activities. Submitted.

34. Depla, M.F.I., de Graaf, R., van Weeghel, J., Heeren, T.J. (2005). The role of stigma in the quality of life of older adults with severe mental illness. *International Journal of Geriatric Psychiatry*, 20, 146–53.

35. Berry, K., Purandare, N., Drake, R., et al. (2013). A mixed-methods evaluation of a pilot psychosocial intervention group for older people with schizophrenia. *Behavioural and Cognitive Psychotherapy*, 42(2), 199–210.

36. Granholm, E., Holden, J., Link, P.C., McQuaid, J.R., Jeste, D.V. (2013). Randomized controlled trial of cognitive behavioral social skills training for older consumers with schizophrenia: defeatist performance attitudes and functional outcome. *American Journal of Geriatric Psychiatry*, 21(3), 251–62.

37. Patterson, T.L., Mausbach, B.T., McKibbin, C., et al. (2006). Functional adaptation skills training (FAST): a randomized trial of a psychosocial intervention for middle-aged and older patients with chronic psychotic disorders. *Schizophrenia Research*, 86(1–3), 291–9.

38. Mueser, K.T., Bartels, S.J., Santos, M., Pratt, S.I., Riera, E.G. (2012). Integrated illness management and recovery: a program for integrating physical and psychiatric illness self-management in older persons with severe mental illness. *American Journal of Psychiatric Rehabilitation*, 15, 131–56.

39. Kreyenbuhl, J., Nossel, I.R., Dixon, L.B. (2009). Disengagement from mental health treatment among individuals with schizophrenia and strategies for facilitating connections to care: a review of the literature. *Schizophrenia Bulletin*, 35(4), 696–703.

40. Mojtabai, R., Fochtmann, L., Chang, S.-W., et al. (2009). Unmet need for mental health care in schizophrenia: an overview of literature and new data from a first-admission study. *Schizophrenia Bulletin*, 35(4), 679–95.

41. Stobbe, J., Wiersma, A.I., Kok, R.M., et al. (2013). Lack of motivation for treatment associated with greater care needs and psychosocial problems. *Aging and Mental Health*, 17(8), 1052–8.

42. Stobbe, J., Wiersma, A.I., Kok, R.M., et al. (2014). Decrease in unmet needs contributes to improved motivation for treatment in elderly patients with severe mental illness. *Social Psychiatry and Psychiatric Epidemiology*, 50(1), 125–32.

Chapter 13

Treatment of Schizophrenia and Psychoses in Older Adults: Psychopharmacological Approaches

Subramoniam Madhusoodanan, M.D.
and Alisa Coleman, M.D.

Introduction

The psychopharmacological treatment of schizophrenia and psychosis in older adults can be challenging. This is because dosing and selection of the appropriate medication are governed by a combination of age-related pharmacokinetic and pharmacodynamic changes, medical comorbidities, concurrent use of medications that increases the potential for drug–drug and drug–disease interactions, and psychosocial factors. Moreover, the treatment of psychosis associated with dementia in the elderly is complicated by the lack of approved pharmacological agents and the potential for serious adverse effects, such as increased mortality and morbidity. The aim of this chapter is to review these issues with respect to the treatment of schizophrenia and non-affective psychosis.

Psychosis in the elderly and neuropsychiatric syndromes

Psychotic symptoms in the elderly may be caused by either primary or secondary psychotic disorders. Primary psychotic disorders include schizophrenia, schizoaffective disorder, schizophreniform disorder, brief psychotic disorder, delusional disorder, or a mood disorder with psychotic features. Secondary psychotic disorders include dementia and delirium. These disorders are described in detail in Chapter 3 of this volume.

Antipsychotics as first-line treatment

Antipsychotic medications are the first line of treatment for psychotic disorders in all age groups, but it is important to consider that many drug trials have excluded geriatric patients [1]. Antipsychotics have been approved for use in adults, although there are no drugs specifically approved for older adults. Antipsychotics generally act through dopamine blockade in the brain. These drugs target the positive and negative symptoms of schizophrenia, and associated agitation. Antipsychotics are thought to ameliorate the positive symptoms of schizophrenia by binding to postsynaptic dopamine D2 receptors in the mesolimbic dopamine tracts of the brain. Their action on the tuberoinfundibular and nigrostriatal dopamine tracts leads to hyperprolactinemia and drug-induced movement disorders, respectively [2]. In young adults, a clinical response to antipsychotics is seen at blockade of 65–80% of striatal dopamine D2/D3 receptors, with extra-pyramidal symptoms (EPS) becoming evident when blockade is more than 80% [3]. In older adults, however, studies have shown that a clinical response may be seen at dopamine blockade as low as 50–60% [4]. In addition, EPS are more likely to occur at lower receptor occupancy in older adults. EPS become evident at as low as 60% dopamine blockade in older adults, compared to 80% in younger adults [4]. Imaging studies have shown that striatal D2/D3 receptor availability decreases with age [5].

The first available antipsychotics, or first-generation antipsychotics (FGAs), are considered to be as effective as the newer, or second-generation antipsychotics. The exception is clozapine, which may be more effective than other agents and is generally reserved for use in treatment-resistant individuals, although as described below, this has not been demonstrated conclusively in older adults. One of the largest and best designed studies of the use of antipsychotic agents in schizophrenia, the Clinical Antipsychotic Trials of Intervention Effectiveness (CATIE) study, compared several second-generation antipsychotics to a first-generation antipsychotic for the treatment of schizophrenia over the course of 18 months [6]. Included in the study were the second-generation antipsychotics olanzapine, quetiapine, risperidone, and ziprasidone, which were compared to the first-generation antipsychotic perphenazine. All the antipsychotics agents were found to have comparable efficacy, with olanzapine being only slightly more effective but with an increased cardiovascular risk [6]. However, the mean age of CATIE study participants was 40.3 years, and individuals over age 65 were excluded from the study [6,7]. It is important to consider that some individuals may have no or poor response to these medications, and in others the drugs may take months before an adequate clinical response is seen. A large meta-analysis by Leucht and colleagues [8] of the short-term effects of first- and second-generation antipsychotic medications in a broad age range of patients found that there were substantial differences in side effects and small, possibly meaningful, differences in efficacy. The findings suggested selecting (or conversely, avoiding) medications based on their potential for certain adverse effects.

Antipsychotic drugs

Like in younger persons, antipsychotics are prescribed as first-line drugs for the treatment of psychotic symptoms of any etiology. As seen in Table 13.1, there have been few controlled studies of antipsychotic agents in older adults and there are little data concerning late-onset schizophrenia, especially very late-onset schizophrenia-like psychosis that develops after age 60. Based on a limited number of comparison studies, there appears to be no appreciable differences in the efficacy of the either first- or second-generation drugs in treating psychotic symptoms in older adults, including clozapine. However, consistent with Leucht and coauthor's study [8], their side effect profiles and metabolism may be relevant to selecting a medication, especially because of the elderly's comorbid physical conditions and use of multiple medications. As a practical matter, most geriatric psychiatrists rarely use FGAs [9].

In summarizing the findings described in Table 13.1, it was surprising to see that trials with first-generation medications were mostly negative to mixed in older adults. Haloperidol did not improve positive symptoms in two small studies; however, in a larger comparison study with risperidone, not only did both drugs improve psychotic symptoms, but haloperidol outperformed risperidone. In several other small studies, fluphenazine decanoate improved negative symptoms and suspiciousness, but failed to improve

Table 13.1 Selected studies of antipsychotic drugs in elderly patients with schizophrenia and other psychoses

Study drug and reference	Total no. of subjects	Mean age in years (range)	Mean daily dose in mg (range)	Efficacy	Tolerability	Conclusion
Chlorpromazine (as comparison drug)						
Howanitz et al. [10] Double-blind comparison study	42 (18 chlorpromazine) S-42	68.5	600 mg/day chlorpromazine	Chlorpromazine and clozapine are equally effective	Both agents had similar incidence of side effects: hematological, hypotension, sialorrhea	Both agents are effective in the treatment of psychosis in the elderly, both are fairly well tolerated with careful monitoring and titration
Fluphenazine (decanoate)						
Altamura et al. [11] Prospective study	20 S-20	63 ± 0.81	12.5 IM Q21 days	Effective in improving negative symptoms and paranoia, but not positive symptoms	Most side effects – EPS – occurred within two days following administration and decreased after fifth injection	Fluphenazine was effective in treating symptoms such as emotional withdrawal, blunted affect, suspiciousness, thought disturbances, but not hallucinations
Haloperidol						
Weisbard et al. [12] Prospective study	19 S-19	67.5 ± 6.4	Unavailable	Haloperidol dose was negatively associated with improvement in positive symptoms	Unavailable	May indicate that elderly patients with schizophrenia do not respond in the same way as younger patients
Thiothixene						
Mohler [13] Prospective study	11 S-11	69.9 (60–76)	(2–105)	No improvement in behavior or delusions. Patients would not cooperate for BPRS	Pneumonia 2, tremor 2, confusion 1, seizure 1, akathisia 1, pigmented lenticular deposits 1	No permanent significant or meaningful change in any of the usual categories of psychotic symptomatology
Loxapine						
Branchey et al. [14] Prospective study	26 S-14 D-12	77.7	(20–150)	Moderate degree of improvement	Sedation, confusion, constipation, EPS, five patients discontinued due to adverse effects	Therapeutic effect similar to that of other neuroleptic drugs in elderly patients with chronic psychosis or with psychosis and organic brain syndrome

Table 13.1 (cont.)

Study drug and reference	Total no. of subjects	Mean age in years (range)	Mean daily dose in mg (range)	Efficacy	Tolerability	Conclusion
Clozapine						
Oberholzer et al. [15] Retrospective study	18 S-2 D-15 O-1	(59–95)	53.2 (12.5–200)	Improvement in NOSIE and SCAG scales	Four patients discontinued due to adverse effects or inefficiency	A low-dose administration of clozapine is an acceptable treatment in geriatric patients with psychosis
O'Connor et al. [16] Retrospective review	75 S-71 B-1 D-2 O-1	74.2 (65–89)	296 (25–800)	Unavailable	Leukopenia 3, constipation, 37 patients discontinued, including 14 due to death and 12 to adverse events	Slow titration is required to minimize adverse events and strict monitoring procedures to prevent hematological complications
Pitner et al. [17] Case studies	4 S-2 O-2	74 (68–83)	26.6 (12.5–400)	Two of four patients (one with schizophrenia) had improved psychosis	All had adverse effects including bradycardia, falls, and delirium	May be used for patients with treatment resistant illness Adverse effects may occur especially on first dose
Pridan et al. [18] Retrospective analysis	43 S-43	69.4 ± 8.7 (>60)	264 ± 110 (25–700)	Re-hospitalization rates were significantly lower on clozapine	Well tolerated, mortality rate was equal to other first- and second-generation antipsychotics	Clozapine appears to be effective and safe for the treatment of elderly schizophrenia patients
Sajatovic et al. [19] Open-label	329 S-267 O-45	59 (55–64) 71 (65–86)	310 ± 223 (12.5–900)	Overall improvement; positive symptom >negative symptom improvement, reduction in aggression	Agranulocytosis 2 (1.9%) Discontinuation rate slightly higher than that for younger adults	Patients 55–64 years old may have better response than those of 65 years or older
Chengappa et al. [20] Retrospective chart review	12 S-11 B-1	69 (61–81)	150 (25–300)	Two of twelve patients had significant improvement in psychosis, five of twelve patients had moderate improvement	Hypotension 7, non-fatal agranulocytosis 1, one patient death due to unrelated causes	Low dose and slow titration suggested
Frankenberg et al. [21] Retrospective chart review	8 S-3 O-5	72 (68–80)	135 (12.5–400)	Six of eight patients had improved psychotic symptoms. All three schizophrenic patients had marked or moderate response	Orthostasis 2, hypotension 1, confusion 1, sedation 2, two patients discontinued due to side effects	Improvement in psychosis A variety of side effects can limit use

(cont.)

Table 13.1 (cont.)

Study drug and reference	Total no. of subjects	Mean age in years (range)	Mean daily dose in mg (range)	Efficacy	Tolerability	Conclusion
Salzman et al. [22] Retrospective chart review	20 S-13 B-1 D-1 O-5	72 (65–84)	208 (75–350)	All patients had significant behavioral improvement with moderate reduction in psychotic symptoms; 11 patients with schizophrenia showed improvement, although 2 did not	Seizure 1, leukopenia 3, sedation 12, two patients discontinued due to respiratory symptoms	Clozapine possibly useful in controlling disruption in older patients, may be greater risk of leukopenia
Sajatovic et al. [23] Open-label	10 S-9 B-1	70.6	204	Seven of ten patients had clinical improvement	Two patients discontinued due to adverse events (atrial fibrillation, systemic lupus erythematosus)	Clozapine is a useful treatment option Inability to tolerate adverse events or weekly blood drawing can limit use
Clozapine as comparison drug						
Howanitz et al. [10] 12-week, double-blind comparison study	42 (24 clozapine) S-42	65	300	Chlorpromazine and clozapine are equally effective	Both agents had similar incidence of side effects – hematological, hypotension, sialorrhea	Both agents are effective in the treatment of psychosis in the elderly, both are fairly well tolerated with careful monitoring and titration
Risperidone						
Madhusoodanan et al. [24] Prospective, multicenter, open-label	103 S-103	71	2.4	50% clinically improved	Dizziness 23, insomnia 17, agitation/somnolence 15, EPS 10, postural hypotension 5	Risperidone was well tolerated and efficacious in elderly patients with schizophrenia or schizoaffective disorder
Madhusoodanan et al. [25] Retrospective chart review	151 (114 Risperidone) S-90 O-24	71	3	78% responded; very much improved in 24%, much improved in 54%	EPS 4, tremor 4, sedation 3, diarrhea 2, chest pain 1, anxiety-restlessness 1, itching 1, insomnia 1, fall 1	Risperidone efficacious and well tolerated in elderly patients with comorbid medical conditions (89% receiving concurrent medications)
Madhusoodanan et al. [26] Case series	11 S-9 B-2	69 (61–79)	4.9 (0.5–3)	Eight responded, one no response. Marked improvement in nine schizophrenia and schizoaffective patients	Orthostatic hypotension 2, hypotension 4 (severe in 1 at 0.5 mg), somnolence 1, EPS/ TD improved in 4, two patients discontinued due to side effects	Risperidone effective and well tolerated Hypotension possible in patients with heart disease

Table 13.1 (cont.)

Study drug and reference	Total no. of subjects	Mean age in years (range)	Mean daily dose in mg (range)	Efficacy	Tolerability	Conclusion
Davidson et al. [27] Long-term, multicenter, open-label study	180 S-180	72 (54–79)	3.7 (2.6–4.5)	54% clinically improved	Pre-existing EPS decreased, no spontaneous TD, assessed TD 4.3%, EPS 40, insomnia 32, agitation 28, UTI 21, constipation 19, dizziness 18	Continuous symptom improvement Decrease in severity of pre-existing EPS and low incidence of TD
Sajatovic et al. [28] Retrospective study	26 S-20 B-2 O-4	70.4 (65–85)	3.8 (1–8)	Clinical improvement in 85%; moderate/marked improvement in 77%	EPS 4, anxiety/restlessness 2, increased LFTs 1, diaphoresis/tachycardia/hypotension 1, two patients discontinued	Risperidone effective and well tolerated
Berman et al. [29] Open label	10 S-10	71 (66–81)	6	Psychotic symptoms and cognition improved	Restlessness, sialorrhea 1, EPS 0, one patient discontinued due to deterioration	Results warrant larger double-blind trial
Berman et al. [30] Pilot study	6 S-6	72 (65–81)	(4–6)	PANSS improvement Changes in positive symptoms correlated to relative activity and reduction in 99m Tc-HMPAO %uptake	None significant	Risperidone improves psychotic symptoms
Bullock and Libretto [31] Case series	12 S-6 O-6	81.1 (66–99)	Unavailable	Marked improvement in patients with late-life psychosis	Side effects not described	Risperidone efficacious and well tolerated in elderly patients
Kiraly et al. [32] Retrospective study	36 S-2 B-1 O-33	79	1.26 maintenance	Greater treatment response at lower dosage Best response in late-onset delusional disorder	Side effects 34.3%, sedation most common	Better response in older patients Strongest effect on psychotic spectrum disorder
Barak et al. [33] Retrospective study	51 (Risperidone group n = 25) S-51	72.7 (65–88)	2.3 (1.0–5.0)	Statistically significant improvement in PANSS scores in risperidone group	EPS 1, agitation 2, hypotension 1	Risperidone more effective and better tolerated compared with typical antipsychotics
Jeste et al. [34] Open label	10 S-10	(47–79)	3.9 (0.5–8)	Marked improvement in seven, moderate in two, one became worse	Daytime sedation 1 (well tolerated)	Risperidone useful first-line agent in elderly

(cont.)

Table 13.1 (cont.)

Study drug and reference	Total no. of subjects	Mean age in years (range)	Mean daily dose in mg (range)	Efficacy	Tolerability	Conclusion
Jeste et al. [34] Open label	19 S-19	65	(0.25–6.0)	MMSE scores improved significantly (24.2–28.2 after treatment)	Not reported	Possible cognitive-enhancing effect of risperidone
Zarate et al. [35] Retrospective review	122 B-35 D-65 O-22	77.5 (65–95)	1.6 (0.25–8)	Treatment effective in 85% of patients	Orthostasis 12, hypotension 35, EPS 12, cardiac arrest 2	Low doses are effective and well tolerated Caution needed in patients with cardiovascular disease or patients receiving SSRIs or valproate
Risperidone long-acting injectable						
Tadger et al. [36] Retrospective chart review	25 S-25	(>60)	36 IM Q 2 weeks	18 patients improved on CGI-global improvement item scale (60%), patients achieved symptomatic remission	Tolerability was high, six patients discontinued due to insufficient response	LAI may be effective in achieving remission among elderly schizophrenia patients
Lasser et al. [37] Subanalysis of open-label study	57 S-57	70.9 ± 0.7	(25–75) Q 2 weeks	Reduction in PANSS in 49% of patients, 55% improved on the CGI	Insomnia (14%), constipation (12%), and bronchitis (12%), EPS was reduced significantly	Long-acting risperidone appears to be effective and well tolerated in stable elderly patients with schizophrenia or schizoaffective disorder
Risperidone as comparison drug						
Madhusoodanan et al. [38] Retrospective study	114 S-114	71	3 risperidone	78% of patients treated with risperidone improved	Discontinuation rates for both medications were the same, adverse events 18% in risperidone group	Both olanzapine and risperidone are effective in elderly patients
Verma et al. [39] Retrospective study	34 (17 risperidone) S-13 B-7 D-10 O-4	71.44 (65–77)	2.2 (0.5-5) risperidone	Improvement on PANSS scores: total and positive subscale scores ESRS and RSSE scores decreased	Side effects not described	No differences between risperidone and olanzapine Daily cost of risperidone one-third that of olanzapine

Study drug and reference	Total no. of subjects	Mean age in years (range)	Mean daily dose in mg (range)	Efficacy	Tolerability	Conclusion
Jeste et al. [40] Prospective double-blind study	176 S-176	70	2 risperidone	Significant improvement in both groups PANSS and CGI scores decreased	Risperidone and olanzapine did not differ in the incidence of side effects Risperidone patients showed more improvement on ESRS scores	Both medications are safe and effective
Frenchman et al. [41] Retrospective analysis	202 (risperidone n = 105) S-32 D-123 O-47	69.4	(2.8–3.1)	Psychotic symptoms improved	Not specified, no discontinuations	More patients treated with risperidone improved compared with haloperidol and olanzapine
Olanzapine						
Madhusoodanan et al. [42] Retrospective chart review	151 (olanzapine n = 37) S-30 O-7	71 (60–87)	10	75% appear to have responded	16% adverse effects, sedation 11%, EPS 3%, postural hypotension 3%, mean weight gain 0.9 kg, 22% patients discontinued due to poor response and compliance	Safe and effective in geropsychiatric patients with comorbid medical illnesses
Madhusoodanan et al. [43] Prospective open label	11 S-11	75 (60–85)	11 (5–20)	64% showed >20% reduction in PANSS total scores at endpoint; 82.5% improved on CGI scale	Postural hypotension 1, dizziness 2, diarrhea 1, sedation 1, rash 1, mean weight gain 1.5 kg	Safe and effective in elderly patients with schizophrenia/ schizoaffective disorder and comorbid medical illnesses
Barak et al. [44] Prospective study	20 S-20	(60–88)	12.9	Significant improvement in PANSS, GDS, and CGI-S	No significant change in weight, three patients discontinued treatment	Clinically meaningful change in positive and negative psychotic symptoms but not in depressive symptoms
Sajatovic et al. [45] Open label	27 S-27	71 (65–80)	8.5 (2.5–20)	Minimal change in BPRS scores from baseline to endpoint in conventional neuroleptic responders Significant improvement in EPS scales (SAS, AIMS, BAS)	Hypotension, agitation, disorientation, mean weight gain 1 kg, 3 patients discontinued due to adverse effects	Effective and well tolerated in elderly veterans. Significant improvement in EPS

(cont.)

Table 13.1 (cont.)

Study drug and reference	Total no. of subjects	Mean age in years (range)	Mean daily dose in mg (range)	Efficacy	Tolerability	Conclusion
Street et al. [46] Double-blind (post hoc analysis)	59 S-59	69 ± 4 (>65)	12 modal dose (5–20)	Greater numerical improvement in efficacy scales, but not statistically significant	Insomnia 16%, somnolence 14%, accidental injury 11%, mean weight gain 1.3 kg	Excellent efficacy and tolerability profile Mode dose and response rate similar to non-geriatric patients Superior adverse event profile versus haloperidol
Solomons et al. [47] Retrospective review	58 S+O-43 D-15	(60–99)	3.9 (1.25–10)	60.3% rate of improvement	Delirium 7, EPS 5, drowsiness 4	Safe and effective medication in elderly refractory psychosis patients
Olanzapine as comparison drug						
Madhusoodanan et al. [48] Retrospective study	37 S-37	71	10	75% of patients treated with olanzapine improved	Discontinuation rates for both medications were the same, adverse events 15% in olanzapine group	Both olanzapine and risperidone are effective in elderly patients
Jeste et al. [40] Prospective double-blind study	176 S-176	70	2 risperidone	Significant improvement in both groups PANSS and CGI scores decreased	Risperidone and olanzapine did not differ in the incidence of side effects Risperidone patients showed more improvement on ESRS scores	Both medications are safe and effective
Verma et al. [39] Retrospective study	34 (17 olanzapine) S-13 B-7 D-10 O-4	71.44 (65–77)	13.2 (5–20) olanzapine	Improvement on PANSS scores: total and positive subscale scores ESRS and RSSE scores decreased	Side effects not described	No differences between risperidone and olanzapine Daily cost of risperidone one-third that of olanzapine
Quetiapine						
Madhusoodanan et al. [48] Case series	7 S-6 B-1	65 (61–72)	325 (mean discharge dose for responders)	Four patients responded to treatment Positive symptoms decreased in four patients, negative symptoms decreased in three	Transient hypotension (dizziness and sedation) in three, pre-existing EPS diminished in three, new onset mild EPS in one	Appears to be effective in reducing positive and negative symptoms and well tolerated in elderly patients

Study drug and reference	Total no. of subjects	Mean age in years (range)	Mean daily dose in mg (range)	Efficacy	Tolerability	Conclusion
McManus et al. [49] Open label (interim analysis)	151 S-33 B-4 D-106 O-8	77 (62–94)	75 (median total daily dose (25–400))	BPRS total and CGI severity of illness scores showed significant improvement at endpoint	Somnolence 32%, dizziness 14%, postural hypotension 13%, agitation 11%, EPS 6%	Well tolerated Associated with improvement in symptoms
Tariot et al. [50] 52-week analysis	184 S-38 B-5 D-132 O-9	76.1 (>65)	137.5	Significant decrease in BPRS in total and CGI severity of illness scores	Somnolence 31%, dizziness 17%, postural hypotension 15%, EPS 13%	Results provide preliminary information regarding safety and efficacy in elderly patients with psychotic disorder
Yang et al. [51] Open-label naturalistic study	91 S-8 B-6 D-45 O-32	(>65)	276 (50–800)			Efficacious and safe for geriatric patients with psychosis Dosage is within a wide range and is diagnosis-dependent
Ziprasidone						
Barak et al. [52] Prospective study	21 S-21	71.4 ± 1.3	(10–20)	Reduction in BPRS and BARS scores	Urinary retention 1, blurred vision 1, sedation 1	Acceptable safety and efficacy in the management of acute psychotic agitation among elderly patients with schizophrenia
Aripiprazole						
Madhusoodanan et al. [53] Retrospective review	10 S-10	70.3 (62–85)	17.5 (15–20)	Seven patients responded to treatment, one showed partial improvement, two did not improve Of those that improved, mean CGI scores improved from 6 to 2.3	Postural hypotension 4, hypotension 1, sleepiness 1, vomiting 2, diarrhea 2, urinary frequency 1, two discontinued due to poor response and compliance	Aripiprazole treatment was associated with a reduction of both positive and negative symptoms of schizophrenia and schizoaffective disorder May be a safe and effective medication for use in elderly with these diagnoses
Paliperidone						
Madhusoodanan et al. [54] Prospective open-label short-term pilot study	11 S-11	68.27 (>60)	6.91 (3–12)	Significant improvement in PANSS and CGI scales	Postural hypotension 27%, elevated prolactin 100%, one patient discontinued secondary to lack of efficacy	May be effective in controlling acute symptoms of schizophrenia/schizoaffective disorder but caution should be used in patients with cardiovascular disease

(cont.)

Table 13.1 (cont.)

Study drug and reference	Total no. of subjects	Mean age in years (range)	Mean daily dose in mg (range)	Efficacy	Tolerability	Conclusion
Tzimos et al. [55] Double-blind, randomized, placebo-controlled	114 S–114	70	(3–12)	Efficacy measures did not show consistent statistical improvement between treatment groups	Elevated prolactin 50%, serious adverse events 3%, 7% patients discontinued treatment	Well tolerated and may improve symptom severity in elderly patients with schizophrenia
Asenapine						
Barak et al. [56] Open-label	34 O–34	67.2 (>60)	(10–20)	YMRS score decreased with 14% achieving remission, sleep duration increased	Seven patients discontinued treatment because of adverse events, two patient deaths after study completion	Asenapine may reduce acute manic symptoms and achieve remission in the elderly, caution should be used in patients with comorbid medical conditions
Sajatovic et al. [57] 12-week prospective, open-label study	15 B–15	68.6 (>60)	11.2 (5–25)	Unavailable	GI discomfort 33%, restlessness 13%, tremors 13%, cognitive difficulties 13%, sedation 13%, four patients discontinued	May be a treatment consideration for geriatric patients with bipolar disorder who were poor responders to other treatments
Lurasidone						
Sajatovic et al. [58] Post hoc analysis	142 B–142	(>55)	(20–120)	Mean change in MADRS was significantly increased	Minimal effects on metabolic panel Discontinuation rates were similar for lurasidone and placebo	Both monotherapy and adjunctive therapy were safe and well tolerated in older adults with bipolar depression

S: Schizophrenia and schizoaffective disorders, B: Bipolar disorder, MDD: Major depressive disorder with psychotic features, D: Dementia, O: other (including delusional disorder, organic psychosis, Korsakoff's syndrome, delirium, TBI, Parkinson's-related psychosis, functional psychosis, mania, and others)

Adapted from Madhusoodanan et al. Use of atypical antipsychotics in elderly patients with schizophrenia and schizoaffective disorder, *Journal of Advances in Schizophrenia and Brain Research*, 4(4), 2002 with permission from Remedico Publishers.

positive symptoms. Likewise, thiothixene failed to diminish psychotic symptoms. On the other hand, loxapine produced improvement in psychotic symptoms. Finally, when chlorpromazine was compared to clozapine, both agents were equally effective in improving symptoms.

The second generation generally showed more favorable results with larger samples. The most commonly studied drugs were clozapine and risperidone. Clozapine had a mixed picture, with improvements in psychotic symptoms in about half of studies; however, the drug often produced adverse side effects that were sometimes severe. Results with risperidone were generally favorable and the medication was well-tolerated; the long-acting injectable of risperidone was also found to be effective and well-tolerated. In comparison studies, risperidone was found to be equivalent to olanzapine but, as noted above, it was less effective than haloperidol. Based on a few studies, olanzapine and quetiapine yielded favorable results and were well-tolerated, except for excessive sedation with the latter. Finally, in a few small investigations, aripriprazole, paliperidone, and asenapine all showed promising results.

Side effects

Increased susceptibility to various adverse side effects may be the result of the pharmacokinetic and pharmacodynamic alterations associated with aging. Pharmacokinetic changes affect the absorption, distribution, and elimination (metabolism and excretion) of drugs. The most important changes with aging are delayed gastric emptying, decreased levels of plasma proteins, primarily albumin, reduced hepatic and renal blood flow, increased fat content, which is important because antipsychotic drugs are lipophilic, decreased body water, and decreased glomerular filtration rate. An increased volume of distribution causes lipid-soluble drugs to have a more prolonged half-life. Decreased albumin and other proteins, also seen in malnutrition and other medical conditions, lead to an increase in the amount of unbound drug. All these factors affect the distribution of the psychotropic drugs, resulting in higher plasma levels compared to younger adults. Pharmacodynamic changes with aging may result in increased sensitivity to medications due to one or more of the following: decline in the density of receptors, alterations in receptor affinity, postreceptor changes, and age-related impairment of homeostatic mechanisms (e.g., diminished baroreceptor responses).

Table 13.2 summarizes the side effects of the antipsychotic medications as well as their impact on various receptors. There are several key take-away points. Among first-generation antipsychotic agents, the low-potency drugs (e.g., chlorpromazine, thioridazine) have less affinity for and bind more loosely to dopamine receptors, are more anticholinergic, and have varying degrees of antiadrenergic and antihistaminic activity. While there is less potential for acute EPS, there is an increased risk of falls secondary to orthostatic hypotension, as well as anticholinergic side effects, such as cognitive impairment, urinary retention, and constipation. They are also associated with prolonged QT intervals and potential for fatal arrhythmias. The high-potency drugs (e.g., haloperidol, fluphenazine, thiothixene) bind more tightly to dopamine receptors and are more likely to cause hyperprolactinemia and EPS. The occurrence of EPS from first-generation antipsychotics in older individuals is over 60% [59].

The second-generation antipsychotic drugs also bind to dopamine receptors; however, they have greater affinity for 5HT2A receptors [60]. Mesocortical and nigrostriatal

Table 13.2 Summary of side effects and receptor blockades for antipsychotic agents

	1st gen high pot.	1st gen low pot.	Ari	Ase	Clo	Ilo	Lur	Ola	Pal	Que	Ris	Zip
Weight gain	low	med	low	med	high	med	low	high	med	med	med	low
Diabetes	low	low	low	low	med	low	low	high	low	med	med	low
Dyslipidemia	low	medium	low	low	high	low	low	high	low	med	low	low
Sedation	low	high	low	med	high	low	med	med	low	med	low	low
Prolactin elevation	high	med	low	med	low	low	low	low	high	low	high	low
Orthostatic hypotension	low	high	low	low	low	high	low	low	med	med	med	low
Prolonged QT interval	low	med	low	low	low	med	low	low	low	low	low	med
Extrapyramidal symptoms	high	low	low	med	low	low	low	low	high	low	high	low
Anticholinergic effects	low	high	low	low	high	low	low	med	low	med	low	low
D2 blockade	high	high	low	high	low	high	high	med	high	low	high	med
5-HT2 blockade	med	high	med	high	med	high	med	high	high	med	high	med
M1 blockade	low	high	low	low	high	low	low	med	low	low	low	low
α1 blockade	low	high	low	high	low	high	medium	low	medium	low	high	low

Ari: aripiprazole; Ase: asenapine; Clo: clozapine; Ilo: iloperidone; Lur: lurasidone; Ola: olanzapine; Pal: paliperidone; Que: quetiapine; Ris: risperidone; Zip: ziprasidone
Information from: [74,75,76,77] and www.uptodate.com/contents/Image?imageKey=PSYCH%2F82533

5HT2 receptors cause presynaptic inhibition of dopamine release. The blockade of these receptors by the antipsychotic agents allows for increased dopamine in these tracts, which is thought to exert an effect on the negative symptoms of schizophrenia as well as EPS caused by dopamine blockade [60]. Side effects most commonly associated with second-generation antipsychotics include weight gain, sedation, hypotension, hyperprolactinemia, EPS, cardiac effects, sexual dysfunction, and anticholinergic effects. QTc prolongation occurs more frequently with ziprasidone, iloperidone, and possibly quetiapine. QTc prolongation of more than 500 milliseconds (ms) or an increase of 60 ms from baseline puts an individual at increased risk of developing torsades de pointes and possibly fatal cardiac arrhythmias.

Medical conditions and eating habits that affect absorption, and hepatic and renal function must be considered. The bioavailability, metabolism, and clearance of the drugs vary greatly. Asenapine is formulated as a sublingual tablet, as the oral bioavailability of the drug is less than 2% [61]. Both lurasidone and ziprasidone should be given with a meal of at least 350 calories as the bioavailability of the drugs increases two to three times when given with food [62,63]. In contrast, the absorption of the XR formulation of quetiapine is increased by 50% when given with a high-fat meal, which should be avoided [64]. Elderly individuals are much more likely to be on multiple medications, which may lead to dangerous drug–drug interactions. Studies have shown a negative relationship between polypharmacy and clinical outcomes [65]. Individuals in nursing homes may be on as many as 10 different drugs, which increases the probability of a drug–drug interaction to nearly 100% [66]. Polypharmacy also increases the risk of a prescribing cascade, in which new medications are prescribed to manage adverse drug reactions [67]. Drugs most commonly involved in interactions are cardiovascular drugs, antibiotics, sulfonylureas, theophylline, warfarin, and non-steroidal anti-inflammatory drugs (NSAIDs) [68]. A study of older adults residing in nursing homes who were potentially exposed to drug–drug interactions involving antipsychotics showed a 70% increase in risk of death compared to individuals receiving antipsychotics without any exposure to potentially interacting medications [68]. In addition, more than 63% of older adults use herbal supplements, many of which can be implicated in drug–drug interactions [69].

Hepatic function declines with age and may have an adverse effect on drug metabolism [70]. Those drugs that rely on cytochrome P450 (CYP) enzymes for metabolism are most likely to be involved in drug–drug interactions when an inducer or inhibitor of the enzyme is also administered. Most first-generation antipsychotics are metabolized by CYP2D6 of the hepatic P450 enzyme system, while second-generation antipsychotics primarily involve CYP3A4, CYP1A2, and CYP2D6 [71]. Exceptions are paliperidone and ziprasidone. Paliperidone is excreted 80% unchanged in the renal system [72]. Ziprasidone undergoes extensive metabolism, only one-third of which occurs via CYP3A4, with the remainder occurring via aldehyde oxidase enzymes [73]. Both CYP1A2 and CYP3A4 enzymes appear to decline meaningfully with aging, and all enzyme systems are affected by the interactions of various drugs on this metabolism; thus, older people who are typically on multiple medications are at increased risk for experiencing drug–drug interactions on liver metabolism. Induction of CYP1A2 occurs with smoking, and can affect the plasma levels of clozapine, olanzapine, thiothixene, and trifluoperazine. Fluphenazine is metabolized almost exclusively via CYP2D6, and its use with inhibitors is not recommended. Carbamazepine, which is a CYP3A4 inducer, can reduce the levels of aripiprazole and to a lesser extent olanzapine and clozapine.

Table 13.3 Potential drug–drug interactions involving antipsychotics and their implications with respect to older adults

Interacting drugs	Potential complications	Implications in the elderly
CNS depressants, alcohol, tricyclic antidepressants	Increased risk of seizures, sedation, and cardiac effects	Increased risk of falls, cardiac mortality
Benzodiazepines	Increased risk of orthostatic hypotension, syncope, respiratory depression	Increased risk of falls
Levodopa and dopamine agonists	Antagonistic effects	May lead to worsening of psychosis
Carbamazepine, phenytoin	May decrease the plasma level of antipsychotics metabolized by CYP3A4	Lower efficacy if dose is not increased and potential for side effects when dose is increased
Lithium	Increased risk of seizures, movement disorders, confusion	Increased risk of falls, cognitive impairment
Paroxetine, fluoxetine	Increased plasma levels of drugs that are metabolized by CYP2D6	Increased risk of side effects, including EPS
Fluvoxamine	Increased plasma levels of drugs that are metabolized by CYP1A2	Increased risk of side effects, including EPS
QT_c prolonging agents	May have additive effect on QT_c prolongation	Increased risk of cardiac conduction defects, cardiac mortality
Anticholinergic agents	May augment anti-muscarinic receptor effects	Constipation, urinary retention, cognitive impairment, dry mouth, tachycardia, blurred vision, increased intraocular pressure

Note: There are limited data on cariprazine and brexpiprazole

Table 13.2 lists the differences in side effects among the drugs and Table 13.3 describes the adverse effects of some of the more common drug–drug interactions. Older adults are especially at risk for such side effects because of a combination of pharmacodynamic and pharmacokinetics changes, comorbid medical disorders, and their use of multiple medications. The decision to use first- or second-generation antipsychotics is largely influenced by the side effect profile, patient preference, presence of a pre-existing movement disorder or increased susceptibility, and the availability of long-acting formulations. Assuming that all the agents are more or less equally effective in older adults (which is likely, but not proven), clinicians must decide which side effects must be avoided. For example, one would not use an agent that has a high risk of extrapyramidal symptoms in a person with Parkinson's disease or use a drug that is likely to increase serum glucose in a pre-diabetic individual. Alternatively, some side effects may benefit a person, e.g., sedation in person with insomnia or weight gain in a person with diminished appetite.

Serious side effects and safety concerns

Although the focus of this chapter is the treatment of schizophrenia and non-affective psychoses, the findings of a possible increase in all-cause mortality risk in elderly patients with dementia using antipsychotic agents may be instructive [78]. The Beers Criteria published by the American Geriatric Society is a set of guidelines aimed at increasing the safety of prescribed medications in the geriatric population by identifying drugs that may be potentially inappropriate for older adults. The Beers Criteria recommends that all antipsychotic drugs be used with caution and to avoid the use of antipsychotics to treat behavioral problems in older adults with neurocognitive disorders unless all non-pharmacological interventions have failed and the person is an immediate threat to self or others [79]. The FDA issued black box warnings for both first- and second-generation antipsychotics, citing increased risk of mortality in elderly patients with dementia-related psychosis. Importantly, a recent Danish study of individuals aged 70+ years with and without dementia who were naïve to antipsychotics showed an increased rate of major adverse cardiovascular events, as well as non-cardiac mortality, which was highest within the first month after starting the drug for both first- and second-generation antipsychotics [80]. Moreover, sudden death caused by cardiovascular effects has been reported to be more than twice that of age-matched controls, and is usually due to fatal arrhythmias caused by QT prolongation and cardiac conduction effects [81]. However, studies have produced contradictory results on the increased risk of mortality in elderly individuals taking antipsychotic drugs. A 2015 meta-analysis of 17 placebo-controlled randomized controlled trials did not show an increased mortality risk in elderly dementia patients taking typical antipsychotics [82].

Neuroleptic malignant syndrome (NMS), a life-threatening reaction to antipsychotic exposure, occurs in 0.01–0.02% of those taking an antipsychotic [83] and has a mortality rate of about 10% [84]. The elderly may be more vulnerable to the development of NMS because of the higher prevalence of medical comorbidity, organic brain syndrome, dehydration, and malnutrition.

Severe neurological side effects of antipsychotics include movement disorders such as akathisia, acute dystonias, and tardive dyskinesia. Jeste and colleagues reported that the one-year incidence of tardive dyskinesia in elderly individuals treated with first-generation antipsychotics ranged from 22.3% to 36.9%, depending on previous exposure [85]. The prevalence of tardive dyskinesia among individuals who have been on long-term antipsychotic therapy is 24%, and as high as 68% after 25 years of antipsychotic drug exposure [86,87]. There are compelling data that the second-generation antipsychotic agents cause substantially less TD than first-generation drugs, e.g., roughly three times lower after one year, although systematic long-term evidence is lacking. The FDA has recently approved two medications, valbenazine and deutetrabenazine, for the treatment of tardive dyskinesia, although specific studies in older adults are lacking.

DRESS syndrome (drug reaction with eosinophilia and systemic symptoms) has been associated with ziprasidone and hypersensitivity reactions have been reported with asenapine [88,89]. High doses of thioridazine (greater than 800 mg/day) have been associated with retinitis pigmentosa [6].

Dosing of antipsychotic drugs

Due to increased receptor sensitivity and potential for adverse side effects in older persons, starting doses in the elderly should generally be 25% of the normal adult dose, with maintenance doses generally about 30–50% of the normal adult dose [90]. The phrase "start low and go slow" is frequently referenced in geriatric pharmacology. Medications should be titrated slowly and carefully to account for age-related changes and decline in hepatic and renal function to avoid adverse drug effects. The following maximum daily dosage guidelines have been suggested by Khan and coauthors [91], which is updated from an earlier expert consensus by Alexopoulos et al. [92]:

- Risperidone 2–3 mg (starting dose: 0.25–0.5 mg)
- Risperidone Consta 50 mg every two weeks (starting dose: 25–50 mg IM every two weeks)
- Quetiapine 100–200 mg (starting dose: 12.5–25 mg)
- Olanzapine 5–15 mg (starting dose: 1–5 mg)
- Aripiprazole 10–15 mg (starting dose: 2.5–5 mg)
- Clozapine 50–100 mg (starting dose: 6.25 mg)
- Ziprasidone 80–160 mg (starting dose: 20 mg)

Note: limited data are available for other antipsychotic agents in older adults.

Somatic and alternative treatments

Liu and colleagues' extensive review of electroconvulsive therapy (ECT) in OAS identified six prospective studies and one case series; participants were between 49 years and 96 years old [93]. The authors concluded that bilateral ECT appeared effective as an acute and maintenance treatment for older persons with early-onset schizophrenia. ECT was not effective in those with very-late-onset psychosis, possibly due to the high prevalence of comorbid brain pathology.

In postmenopausal women with schizophrenia, two studies of raloxifene were found to diminish general psychopathology and total Positive and Negative Syndrome Scale (PANSS) score (but not positive symptoms) versus placebo [26,27]; negative symptoms improved in one of the studies [27]. A controlled trial of citalopram was effective for treating middle-aged and older schizophrenia adults with subsyndromal depression [28]. Adjunctive treatments with multiple antipsychotics, antidepressants, mood stabilizers, and benzodiazepines are not uncommon; however, neither the safety nor efficacy of these treatments in older adults has been established.

Treatment strategies to maximize compliance

To improve compliance, several antipsychotic medications, both first and second generation, are available as long-acting injectable preparations. Orally dissolving tablets are available for aripiprazole, asenapine, clozapine, olanzapine, and risperidone. Immediate-acting injections are available for haloperidol, fluphenazine, chlorpromazine, aripiprazole, olanzapine, and ziprasidone. Long-acting injections are available for haloperidol, fluphenazine, aripiprazole, olanzapine, paliperidone, and risperidone.

Antipsychotic drugs should be used in conjunction with supportive psychosocial interventions to maximize compliance and response. It has been estimated that fewer than 60% of individuals with schizophrenia are compliant with oral treatment [94]. This may require enlisting the help of a family member or caretaker to help monitor medication use. These strategies are described in Chapter 14.

Possibility of reducing or discontinuing medications

In light of the higher risks for adverse events in older persons, several investigators have proposed that patients who have been stably maintained on antipsychotic medications should be given a trial to gradually taper or discontinue medications [95]. A review by

Suzuki and Uchida [96] identified a subgroup of OAS who need little or no medication, either because symptoms had been stable or it was ineffective. Graff-Guerrero and colleagues' [97] study of older adults with schizophrenia (aged 50 and over) found antipsychotic dose reduction was feasible in patients with stable illness and was accompanied by diminished adverse effects and improved illness severity measures. Importantly, from a clinical standpoint, lower doses may be more feasible, since the therapeutic window of D2/3 receptor occupancy in OAS (50–60%) was lower than reported results for younger patients (65–80%).

Conclusion

The psychopharmacological treatment of psychoses has evolved over the past couple of decades. The availability of newer medications with different receptor affinities and side effect profiles is facilitating the treatment. Elderly persons are vulnerable to medication side effects and toxicity because of age-related biological and psychosocial factors. Treatment of psychosis associated with dementia is complicated by the mortality and morbidity risk. Selection of appropriate medications based on the patient's clinical profile, discussion and documentation of risks, benefits, and alternative treatments with patient and family, use of minimum required dose and gradual dose reductions as needed, and behavioral interventions will assist the physician in achieving an optimal outcome.

References

1. Cho S, Lau SW, Tandon V, et al. Geriatric drug evaluation. *Archives of Internal Medicine*. 2011; 171(10): 937–40.

2. Wecker L, Crespo L, Dunway G. Treatment of psychotic disorders. In *Brody's Human Pharmacology*, ed. L Wecker, DA Taylor, RJ Theobald, Jr. Philadelphia, PA: Elsevier, 2012: 324–31.

3. Uchida H, Suzuki T, Graff-Guerrero A, et al. Therapeutic window for striatal dopamine D2/3 receptor occupancy in older patients with schizophrenia. *American Journal of Geriatric Psychiatry*. 2014; 22(10): 1007–16.

4. Graff-Guerrero A, Rajji TK, Mulsant BH, et al. Evaluation of antipsychotic dose reduction in late-life schizophrenia. *JAMA Psychiatry*. 2015; 72(9): 927.

5. Nakajima S, Caravaggio F, Mamo DC, et al. Dopamine D2/3 receptor availability in the striatum of antipsychotic-free older patients with schizophrenia: a [11C]-raclopride PET study. *Schizophrenia Research*. 2015; 164(1–3): 263–7.

6. Questions and answers about the NIMH Clinical Antipsychotic Trials of Intervention Effectiveness Study (CATIE): Phase 1 results. www.nimh.nih.gov/ funding/clinical-research/practical/catie/ phase1results.shtml (accessed October 2018).

7. Swartz MS, Stroup TS, Mcevoy JP, et al. Special section on implications of CATIE: What CATIE found: results from the schizophrenia trial. *Psychiatric Services*. 2008; 59(5): 500–6.

8. Leucht S, Cipriani A, Spineli L, et al. Comparative efficacy and tolerability of 15 antipsychotic drugs in schizophrenia: a multiple-treatments meta-analysis *Lancet*. 2013; 382(9896): 951–62.

9. Sakauye K. *Geriatric Psychiatry Basics*. New York: WW Norton, 2008.

10. Howanitz E, Pardo M, Smelson DA, et al. The efficacy and safety of clozapine versus chlorpromazine in geriatric schizophrenia. *Journal of Clinical Psychiatry*. 1999; 60(1): 41–4.

11. Altamura AC, Mauri MC, Girardi T, Panetta B. Clinical and toxicological profile of fluphenazine decanoate in elderly chronic schizophrenia. *International Journal of Clinical Pharmacology Research*. 1990; 10(4): 223–8.

12. Weisbard JJ, Pardo M, Pollack S. Symptom change and extrapyramidal side effects during acute haloperidol treatment in chronic geriatric schizophrenics. *Psychopharmacology Bulletin.* 1997; 33(1): 119–22.

13. Mohler G. Clinical trial of thiothixene (Navane) in elderly chronic schizophrenics. *Current Therapeutic Research.* 1970; 12(6): 377–86.

14. Branchey MH, Lee JH, Simpson GM, Elgart B, Vicencio A. Loxapine succinate as a neuroleptic agent: evaluation in two populations of elderly psychiatric patients. *Journal of the American Geriatric Society.* 1978; 26(6): 263–7.

15. Oberholzer AF, Hendriksen C, Monsch AU, Heierli B, Sthelin HB. Safety and effectiveness of low-dose clozapine in psychogeriatric patients: a preliminary study. *International Psychogeriatrics.* 1992; 4(2): 187–95.

16. O'Connor D, Sierakowski C, Chin L, Singh D. The safety and tolerability of clozapine in aged patients: a retrospective clinical file review. *World Journal of Biological Psychiatry.* 2010; 11(6): 788–91.

17. Pitner JK, Mintzer JE, Pennypacker LC, Jackson CW. Efficacy and adverse effects of clozapine in four elderly psychotic patients. *Journal of Clinical Psychiatry.* 1995; 56(5): 180–5.

18. Pridan S, Swartz M, Baruch Y, et al. Effectiveness and safety of clozapine in elderly patients with chronic resistant schizophrenia. *International Psychogeriatrics.* 2015; 27(1): 131–4.

19. Sajatovic M, Ramirez LF, Garver D, et al. Clozapine therapy for older veterans. *Psychiatric Services.* 1998; 49(3): 340–4.

20. Chengappa KN, Baker RW, Kreinbrook SB, Adair D. Clozapine use in female geriatric patients with psychoses. *Journal of Geriatric Psychiatry and Neurology.* 1995; 8(1): 12–15.

21. Frankenburg F, Kalunian D. Clozapine in the elderly. *Journal of Geriatric Psychiatry and Neurology.* 1994; 7(2): 129–32.

22. Salzman C, Vaccaro B, Lieff J, Weiner A. Clozapine in older patients with psychosis and behavioral disruption. *American Journal of Geriatric Psychiatry.* 1995; 3(1): 26–33.

23. Sajatovic M, Jaskiw G, Konicki PE, et al. Outcome of clozapine therapy for elderly patients with refractory primary psychosis. *International Journal of Geriatric Psychiatry.* 1997; 12(5): 553–8.

24. Madhusoodanan S, Brecher M, Brenner R, et al. Risperidone in the treatment of elderly patients with psychotic disorders. *American Journal of Geriatric Psychiatry.* 1999; 7(2): 132–8.

25. Madhusoodanan S, Suresh P, Brenner R, Pillai R. Experience with the atypical antipsychotics risperidone and olanzapine in the elderly. *Annals of Clinical Psychiatry.* 1999; 11(3): 113–18.

26. Madhusoodanan S, Brenner R, Araujo L, Abaza A. Efficacy of risperidone treatment for psychoses associated with schizophrenia, schizoaffective disorder, bipolar disorder, or senile dementia in 11 geriatric patients: a case series. *Journal of Clinical Psychiatry.* 1995; 56(11): 514–18.

27. Davidson M, Harvey PD, Vervarcke J, et al. A long-term, multicenter, open-label study of risperidone in elderly patients with psychosis. *International Journal of Geriatric Psychiatry.* 2000; 15(6): 506–14.

28. Sajatovic M, Ramirez LF, Vernon L, et al. Outcome of risperidone therapy in elderly patients with chronic psychosis. *International Journal of Psychiatry in Medicine.* 1996; 26(3): 309–17.

29. Berman I, Merson A, Rachov-Pavlov J, et al. Risperidone in elderly schizophrenic patients: an open-label trial. *American Journal of Geriatric Psychiatry.* 1996; 4(2): 173–9.

30. Berman I, Merson A, Sison C, et al. Regional cerebral blood flow changes associated with risperidone treatment in elderly schizophrenia patients: a pilot study. *Psychopharmacology Bulletin.* 1996; 32(1): 95–100.

31. Bullock R, Libretto S. Risperidone in the treatment of psychoses in the elderly: a case report series. *European Psychiatry.* 2002; 17(2): 96–103.

32. Kiraly SJ, Gibson RE, Ancill RJ, Holliday SG. Risperidone: treatment response in adult and geriatric patients. *International Journal of Psychiatry in Medicine.* 1998; 28(2): 255–63.

33. Barak Y, Shamir E, Weizman R. Would a switch from typical antipsychotics to risperidone be beneficial for elderly schizophrenic patients? A naturalistic, long-term, retrospective, comparative study. *Journal of Clinical Psychopharmacology.* 2002; 22(2): 115–20.

34. Jeste DV, Eastham JH, Lacro JP, et al. Management of late-life psychosis. *Journal of Clinical Psychiatry.* 1996; 57(Suppl 3): 39–45; discussion 49–50.

35. Zarate CA Jr, Baldessarini RJ, Siegel AJ, et al. Risperidone in the elderly: a pharmacoepidemiologic study. *Journal of Clinical Psychiatry.* 1997; 58(7): 311–17.

36. Tadger S, Baruch Y, Barak Y. Symptomatic remission in elderly schizophrenia patients treated with long-acting risperidone. *International Psychogeriatrics.* 2008; 20(6): 1245–50.

37. Lasser RA, Bossie CA, Zhu Y, et al. Efficacy and safety of long-acting risperidone in elderly patients with schizophrenia and schizoaffective disorder. *International Journal of Geriatric Psychiatry.* 2004; 19(9): 898–905.

38. Madhusoodanan S, Brecher M, Brenner R, et al. Risperidone in the treatment of elderly patients with psychotic disorders. *American Journal of Geriatric Psychiatry.* 1999; 7(2): 132–8.

39. Verma S, Orengo C, Kunik M, Hale D, Molinari V. Tolerability and effectiveness of atypical antipsychotics in male geriatric inpatients. *International Journal of Geriatric Psychiatry.* 2001; 16(2): 223–7.

40. Jeste DV, Barak Y, Madhusoodanan S, Grossman F, Gharabawi G. International multisite double-blind trial of the atypical antipsychotics risperidone and olanzapine in 175 elderly patients with chronic schizophrenia. *American Journal of Geriatric Psychiatry.* 2003; 11(6): 638–47.

41. Frenchman I. Risperidone, haloperidol, and olanzapine for the treatment of behavioral disturbances in nursing home patients: a retrospective analysis. *Current Therapeutic Research.* 2000; 61(10): 742–50.

42. Madhusoodanan S, Suresh P, Brenner R, Pillai R. Experience with the atypical antipsychotics risperidone and olanzapine in the elderly. *Annals of Clinical Psychiatry.* 1999; 11(3): 113–18.

43. Madhusoodanan S, Brenner R, Suresh P, et al. Efficacy and tolerability of olanzapine in elderly patients with psychotic disorders: a prospective study. *Annals of Clinical Psychiatry.* 2000; 12(1): 11–18.

44. Barak Y, Shamir E, Mirecki I, Weizman R, Aizenberg D. Switching elderly chronic psychotic patients to olanzapine. *International Journal of Neuropsychopharmacology.* 2004; 7(2): 165–9.

45. Sajatovic M, Perez D, Brescan D, Ramirez LF. Olanzapine therapy in elderly patients with schizophrenia. *Psychopharmacology Bulletin.* 1998; 34(4): 819–23.

46. Street S, Tollefson G, Tohen M, et al. Olanzapine for psychotic conditions in the elderly. *Psychiatric Annals.* 2000; 30(3): 191–6.

47. Solomons K, Geiger O. Olanzapine use in the elderly: a retrospective analysis. *Canadian Journal of Psychiatry.* 2000; 45(2): 151–5.

48. Madhusoodanan S, Brenner R, Alcantra A. Clinical experience with quetiapine in elderly patients with psychotic disorders. *Journal of Geriatric Psychiatry and Neurology.* 2000; 13(1): 28–32.

49. McManus DQ, Arvanitis LA, Kowalcyk BB. Quetiapine, a novel antipsychotic: experience in elderly patients with psychotic disorders. *Journal of Clinical Psychiatry.* 1999; 60(5): 292–8.

50. Tariot PN, Salzman C, Yeung PP, Pultz J, Rak IW. Long-term use of quetiapine in elderly patients with psychotic disorders. *Clinical Therapeutics.* 2000; 22(9): 1068–84.

51. Yang CH, Tsai SJ, Hwang JP. The efficacy and safety of quetiapine for treatment

of geriatric psychosis. *Journal of Psychopharmacology*. 2005; 19(6): 661–6.

52. Barak Y, Mazeh D, Plopski I, Baruch Y. Intramuscular ziprasidone treatment of acute psychotic agitation in elderly patients with schizophrenia. *American Journal of Geriatric Psychiatry*. 2006; 14(7): 629–33.

53. Madhusoodanan S, Brenner R, Gupta S, Reddy H, Bogunovic O. Clinical experience with aripiprazole treatment in ten elderly patients with schizophrenia or schizoaffective disorder: retrospective case studies. *CNS Spectrums*. 2004; 9(11): 862–7.

54. Madhusoodanan S, Brenner R, Serper MR, Adelsky M, Adler DN. Use of paliperidone in elderly patients with schizophrenia and schizoaffective disorder: a prospective open-label short-term pilot study. *Journal of Clinical Psychopharmacology*. 2011; 31(3): 380–2.

55. Tzimos A, Samokhvalov V, Kramer M, et al. Safety and tolerability of oral paliperidone extended-release tablets in elderly patients with schizophrenia: a double-blind, placebo-controlled study with six-month open-label extension. *American Journal of Geriatric Psychiatry*. 2008; 16(1): 31–43.

56. Barak Y, Finkelstein I, Pridan S. The geriatric mania asenapine study (GeMS). *Archives of Gerontology and Geriatrics*. 2016; 64: 111–14.

57. Sajatovic M, Dines P, Fuentes-Casiano E, et al. Asenapine in the treatment of older adults with bipolar disorder. *International Journal of Geriatric Psychiatry*. 2015; 30(7): 710–19.

58. Sajatovic M, Forester BP, Tsai J, et al. Efficacy of lurasidone in adults aged 55 years and older with bipolar depression: post hoc analysis of 2 double-blind, placebo-controlled studies. *Journal of Clinical Psychiatry*. 2016; 77(10): e1324–e1331.

59. Hoffman WF, Ballard L, Turner EH, et al. Three-year follow up of older schizophrenics: extrapyramidal syndromes, psychiatric symptoms, and ventricular brain ratio. *Biological Psychiatry*. 1991; 30(9): 913–26.

60. Brenner GM, Stevens C. Psychotherapeutic drugs. In *Pharmacology*. Philadelphia, PA: Saunders, 2013: 221–37.

61. Balaraman R, Gandhi H. Asenapine, a new sublingual atypical antipsychotic. *Journal of Pharmacology and Pharmacotherapeutics*. 2010; 1(1): 60.

62. Highlights of prescribing information: Latuda. www.accessdata.fda.gov/drugsatfda_docs/label/2017/200603s26s27lbl.pdf (accessed October 2018).

63. Highlights of prescribing information: Geodon. www.labeling.pfizer.com/ShowLabeling.aspx?id=584 (accessed October 2018).

64. Highlights of prescribing information: Seroquel XR. www.accessdata.fda.gov/drugsatfda_docs/label/2009/022047s011s016s017s019s022lbl.pdf (accessed October 2018).

65. Maher RL, Hanlon J, Hajjar ER. Clinical consequences of polypharmacy in elderly. *Expert Opinion on Drug Safety*. 2013; 13(1): 57–65.

66. Gupta S, Masand P, Madhusoodanan S. Side effects of atypical antipsychotics in the geriatric population. *Current Psychosis and Therapeutics Reports*. 2005; 3(1): 26–31.

67. Rochon PA, Gurwitz JH. Optimising drug treatment for elderly people: the prescribing cascade. *British Medical Journal*. 1997; 315(7115): 1096–9.

68. Liperoti R, Sganga F, Landi F, et al. Antipsychotic drug interactions and mortality among nursing home residents with cognitive impairment. *Journal of Clinical Psychiatry*. 2017; 78(1): e76–e82.

69. Qato DM, Wilder J, Schumm LP, Gillet V, Alexander GC. Changes in prescription and over-the-counter medication and dietary supplement use among older adults in the United States, 2005 vs 2011. *JAMA Internal Medicine*. 2016; 176(4): 473.

70. Tan JL, Eastment JG, Poudel A, Hubbard RE. Age-related changes in hepatic function: an update on implications for drug therapy. *Drugs and Aging*. 2015; 32(12): 999–1008.

71. Madhusoodanan S, Velama U, Parmar J, Goia D, Brenner R. A current review of cytochrome P450 interactions of psychotropic drugs. *Annals of Clinical Psychiatry*. 2014; 26(2):120–38.

72. Highlights of prescribing information: Invega. www.invega.com/prescribing-information (accessed October 2018).

73. Beedham C, Miceli JJ, Obach RS. Ziprasidone metabolism, aldehyde oxidase, and clinical implications. *Journal of Clinical Psychopharmacology*. 2003; 23(3): 229–32.

74. Ayano G. First generation antipsychotics: pharmacokinetics, pharmacodynamics, therapeutic effects and side effects: a review. *Research and Reviews: Journal of Chemistry* 2016; 5(3): 53–63.

75. Muench J, Hamer, AM Adverse effects of antipsychotic medications. *American Family Physician*. 2010; 81: 617–22.

76. Mulsant B, Pollack BG. Psychopharmacology. In *American Psychiatric Publishing Textbook of Geriatric Psychiatry*, ed. DC Steffens, DG Blazer, ME Thakur. Washington DC: American Psychiatric Publishing, 2015: 527–88.

77. Kusumi I, Boku S, Takahashi Y. Psychopharmacology of atypical antipsychotic drugs: from the receptor binding profile to neuroprotection and neurogenesis. *Psychiatry and Clinical Neurosciences*. 2015; 69: 243–58.

78. Liperoti R, Onder G, Landi F, et al. All-cause mortality associated with atypical and conventional antipsychotics among nursing home residents with dementia. *Journal of Clinical Psychiatry*. 2009; 70(10): 1340–7.

79. American Geriatrics Society 2015 Beers Criteria Update Expert Panel. American Geriatrics Society 2015 updated Beers criteria for potentially inappropriate medication use in older adults. *Journal of the American Geriatrics Society*. 2015; 63(11): 2227–46.

80. Sahlberg M, Holm E, Gislason GH, et al. Association of selected antipsychotic agents with major adverse cardiovascular events and noncardiovascular mortality in elderly persons. *Journal of the American Heart Association*. 2015; 4(9): e001666.

81. Nielsen J, Graff C, Kanters JK, et al. Assessing QT interval prolongation and its associated risks with antipsychotics. *CNS Drugs*. 2011; 25(6): 473–90.

82. Hulshof TA, Zuidema SU, Ostelo RW, Luijendijk HJ. The mortality risk of conventional antipsychotics in elderly patients: a systematic review and meta-analysis of randomized placebo-controlled trials. *Journal of the American Medical Directors Association*. 2015; 16(10): 817–24.

83. Stübner S, Rustenbeck E, Grohmann R, et al. Severe and uncommon involuntary movement disorders due to psychotropic drugs. *Pharmacopsychiatry*. 2004; 37(Suppl 1): S54–64.

84. Shalev A, Hermesh H, Munitz H. Mortality from neuroleptic malignant syndrome. *Journal of Clinical Psychiatry*. 1989; 50(1): 18–25.

85. Jeste DV, Lacro JP, Palmer B. Incidence of tardive dyskinesia in early stages of low-dose treatment with typical neuroleptics in older patients. *American Journal of Psychiatry*. 1998; 155: 1521–9.

86. Jeste DV, Caligiuri MP. Tardive dyskinesia. *Schizophrenia Bulletin*. 1993; 19(2): 303–15.

87. Glazer WM, Morgenstern H, Doucette JT. Predicting the long-term risk of tardive dyskinesia in outpatients maintained on neuroleptic medications. *Journal of Clinical Psychiatry*. 1993; 54(4): 133–9.

88. Center for Drug Evaluation and Research. Drug Safety and Availability. FDA Drug Safety Communication: FDA reporting mental health drug ziprasidone (Geodon) associated with rare but potentially fatal skin reactions. www.fda.gov/Drugs/DrugSafety/ucm426391.htm

89. Center for Drug Evaluation and Research. Drug Safety and Availability. FDA Drug Safety Communication: Serious allergic reactions reported with the use of Saphris (asenapine maleate). www.fda.gov/Drugs/DrugSafety/ucm270243.htm (accessed October 2018).

90. Sajatovic M, Madhusoodanan S, Brenner R. Schizophrenia in the elderly. *CNS Drugs.* 2000; 13(2): 103–15.

91. Khan AY, Redden W, Ovais M, et al. Current concepts in the diagnosis and treatment of schizophrenia in later life. *Current Geriatric Reports.* 2015; 4(4): 290–300.

92. Alexopoulos GS, Streim J, Carpenter D, et al. Using antipsychotic agents in older patients. *Journal of Clinical Psychiatry* 2004; 65(Suppl 2): 5–99; discussion: 100–2; quiz: 103–4.

93. Liu AY, Rajji TK, Blumberger DM, Daskalakis ZJ, Mulsant BH. Brain stimulation in the treatment of late-life severe mental illness other than unipolar nonpsychotic depression. *American Journal of Geriatric Psychiatry.* 2014; 22(3): 216–40.

94. Valenstein M, Blow FC, Copeland LA, et al. Poor antipsychotic adherence among patients with schizophrenia: medication and patient factors. *Schizophrenia Bulletin.* 2004; 30(2): 255–64.

95. Jeste DV, Maglione JE. Treating older adults with schizophrenia: challenges and opportunities. *Schizophrenia Bulletin.* 2013; 39(5): 966–8.

96. Suzuki T, Uchida H. Successful withdrawal from antipsychotic treatment in elderly male inpatients with schizophrenia: description of four cases and review of the literature. *Psychiatry Research.* 2014; 220(1–2): 152–7.

97. Graff-Guerrero A, Rajji TK, Mulsant BH, et al. Evaluation of antipsychotic dose reduction in late-life schizophrenia: a prospective dopamine D2/3 receptor occupancy study. *JAMA Psychiatry.* 2015; 72(9): 927–34.

Model Programs and Interventions for Older Adults with Schizophrenia

Stephen J. Bartels, M.D., M.S., Peter R. DiMilia, M.P.H., and Heather Leutwyler, R.N., Ph.D., N.P.

Over the next 10–12 years, the proportion of U.S. residents aged 65 and over is projected to increase from 13% in 2010 to greater than 20% by 2030 [1]. This growth in the older adult population is anticipated to include a disproportionately larger growth in the number of older adults with schizophrenia spectrum disorder and other serious mental illnesses [2,3]. The burgeoning population of older adults with schizophrenia spectrum disorder and other serious mental illnesses will overwhelm an already strained mental health care, medical care, and long-term care system in the U.S., in the absence of preventive interventions and reforms in care for this high-risk population. As the number of older adults with serious mental illness expected to dwell in the community increases, it will become imperative to provide effective rehabilitative, self-management, and health promotion programs that address the unique needs of this population.

The growing number of older adults with serious mental illness presents numerous challenges to health care delivery in the United States. According to recent studies, as people with serious mental illness enter their fifth decade of life, they become exceptionally vulnerable to experiencing adverse health events and institutionalization in nursing homes. For instance, adults with serious mental illness between the ages of 50 and 65 are three and a half times more likely to be admitted to nursing homes compared to similarly aged Medicaid beneficiaries with other disabilities or financial challenges. Compared to the general population, people with schizophrenia and other serious mental illnesses experience mortality rates up to four times greater [4] and die upwards of 32 years earlier [5]. The early mortality and institutionalization affecting people with serious mental illnesses reflect a major health disparity in our nation, largely due to greater rates of preventable chronic health conditions. Adults with schizophrenia and other serious mental illness have an average life expectancy of approximately 54 years, with early mortality largely due to cardiovascular disease [6], as well as diabetes and respiratory disorders [7].

It is estimated that as many as 75% of persons with schizophrenia have a co-occurring medical disorder [8]. Medical disorders co-occurring with debilitating mental illness are associated with limitations in independent functioning for community-dwelling older adults. Functional deficits in community living, self-care, and illness self-management skills are strongly associated with placement in restrictive residential settings such as nursing homes [9], despite the majority of older adults with serious mental illness preferring to live in community-based settings [10]. In this chapter, we provide an overview of the research supporting three key approaches to addressing these challenges: psychosocial rehabilitation, illness self-management, and health promotion.

Illness self-management

Older adults with schizophrenia spectrum disorder are disproportionately affected by chronic, co-morbid physical health conditions that contribute to high rates of morbidity and increased risk of early mortality [5,11]. The combined impact of serious mental illness and comorbid physical health conditions challenges conventional approaches to health care delivery, underscoring the need for illness self-management interventions. However, illness self-management programs traditionally address either chronic physical health or mental health conditions, but not both. As mental health disorders may adversely affect outcomes of common medical disorders, conversely, chronic health conditions or acute medical events may worsen mental health symptoms. Hence, improving self-management of both mental and physical health domains is most likely to improve functioning and long-term outcomes for older adults with schizophrenia and co-morbid chronic health conditions. Integrated medical and psychiatric self-management programs focus on a combination of three domains: medical management, role management, and emotional management [12]. A recent systematic review by Whiteman and colleagues identified nine interventions, of which three are discussed within this chapter [13]. Health and Recovery Peer (HARP), Targeted Training in Illness Management (TTIM), and Integrated-Illness Management and Recovery (I-IMR) are programs that integrate techniques of mental illness and physical health self-management. The overall goal of these programs is to impart the skills and knowledge necessary for community-dwelling adults with serious mental illness to continue to function and live in their respective communities. Designed specifically for adults with serious mental illness and co-morbid physical health conditions, these programs hold the greatest promise for improving functional outcomes and for reducing excess morbidity and early mortality.

Health and Recovery Peer: HARP

The Health and Recovery Peer (HARP) program developed by Druss and colleagues consists of an illness self-management intervention adapted from the Chronic Disease Self-Management Program (CDSMP) [14,15]. While CDSMP is aimed at illness self-management programs for people with chronic physical health conditions, the HARP program incorporates self-management into the specific health-related needs of adults with serious mental illness. To facilitate adaptation of CDSMP to persons with serious mental illness, Druss and colleagues followed the ADAPT-ITT method [14,16]. Additionally, peer leaders and an expert panel were consulted in the adaptation process to ensure the HARP program meets the unique needs of patients with serious mental illness and chronic physical health conditions.

In modifying CDSMP for adults with serious mental illness, Druss and colleagues enhanced the model for low health literacy populations such as individuals with serious mental illness by ensuring that written materials were at a sixth-grade reading level, as well as providing a greater emphasis on the relationship between body and mind. In developing the intervention, a method of tracking disease-specific self-management tasks was added to further enhance the HARP program. HARP is designed to be delivered to persons with serious mental illness by certified mental health peer specialists that have received extensive training in both CDSMP and HARP. Over the duration of the HARP program, participants meet with peer specialists in group sessions up to six times. Keeping the core structure of CDSMP intact, the HARP program follows six sessions intended to improve illness self-management among persons with serious mental illness and chronic physical health conditions: (1) an overview of illness self-management, (2) exercise and physical activity, (3) pain and fatigue management, (4) healthy eating with a limited budget, (5) medication management, and (6) finding and working with a consistent physician. Peer specialists further promote health behavior change by encouraging participants to identify negative health behaviors and establish short-term goals to reach potential manageable ways to improve.

The effectiveness of HARP has been evaluated in a randomized controlled pilot study comparing HARP to usual care in a community mental health center [14]. Among a cohort of middle-aged and older adults (mean age 48 years) with serious mental illness (schizophrenia 29%, bipolar disorder 33%) and co-occurring physical health conditions (hypertension 63%, arthritis 50%, heart disease 23%), 41 participants were assigned to the HARP intervention and 39 received usual care. Participants were evaluated by the study investigators in terms of the ability to self-manage illnesses, patient activation, quality of life, physical health, and mental health. After six months, the HARP program participants attended an average of 4.75 out of 6 possible group sessions and reported significantly higher patient activation, indicating greater perceptions of their abilities to manage their own illnesses, and a greater proportion of participants utilizing a primary care provider compared to the usual care group. A subsequent large study randomized 400 participants with a serious mental illness and chronic general medical conditions to either the HARP self-management program led by certified peer specialists or to usual care [17]. At six-month follow-up, participants receiving HARP demonstrated a significant improvement in health-related quality of life in the Short-Form Health Survey physical and mental component subscales and greater improvements in mental health recovery, but no other between-group differences were significant [17]. These studies suggest that adapting CDSMP to respond to the special needs of middle-aged and older adults with serious mental illness and co-morbid physical health conditions holds promise as an effective means of improving outcomes and community tenure for this high-risk population.

Targeted Training in Illness Management: TTIM

Developed by Sajatovic and colleagues, the Targeted Training in Illness Management (TTIM) program is a group-based program for community-dwelling adults with serious mental illness and comorbid diabetes mellitus [18]. The TTIM program incorporates peer educators and illness self-management principles for adults with serious mental illness into the Life Goals Program [19] and the Diabetes Awareness Rehabilitation Training [20] models. TTIM integrates aspects of both mental health and diabetes care with social support from peer educators by blending psychoeducation, problem identification, goal setting, behavioral modeling, and care co-ordination. Intended to be delivered in primary care settings, the TTIM program is co-led by a nurse educator with expertise in diabetes management and a peer specialist with serious mental illness and diabetes in a safety-net primary care system. TTIM is provided in two phases in a program lasting approximately 60 weeks.

In the first phase of TTIM, participants engage in 12 weekly small-group sessions of six to ten participants, a nurse educator, and a peer specialist. These weekly group sessions typically last for 60 to 90 minutes and focus on different physical and mental health topics, health behaviors, and self-management skills. For example, some sessions emphasize medications, nutrition, exercise, and substance use, while others promote problem-solving skills, engaging social support systems, and setting personal goals. After the participants have completed the 12 weekly group sessions, they advance to the second phase of the TTIM program. In the second phase, participants consult with the nurse educator and peer specialist over the telephone for brief maintenance sessions. For the first three months these 10–15-minute telephone sessions occur bi-weekly, then monthly for 48 total weeks of the second phase of the program.

Sajatovic and colleagues conducted a randomized controlled trial of TTIM to determine if participants experience improvements in mental health symptoms, functional status, general health status, and outcomes specific to diabetes [21]. In a safety-net primary care setting, 200 adults (mean age 53 years) with serious mental illness (schizophrenia 25%, major depressive disorder 48%) and diabetes mellitus were randomly assigned to receive treatment as usual or participate in the TTIM program [21]. Study investigators assessed the effectiveness of the TTIM program in terms of serious mental illness symptom severity, functional status, general health status, diabetes control, and diabetes knowledge observed among study participants. Systolic blood pressure and body mass index were also observed during the study. Compared to the treatment-as-usual group, TTIM participants experienced significantly improved psychiatric symptoms and functional status after 60 weeks. TTIM participants displayed a significantly greater knowledge of diabetes compared to the control group. However, there were no differences between TTIM and treatment-as-usual in outcomes of general health status, management of diabetes, systolic blood pressure, or body mass index. Remarkably, over the course of the 60-week intervention, both groups experienced an increase in body mass index compared to baseline. Of the participants that completed the program and responded to the satisfaction survey (84 out of 100), 98% of TTIM participants considered the program to be useful and 92% agreed or strongly agreed that TTIM addressed issues important to them.

A strength of the TTIM program stems from its ability to simultaneously provide instruction in illness self-management of serious mental illness and diabetes as a common co-morbid, chronic physical health condition, while providing strong social support through the integration of peer specialists. Additionally, providing the program in a primary care setting allows health systems to leverage existing resources and provide a more integrated approach to managing mental and physical health conditions.

Integrated Illness Management and Recovery: I-IMR

Integrated Illness Management and Recovery (I-IMR) was developed with the goal of providing older adults with serious mental illness and co-morbid chronic health conditions training in illness self-management and support to effectively self-manage both medical and psychiatric illness. I-IMR provides concurrent training and coaching in both psychiatric and medical illness self-management to minimize symptoms and their disruptive effects on functioning, and to prevent unnecessary use of emergency room visits and acute hospitalizations [22,23]. I-IMR builds on principles from the evidence-based practice of mental illness management and recovery (IMR) [24], and adds the critical element of medical illness self-management training [22]. I-IMR combines medical illness self-management with four evidence-based psychosocial interventions shown to be effective among people with serious mental illness: (1) psychoeducation, which improves knowledge about mental illness management, (2) behavioral tailoring, which improves medication adherence, (3) relapse prevention training, which decreases relapses and rehospitalizations, and (4) coping skills training, which reduces distress related to symptoms. For each psychiatric self-management skill module in the I-IMR program, there is a corresponding medical illness self-management training component. For instance, psychiatric and medical illness self-management modules include: coping with symptoms of mental and physical distress, stress vulnerability, common mental and physical health conditions, social supports, medication adherence, relapse prevention, coping with stress, substance and medication misuse, navigating mental health and medical health care delivery systems, and recovery and wellness. In I-IMR, a specialist guided by modules provides participants with skills training, which is augmented by health care management offered by a registered nurse. In addition to providing skills training, I-IMR specialists meet with participants on a weekly basis over the course of eight months to offer support as participants work toward personalized goals that were established at the beginning of the program [22].

In a pilot study conducted by Bartels and colleagues [23], the feasibility, acceptability, and preliminary effectiveness of I-IMR was evaluated in adults with serious mental illness aged 50 and over (mean age 60.3 ± 6.5 years) randomized to either I-IMR (n = 36) or usual care (n = 35). Among the participants, 38% had schizophrenia spectrum disorder and 44% had major depression, while all suffered from co-occurring chronic medical illnesses (48% diabetes, 47% hyperlipidemia, and 44% hypertension). Compared to usual care, I-IMR was associated with greater psychiatric illness and diabetes self-management skills, suggesting preliminary effectiveness in improving self-management abilities for psychiatric and medical illness. As a result of enhanced illness self-management ability, I-IMR participants demonstrated a significant reduction in hospitalizations compared to usual care, which was sustained at 14-month follow-up. Participants also demonstrated an increased preference for detailed treatment information during encounters with their primary care providers. Three-quarters of I-IMR participants attended ten or more program sessions, indicating the feasibility of I-IMR among older adults with serious mental illness and co-occurring medical illness. In contrast to HARP and TTIM, which primarily focus on medical illness self-management, I-IMR provides a balanced curriculum of both psychiatric and medical self-management specifically for older adults.

Psychosocial rehabilitation

Psychosocial rehabilitation aims to enrich functioning and recovery for persons with serious mental illness through a combination of social, educational, occupational, behavioral, and cognitive interventions [25–27]. Psychosocial rehabilitation programs were initially developed to address the needs of younger adults with serious mental illness. Examples of these programs include assertive community treatment, social skills training, integrated dual diagnosis treatment of mental illness and substance abuse disorder, family psychoeducation, and supported employment. More recently, psychosocial rehabilitation programs for older adults with serious mental illness have emerged, which focus on developing or enhancing independent living skills, improving quality of life, and engaging in meaningful activities in an attempt to increase community tenure.

Three psychosocial rehabilitation programs for middle-aged to older adults with serious mental illness are highlighted in this section: Helping Older People Experience Success (HOPES), Functional Adaptation Skills Training (FAST), and Cognitive-Behavioral Social Skills Training (CBSST). HOPES is a two-year, integrated social rehabilitation and health management program for older adults with serious mental illness [28]. FAST consists of a 24-week social skills training program to improve community functioning for middle-aged and older adults with persistent psychotic disorders [29]. CBSST combines cognitive behavioral treatment and skills training in a program for older adults with schizophrenia [30]. All three of these psychosocial rehabilitation programs are designed to improve independent living skills and quality of life.

Helping Older People Experience Success: HOPES

The Helping Older People Experience Success (HOPES) program combines elements of psychosocial and preventive health care to improve independent functioning and community tenure for older adults with serious mental illness [31]. The social rehabilitation component of HOPES aims to teach older adults with serious mental illness social skills, community living skills, and healthy living. In addition to social rehabilitation, the HOPES program includes an integrated health management component with nurse coordination of preventive health care. The HOPES program is designed to be delivered over a one-year period of intensive skills training, followed by a second year reinforcing skills. The first, intensive year of the HOPES program includes weekly skills classes, twice-monthly community practice trips, and monthly one-on-one meetings with a nurse. The second year of HOPES is considered primarily a maintenance year and the meeting frequencies are reduced to monthly skills classes, community practice trips, and nurse meetings. Principles of social skills training were used to inform HOPES classes, which include modeling, role-playing, positive and corrective feedback, and homework assignments.

The HOPES program weekly skills class curriculum consists of seven modules: Communicating Effectively, Making and Keeping Friends, Making the Most of Leisure Time, Healthy Living, Using Medications Effectively, and Making the Most of a Health Care Visit. Each of the seven modules includes six to eight skills, with one skill taught each week. The weekly HOPES skills training sessions are usually conducted at community mental health centers or local senior citizens centers and are co-led by rehabilitation specialists (one masters- and one bachelors-level clinician). To reinforce skills learned during the weekly training sessions, the community practice trips are intended to involve an outing to a location in which skills related to the module topic could be practiced (e.g., riding the subway or bus to practice using public transportation) and are typically planned by the group leaders in collaboration with group participants. The integrated health management component of HOPES is delivered by a registered nurse (RN) and begins with a medical history and evaluation of health care needs. Working with the RN, participants identify personal techniques for managing chronic medical conditions and obtaining recommended preventive care, and set health-related goals consistent with these techniques.

The effectiveness of HOPES was evaluated by Bartels and colleagues in a randomized controlled trial to determine if the program resulted in long-term improvements in psychosocial functioning, preventive healthcare, and acute service use [32]. A cohort of older adults (mean age of 60 years) with serious mental illness (28% schizophrenia, 28% schizoaffective disorder, 24% depression) were randomized to either participate in HOPES or receive treatment as usual (routine mental health services). To accommodate community-dwelling older adults with mobility issues and limited access to transportation, two skills training sessions were taught in a single day, with a 90-minute morning session and a 60-minute afternoon session separated by a lunch period. The lunch period provided program participants with opportunities for informal socialization among fellow group members and leaders.

To gauge the effectiveness of HOPES, program participants were evaluated on functional skills performance, psychosocial functioning, self-efficacy, severity of negative symptoms, cognitive functioning, depressive symptom severity, and health status. At the end of the two-year program and at three-year follow-up, HOPES program participants compared to those in usual care demonstrated greater improvements in functional skills performance, psychosocial functioning, self-efficacy, and psychiatric symptoms. HOPES participants, compared to those receiving usual care, also demonstrated greater receipt of preventive services, including a greater proportion receiving flu shots, hearing tests, eye exams, visual acuity tests, mammograms, and PAP smears. Further, 100% of HOPES participants received blood pressure screenings and nearly twice as many completed advanced directives compared to control group participants. Though not statistically significant, HOPES participants were associated with fewer psychiatric hospitalizations, medical hospitalizations, or emergency room vists at three-year follow-up. However, no significant differences were observed between HOPES participants and the control group with respect to health status outcomes or social behaviors.

HOPES links skills training and health management, both of which are integral to optimizing independent functioning and health management necessary to maintain community tenure among older adults with schizophrenia spectrum disorder. Of major significance, greater improvement in psychosocial functioning, community living skills, psychiatric symptoms, and preventive health care persisted at three-year follow-up, supporting the long-term effectiveness of HOPES.

Functional Adaptation Skills Training: FAST

Developed by Patterson and colleagues [29], Functional Adaptation Skills Training (FAST) was designed to improve functioning for middle-aged and older adults with schizophrenia spectrum disorder or psychotic mood disorders residing in community-based settings. Based on Social-Cognitive Theory and the Social and Independent Living Skills Program [33], FAST offers group sessions aimed at improving everyday skills: medication management, social skills, communication skills, organization and planning, transportation, and financial management. Each of these six everyday skills is the topic of instruction for four, 120-minute group sessions. These group sessions are co-led by a masters- or doctorate-level therapist and a management or nursing paraprofessional, and occur weekly over the course of 24 weeks.

A standard FAST group session often contains the following components: review of the weekly class agenda, review of the previously assigned homework, discussion of the application of homework exercises to other life domains, introduction to new material or review of the current material (depending on session), in-session skills practice, including behavioral modeling, role-playing, and reinforcement, review of skills learned during the session, assignment and review of homework for the next session. To enhance the value of these sessions for older adult participants with cognitive impairments, the FAST program was designed with integrated repetition, review, and additional skills-building.

A randomized controlled study was conducted by Patterson and colleagues evaluating the effectiveness of the FAST program on the everyday functioning skills of 240 older adults (greater than 40 years old, mean participant age 51 years) with schizophrenia

(80.6%) or schizoaffective disorder (19.4%) residing in 25 board-and-care facilities in San Diego County [34]. Participants randomized to the comparison "Attention Control" condition participated in weekly, 120-minute discussion group sessions for 24 weeks. Results of this study revealed that FAST program participants demonstrated significantly improved functional skills on the UCSD Performance-based Skills Assessment and social and communication skills on the Social Skills Performance Assessment, compared to the control group, after six months. Additionally, FAST program participants were roughly 60% less likely than the control group to use emergency medical services throughout the six-month intervention. However, one-year post-intervention follow-up indicated that emergency service use did not differ between FAST and control participants.

PEDAL

Building on these findings, Patterson and colleagues adapted the FAST psychosocial rehabilitation program for monolingual Spanish speaking, middle-aged and older Latino adults with schizophrenia [35]. Encouraging results were reported from an initial pilot study of the adapted version of the FAST program, Programa de Entrenamiento para el Desarrollo de Aptitudes para Latinos (PEDAL). Construction of the PEDAL program involved cultural tailoring of FAST, including: (1) translating the intervention and assessment materials into Spanish, (2) using bicultural/bilingual group facilitators, (3) including culture specific icons and idioms in the handouts for participants, and (4) altering the format and content based on Mexican cultural values. While results from a larger randomized trial are pending, a preliminary report on PEDAL by Mausbach and colleagues indicated that the program was effective in improving functioning and well-being in middle-aged to older Latinos with persistent psychotic illness [36].

As psychosocial rehabilitation interventions, the strengths of the FAST and PEDAL programs lie in their positive effects on the functional, everyday skills required to improve the community tenure of older adults with schizophrenia spectrum disorder. Additionally, valuable information can be gleaned from evaluations of the PEDAL adaptation of psychosocial rehabilitative approaches for ethnic minority populations.

Cognitive Behavioral Social Skills Training: CBSST

Designed for middle-aged and older adults with schizophrenia, the Cognitive Behavioral Social Skills Training (CBSST) intervention is a group therapy program aimed at helping participants attain personalized goals related to community functioning and self-efficacy. Developed by McQuaid and Granholm, CBSST combines properties of cognitive behavioral therapy (CBT) and social skills training (SST) within the framework of the biopsychosocial stress-vulnerability model of schizophrenia [30]. The CBT components of this model focus on cognitive restructuring and were adapted, based on work by Beck and colleagues [37] and the 1994 book *Cognitive-Behavioral Therapy of Schizophrenia* by Kingdon and colleagues [38], specifically for patients with schizophrenia. Additionally, drawing from SST interventions developed by Liberman and colleagues [39] and from Psychiatric Rehabilitation Consultants [40], CBSST engages self-management, conversation skills, and interpersonal problem-solving techniques to enhance self-efficacy of and improve community tenure for middle-aged and older adults with schizophrenia. Consisting of three modules, each delivered over four weekly sessions, this integrated treatment program is delivered in two-hour group therapy sessions (12 total sessions).

In the first CBSST program module, participants are introduced to "thought-challenging" scenarios, to facilitate identifying "mistakes" or distortions in thinking, along with considering the relationships between thoughts, feelings, and behaviors. In this module, program participants are instructed to recognize and evaluate their own beliefs and "stop and think" before acting. The second module of CBSST aims to improve participants' ability to identify early warning signs of relapse and seek support from appropriate sources when warning signs emerge. Participants engage in role-playing exercises not only to improve communication skills with doctors and other health care professionals, but also to improve social interactions, including expressing positive and negative feelings, assertive sharing in group situations, and everyday leisure activities. The third and final module of CBSST teaches participants skills for coping with the persistent symptoms associated with schizophrenia. Borrowing from the Symptom Management Module, this "solving problems module" of CBSST promotes medication adherence, cognitive, and behavioral strategies for coping with symptoms of mental illness through the "SCALE" acronym: Specify, Consider possible solutions, Assess the best solution, Lay out a plan, and Execute and evaluate the outcome [41]. To reinforce skills learned during the group therapy session, weekly homework exercises are assigned to participants. All group therapy sessions are co-led by two masters- or doctoral-level therapists with clinical CBT experience.

A randomized controlled trial by Granholm and colleagues evaluated the effectiveness of CBSST compared to treatment as usual among a cohort of community-dwelling, middle-aged to older adults (greater than 40 years old, mean participant aged 54 years) with schizophrenia or schizoaffective disorder [41]. Blinded assessors evaluated the effectiveness of CBSST to improve functional outcomes in participants by assessing social functioning, positive and negative symptoms, and cognitive insight. Assessors also evaluated participant performance on a comprehensive module test. While the CBSST program calls for three modules each delivered weekly over a four-week period, Granholm and colleagues explored delivering each module twice, resulting in a 24-week intervention. To attenuate transportation barriers common among older adults with schizophrenia and schizoaffective disorder, participants were provided transportation to the group therapy sessions if requested.

At the end of the six-month intervention, study investigators observed significantly higher engagement in social functioning activities among CBSST participants compared to the treatment-as-usual group. CBSST participants experienced significantly greater cognitive insight and displayed significantly more knowledge of the skills and information taught in the CBSST program. No significant differences between the two study groups were observed among positive or negative symptoms of schizophrenia. The investigators concluded that there was no significant benefit to participants in completing each of the CBSST program modules twice. Rather, the 12-week program may provide adequate exposure to the CBSST program. After a 12-month follow-up, CBSST participants continued to report significantly greater social functioning and comprehension of CBSST skills, but cognitive insight no longer differed significantly from the treatment-as-usual group.

Granholm and colleagues demonstrated that the CBSST approach of blending cognitive restructuring techniques with social skills training within the biopsychosocial stress-vulnerability model of schizophrenia framework is uniquely effective at enhancing social functioning and living skills in middle-aged and older adults with schizophrenia spectrum disorder.

Adaptions to the current models may include further integrating health promotion, health care, and illness self-management interventions into psychosocial rehabilitation interventions in an attempt to address the whole person [9]. Incorporating physical activity programs designed specifically for older adults with schizophrenia [22,23] into programs such as FAST, HOPES, or CBSST could be a way to not only integrate health promotion into social skills training programs, but also provide another venue for acquiring and practicing social skills. Prior research has shown an association between higher levels of physical activity with higher scores on cognitive tests and lower levels of depression [24,25]. Another step towards addressing the needs of the whole person could be achieved through further optimizing social integration and supporting involvement in meaningful activities, such as volunteer work, as well as consistently including these areas as outcome measures in clinical trials. Finally, robust evaluation of programs that have been implemented in routine practice across the country (rural and urban areas) would lend further credibility to these important programs.

Psychosocial rehabilitation models in review

The Functional Adaptation and Skills Training (FAST) program engenders positive effects of the everyday skills necessary for enhanced community tenure among older adults with schizophrenia spectrum disorder. Additionally, the adaptation of FAST for the Latino population provides valuable information for future adaptations of psychosocial rehabilitative approaches for ethnic minority populations. Both the HOPES and CBSST programs demonstrate that blending skills training with either health management (HOPES) or cognitive restructuring (CBSST) optimizes the independent functioning and living skills necessary for the successful community dwelling of older adults with serious mental illness.

Overall, the programs yielded improvement in functional skills (HOPES, FAST), social skills (HOPES, CBSST), engagement in social, recreation and leisure activities (HOPES, CBSST), and reduction in negative symptoms (HOPES, FAST). Self-efficacy improved in the HOPES program. In general, retention in the programs was ideal, especially with a population that can be difficult to recruit and retain in research programs. The programs described were group based, which seemed to enhance both feasibility and the practical application of the programs. Further research could be done to better understand the importance and impact of the group nature of the programs on outcomes. For example, is the group-based aspect of social skills training essential to learning social skills? Does the group-based aspect in and of itself contribute to improved social skills and social cognition?

Another common feature found among the programs was specifically tailoring programs for individuals with physical or cognitive disabilities [2,14,18]. Specifically tailoring to meet physical and/or cognitive disabilities may be important for individuals with schizophrenia at any age, but is particularly important for the older adult who may also be dealing with multiple physical illnesses in addition to serious psychiatric symptoms. In addition, a key strength noted across the programs was a focus on developing skills in incremental steps, which could also bolster learning in individuals with cognitive disabilities [9]. The use of age-appropriate cognitive behavioral principles and skills training to meet the specific needs of older patients may have contributed to the success of the programs [9].

Health promotion models

Middle-aged and older adults with serious mental illness experience a significantly greater risk of early mortality associated with cardiovascular disease compared to the general population. Lifestyle behaviors associated with poor health outcomes, such as poor eating habits and inactivity, have been found to be more prevalent among people with serious mental illness than in the general population. Less than 20% of persons with schizophrenia engage in one or more periods of moderate exercise on a weekly basis and nearly 40% are physically inactive [42]. Poor diet is also relatively common among persons with schizophrenia, including greater consumption of calories and saturated fats and lower consumption of fruits and vegetables than the general population. Low physical activity and poor diet, combined with metabolic side effects of antipsychotic medications, result in the high rates of chronic physical illnesses found in persons with serious mental illness. Despite adverse health outcomes and greater cost associated with concurrent mental illness and poor physical health, few health promotion interventions have been developed to address the needs of this population.

STRIDE, InSHAPE, and ACHIEVE are health promotion programs designed specifically for adults with serious mental illness who have increased cardiometabolic risks and poor health behaviors associated with obesity. The overall goal of these programs is to establish sustainable techniques for a healthy lifestyle. These three health promotion programs incorporate different strategies, from exercise- or diet-only programs to combined exercise and dieting in an attempt to achieve long-term health behavior change and increased community tenure for older adults with serious mental illness.

STRIDE

Developed by Yarborough and colleagues, the STRIDE program is a lifestyle intervention that promotes self-efficacy and long-term behavior change for community-dwelling adults with serious mental illness and elevated cardiometabolic risks – specifically those taking antipsychotic medications [43]. Based on the DASH diet arm of the National Heart, Lung and Blood Institute's PREMIER lifestyle intervention [44] and drawing from motivational and behavior change theories, the STRIDE program incorporates the following eight strategies to foster behavior change, increase activity level, and ultimately stimulate weight loss among adults with serious mental illness:

1. self-monitoring of diet and physical activity,
2. developing personalized dietary and physical activity plans,
3. reducing calories moderately,
4. reducing portion sizes and substituting lower energy density foods for energy dense foods,
5. focusing on increasing intake of fruits, vegetables, fiber, and low-fat dairy products,
6. increasing physical activity,
7. identifying problematic situations for undesired behavior and developing and rehearsing action plans to deal with those situations,
8. graphing individual weight and behavioral progress [43].

To further adapt the PREMIER lifestyle intervention curriculum to more specifically suit persons with mental illness taking antipsychotic medications, Yarborough and colleagues integrated elements of medication management, anticipating episodes of mental illness, sleep hygiene, stress management, and healthy eating with a restricted budget into the STRIDE curriculum.

Designed to be delivered in routine care settings by a team of one mental-health-trained interventionist and one nutritional counselor, the 12-month STRIDE program is comprised of an intensive phase and a maintenance phase. In the first six-month, intensive phase of the program, participants share in weekly, two-hour group meetings, which include 20 minutes of walking. A key point of emphasis in the STRIDE program is increasing physical activity. Didactic segments of the group meetings also include strategies to improve self-monitoring, improve short-term goal setting, construct plans of action, and develop stronger social support. During the didactic portion of group meetings, instructors present examples of behavioral options and instruct participants in decisional balance approaches to move toward taking healthy actions and setting new behavioral goals. Participants are divided into small groups during weekly group meetings to promote individual interaction with other participants and encourage social support during problem solving, goal setting, and application of new information and skills exercises. The initial intensive phase of the STRIDE program is followed by a less-intensive, six-month maintenance phase that incorporates monthly individual meetings via phone or email and reduces group meetings to once per month. During individual meetings, participants review their diet and physical activity with the instructors, who then assist participants in identifying and troubleshooting specific barriers to success.

The STRIDE program was implemented in three publicly funded community mental health centers and a not-for-profit integrated health plan and a study of effectiveness was conducted. Primary outcome measures included weight, BMI, blood pressure, fasting plasma glucose, and cholesterol among 200 overweight or obese adults (mean BMI 38.4; mean age 47.3 years) with serious mental illness (29% schizophrenia spectrum disorder, 69% bipolar or affective disorder) taking antipsychotic medications [45]. Compared to a usual-care control group, participants who were randomly assigned to partake in the STRIDE program lost an average of 4.37 kg after the six-month intensive phase and 2.60 kg at the end of the 12-month program. Similar to weight, BMI and fasting plasma glucose were reduced by an average of 0.97 kg/m^2 and 0.09 mg/dL, respectively. At the conclusion of the six-month intensive phase, weight, BMI, fasting plasma glucose, systolic blood pressure, and cholesterol were reduced. However, in the following six months maintenance phase all but fasting plasma glucose increased [46].

The results of the STRIDE study indicate that a community-based and -run lifestyle intervention for adults with serious mental illness on antipsychotic medication can effectively reduce weight and fasting plasma glucose during the active treatment phase. However, the average increase in many cardiovascular risk factors during the final six months of the program suggests that the STRIDE maintenance may not adequately engage participants to sustain an improved healthy lifestyle.

InSHAPE

InSHAPE is an individualized health-promotion program for overweight middle-aged to older adults with serious mental illness that promotes healthy eating and exercise behaviors through improved access to community-based health and fitness services [47]. The InSHAPE program incorporates principles of social inclusion and community integration, and is designed to be provided in conventional community settings. Each participant in the InSHAPE program is assigned a health mentor that works with them on a weekly basis for roughly one hour to establish individualized fitness and healthy lifestyle progress, a fitness plan with diet and exercise goals, and an individualized approach to healthy eating and exercise. Among these central principles, the InSHAPE program also includes free access to local fitness facilities, group-based fitness and nutritional education, incentives for meeting healthy behavior goals, and group motivation meetings every six weeks to celebrate individual achievements.

Van Citters, Bartels, and colleagues conducted an initial pilot study to evaluate the InSHAPE program in a community mental health center [47]. Adults aged 18 and older (mean age 43.5 ± 11.4 years) with serious mental illness (39.5% major depressive disorder, 25.0% bipolar disorder, and 23.7% schizophrenia or schizoaffective disorder) were enrolled in the InSHAPE program (n = 76) and followed for ninth months. At the nine-month follow-up, participants reported significantly more hours of exercise compared to baseline, with the average participant engaging in 1.1 more hours of exercise each week. Participants also reported engaging in significantly more vigorous activity each week and met dietary objectives for roughly eight weeks. InSHAPE participants demonstrated improved mental health functioning over time and decreased severity of negative psychological symptoms. Baseline waist circumference of InSHAPE participants significantly decreased after nine months. However, no significant changes were observed in weight or blood pressure, but participants with hypertension at baseline demonstrated a 6.3 ± 18.5 mmHg reduction in systolic blood pressure.

Based on the promising results of this pre–post pilot study, two subsequent randomized controlled trials were conducted. The first randomized controlled trial [48] involved 133 overweight/obese adults with serious mental illness; the mean BMI was 37.6 ± 8.2 kg/m², the mean age was 43.8 ± 11.5, 24% were diagnosed with schizophrenia, and 17% had schizoaffective disorder. Of the participants randomized to participate in the InSHAPE program, 49% achieved *either* clinically significant improved fitness (an increase of ≥ 50 m on the 6 Minute Walk Test) *or* clinically significant weight loss (≥5% reduction in body weight), and 24% achieved *both* when assessed after 12 months [48]. Overall, participants achieved a mean level of weekly moderate to vigorous physical activity that has been associated with an 86% reduction in risk of all-cause mortality [49] and a mean increase of 36 m on the 6 Minute Walk Test that contributes to clinically significant reductions in cardiovascular risk [50–52]. A second randomized controlled trial [53] of InSHAPE in an ethnically heterogeneous sample of 210 participants (mean BMI 36.8 ± 8.2, mean age 43.9 ± 11.2, 23% schizophrenia, 32% schizoaffective disorder) in Boston with a longer follow-up (18 months) replicated prior outcomes and strengthened evidence for the program's sustainability. Akin to the first trial, roughly half (51%) of InSHAPE participants achieved a clinically significant improvement in fitness or weight loss associated with reduced cardiovascular risk after 12 months. Further, 46% of InSHAPE participants sustained clinically significant improved fitness or weight loss by the 18-month follow-up.

The results of both the InSHAPE randomized controlled trial and the replication study demonstrated and confirmed the effectiveness of this health coaching intervention in achieving clinically significant reductions in cardiovascular risk for overweight and obese persons with serious mental illness. Additionally, the InSHAPE randomized controlled trials revealed the ability of community mental health centers to provide an evidence-based program to aid community-dwelling overweight and obese adults with serious mental illness in achieving *sustained* weight loss and reduced cardiovascular risk.

ACHIEVE

The Achieving Healthy Lifestyles in Psychiatric Rehabilitation (ACHIEVE) program was derived from previously documented, effective lifestyle interventions for the general population [54,55], but also integrates components of social cognitive theory, behavioral self-management theory, and psychiatric rehabilitation to fit the needs of obese middle-aged to older adults with serious mental illness [56,57]. Developed by Daumit and Casagrande, each session of the ACHIEVE program is structured as either an individual weight-management, a group weight-management, or a group exercise session, with six core components including self-monitoring, goal setting, social support, skills training, environmental supports, and environmental contingencies [57]. During the program sessions, six primary health behaviors are promoted: avoiding sugary drinks, avoiding junk food, eating five servings of fruits and vegetables every day, portion control, developing smart snack habits, and regular physical activity [58]. The 18-month ACHIEVE program is delivered by trained health workers in community mental health centers over two phases: intensive and maintenance.

The intensive phase of the ACHIEVE program occurs over the first six months of the program and sessions are run by trained study staff while community mental health center staff observe. During the intensive phase, the individual weight-management sessions occur monthly, at which participants meet with program staff for a counseling session. Group weight-management classes occur three times per month during the intensive phase and a segment of the class is devoted to didactic information about healthy eating or physical activity education, and participants set individual health behavior goals based on the information presented that week. The group physical activity sessions are held three days per week for 50 minutes and are led by a trained exercise leader during the intensive phase of the program. After the initial six-month intervention phase, the program enters a maintenance phase for the remaining 12 months. In the maintenance phase of the ACHIEVE program, the frequency of sessions is reduced and study interventionists begin to transition away from leading some of the sessions and introduce community mental health center staff as session instructors. To facilitate self-monitoring, a weekly tracker tool is used by participants to help with self-monitoring of health behaviors, which is reviewed during individual and group weight-management sessions by the participant and program staff. The tracker helps participants keep track of their weekly progress with respect to the six core healthy behaviors and provides behavioral cues to participants based on fidelity to their individual health goals.

In a randomized controlled trial conducted by Daumit and colleagues to test the effectiveness of the ACHIEVE program in outpatient psychiatric rehabilitation centers, 291 overweight or obese participants (mean BMI 36.3 kg/m^2; mean age 45.3 years) with a serious mental illness (58.1% schizophrenia or schizoaffective disorder, 22% bipolar disorder, 12% major depressive disorder) were randomized to either participate in the ACHIEVE program or receive standard nutrition information and participate in a quarterly health class unrelated to weight [56]. The primary outcome of the ACHIEVE study was change in weight from baseline, but study investigators also considered other weight-related metrics (e.g. body mass index) and session attendance. ACHIEVE participants experienced a 3.4 kg mean reduction in weight after 18 months compared to a 0.2 kg mean reduction in the comparison group. Furthermore, 63.9% of ACHIEVE participants lost weight after 18 months while only 49.2% of participants receiving enhanced treatment as usual recorded a lesser weight after 18 months compared to baseline. Attendance at program sessions greatly decreased during the maintenance phase of the program compared to the intensive phase, but weight loss progressively increased over the duration of the 18-month program.

The results of the ACHIEVE program, emblematic of a dose-response, suggest the ability of the program to help persons with serious mental illness attain sustained weight loss. By incorporating existing resources to deliver the program in settings that already provide programs to many persons with serious mental illness, the ACHIEVE model demonstrates a cost-effective, sustainable approach to delivering a health promotion intervention for obese persons with psychiatric disorders.

Videogame-based physical activity program

Leutwyler and colleagues conducted a descriptive longitudinal pilot study that assessed the feasibility of an active videogame-based physical activity program among 34 older adults (mean age 61, SD = 4.6) with schizophrenia [59–60]. In the program, participants played an active videogame once a week for 30 minutes for six weeks using the Kinect for Xbox 360 game system. At each weekly session, participants chose from a variety of games and were encouraged to use a different game each week. Participants engaged in the program at the facility the person attended in groups of three to four and rated the games on appeal, ease of use, and graphics. In terms of acceptability, participants found the Kinect for Xbox 360 game system enjoyable and a fun way to be active. Patients with a wide range of psychiatric and physical abilities (e.g., some patients were in wheelchairs or front-wheel walkers) enrolled in the program. Adherence to the program was excellent, the mean number of groups attended was five out of six, and 50% of participants had perfect attendance [59]. Participants reported a significant increase in vigorous physical activity at the end of the six-week program [60]. Findings from this pilot study demonstrate the ability to recruit, retain, and engage older patients with schizophrenia into a physical activity intervention.

Health promotion models in review

Results from the STRIDE, InSHAPE, and ACHIEVE randomized controlled trials confirm the effectiveness of health promotion interventions for overweight and obese adults with serious mental illness in achieving clinically significant reduction in cardiovascular risk, through varying degrees of intensity of exercise and dietary programming and through group or individual coaching. Further, all three of these programs demonstrated the promising ability of local community mental health centers to provide clinically effective health promotion interventions to community-dwelling middle-aged and older adults. Moreover, preliminary work by Leutwyler and her co-workers suggests that new modalities such as videogames and smartphone apps (see section below) may augment the appeal and impact of these interventions.

Discussion: Future directions and recommendations

Over the coming decades, the number of older adults with serious mental illness will continue to increase dramatically, placing a substantial challenge on a mental health service delivery system that lacks the necessary workforce, capacity, competency, and funding to address the special-needs population. Compounding this challenge is the high prevalence of co-morbid chronic health conditions, which add an additional significant burden to the primary care general health care delivery system. Simply providing conventional psychiatric and medical health care services will be unlikely to substantively achieve the needed and desired outcomes supporting independent living in the community in the absence of enhancing living skills and self-management on the part of the older adult with schizophrenia or other serious mental illness. The current status quo is unacceptable: adults with serious mental illness in their fifth and sixth decades of life experience a dramatic health disparity with respect to early cardiovascular mortality and disproportionate premature placement in nursing homes. Effective services will need to incorporate evidence-based practices that directly support and engage older adults with serious mental illness and service providers in preventive and self-management interventions and supports. To achieve this critical goal, new models of care will need to be implemented and disseminated that incorporate evidence-based practices, delivered in the community through novel workforce solutions, augmented by technology. Fortunately, the last decade has witnessed an emerging research literature documenting the development and effectiveness of a variety of psychosocial skills training, self-management, and health promotion interventions.

The first generation of models focused on delivering group-based psychosocial skills training emphasizing the acquisition of living skills and social skills to support independent living in the community. In general, these models adapted existing psychosocial interventions such as social skills training and cognitive behavioral treatments for older adults with serious mental illness. These interventions, including Helping Older Persons Experience Success (HOPES), Functional Adaptation Skills Training (FAST), and Cognitive Behavioral Social Skills Training (CBSST), demonstrated effectiveness in randomized, community-based trials in improving living skills, social skills, and functional outcomes. Of note, the HOPES trial documented persistence of improved functional outcomes at two-year follow-up, demonstrating that older adults with serious mental illness not only have the capacity to learn and acquire new skills, but also are able to retain and maintain these skills well beyond the active period of the intervention to support improved long-term outcomes.

Recognizing the high prevalence and substantial impact of chronic health conditions on functioning and outcomes, a subsequent generation of studies focused on illness self-management and wellness. Health and Recovery Peers (HARP) adapted the Stanford Chronic Disease Self-Management Program (CDSMP) that has been widely disseminated to general populations for specific application to support wellness self-management for persons with serious mental illness. A novel feature of this model is the delivery of the intervention by certified peer specialists. Other models focusing on chronic medical illness self-management include dedicated strategies for specific common health conditions. For example, the Targeted Training in Illness Management (TTIM) program adapted the diabetes self-management programs Life Goals Program and the Diabetes Awareness Rehabilitation Training model for persons with serious mental illness, including group sessions co-led by nurse and peer educators. Although these programs are adapted for individuals with serious mental illness and include components addressing selected related mental health domains, these programs are largely dedicated to addressing the challenges associated with wellness and self-management of chronic health conditions. In contrast, Integrated Illness Management and Recovery (I-IMR) consists of integrated, concurrent, and co-equal training and support in self-management of both mental health and medical conditions. Adapted from the evidence-based intervention "Illness Management and Recovery" (IMR) specifically developed to support illness self-management of serious mental illness and the associated challenges of living independently in the community, I-IMR was developed to fully integrate self-management skill acquisition and support for wellness and chronic medical illness self-management. This approach explicitly embraces the principle that mental and physical health are intrinsically interrelated and that self-management strategies need to address both domains comprehensively and concurrently. Other more recent developments include health promotion and prevention interventions focused on addressing the major risk factors for early cardiovascular mortality, including obesity and tobacco use. Individually tailored health mentor interventions such as InSHAPE and group-based interventions such as ACHIEVE and STRIDE have demonstrated effectiveness in improving physical activity, nutrition, fitness, and reduced weight. This generation of preventive interventions is critical to addressing key risk factors before they evolve into high-cost, complex health conditions that contribute to premature institutionalization, poor health outcomes, and an early mortality health disparity.

Future interventions and services will need to be formulated and delivered with an emphasis on achieving reach and sustainability at the level of "population health." Current approaches that are underway to achieve this goal consist of the use of novel workforce solutions (peers and community health workers) and technology, such as web-based and smartphone delivery, and the use of wearable sensors. Some of the novel technological approaches include automated telehealth devices that deliver self-management training and support, and remote monitoring using individually tailored programs specific to the individual's goals and psychiatric and medical conditions, as well as smartphone apps augmented by peer support. Despite these innovative and important advances in developing new evidence-based practices, a critical area for future research consists of bridging the implementation gap from "what we know" to "what we do." To date, the most of the evidence-based interventions that we have described here for older adults with serious mental illness are not provided by usual care in community mental health and primary care settings. In this respect one of the most crucial agendas rests in the field of implementation and dissemination research. Finally, health policy and financing reforms need to be pursued that align incentives, health indicators, and reimbursement with the capacity to improve outcomes for the rapidly growing population of older adults with serious mental illness by providing evidence-based prevention and models of care specifically tailored to meet the special needs of this high-risk, complex health disparity group.

References

1. U.S. Census Bureau. The next four decades: the older population in the United States: 2010 to 2050. 2010. www.census.gov/prod/2010pubs/p25-1138.pdf (accessed October 2018).

2. Cohen CI. Studies of the course and outcome of schizophrenia in later life. *Psychiatric Services (Washington, DC).* 1995;46(9):877–9, 889.

3. Jeste DV, Alexopoulos GS, Bartels SJ, et al. Consensus statement on the upcoming crisis in geriatric mental health: research agenda for the next 2 decades. *Archives of General Psychiatry.* 1999;56(9):848–53.

4. Cohen CI. Practical geriatrics: directions for research and policy on schizophrenia and older adults: summary of the GAP

committee report. *Psychiatric Services (Washington, DC)*. 2000;**51**(3):299–302.

5. Walker ER, McGee RE, Druss BG. Mortality in mental disorders and global disease burden implications: a systematic review and meta-analysis. *JAMA Psychiatry*. 2015;**72**(4):334–41.

6. Olfson M, Gerhard T, Huang C, Crystal S, Stroup TS. Premature mortality among adults with schizophrenia in the United States. *JAMA Psychiatry*. 2015;**72**(12):1172–81.

7. Jeste DV, Gladsjo JA, Lindamer LA, Lacro JP. Medical comorbidity in schizophrenia. *Schizophrenia Bulletin*. 1996;**22**(3):413–30.

8. Rystedt IB, Bartels SJ. Medical comorbidity. In: Mueser KT, Jeste DV, eds. *Clinical Handbook of Schizophrenia*. New York: Guilford; 2008:424–36.

9. Bartels SJ, Mueser KT, Miles KM. A comparative study of elderly patients with schizophrenia and bipolar disorder in nursing homes and the community. *Schizophrenia Research*. 1997;**27**(2–3):181–90.

10. Horan ME, Muller JJ, Winocur S, Barling N. Quality of life in boarding houses and hostels: a residents' perspective. *Community Mental Health Journal*. 2001;**37**(4):323–34.

11. DE Hert M, Correll CU, Bobes J, et al. Physical illness in patients with severe mental disorders. I. Prevalence, impact of medications and disparities in health care. *World Psychiatry*. 2011;**10**(1):52–77.

12. Corbin JM, Strauss AL. *Unending Work and Care: Managing Chronic Illness at Home*. San Francisco, CA: Jossey-Bass Publishers; 1988.

13. Whiteman KL, Naslund JA, DiNapoli EA, Bruce ML, Bartels SJ. Systematic review of integrated general medical and psychiatric self-management interventions for adults with serious mental illness. *Psychiatric Services (Washington, DC)*. 2016;**67**(11):1213–25.

14. Druss BG, Zhao L, von Esenwein SA, et al. The Health and Recovery Peer (HARP) Program: a peer-led intervention to improve medical

self-management for persons with serious mental illness. *Schizophrenia Research*. 2010;**118**(1–3):264–70.

15. Lorig KR, Sobel DS, Stewart AL, et al. Evidence suggesting that a chronic disease self-management program can improve health status while reducing hospitalization: a randomized trial. *Medical Care*. 1999;**37**(1):5–14.

16. Wingood GM, DiClemente RJ. The ADAPT-ITT model: a novel method of adapting evidence-based HIV Interventions. *Journal of Acquired Immune Deficiency Syndromes*. 2008;**47**(Suppl 1):S40–6.

17. Druss BG, Singh M, von Esenwein SA, et al. Peer-led self-management of general medical conditions for patients with serious mental illnesses: a randomized trial. *Psychiatric Services (Washington, DC)*. 2018;**69**(5):529–35.

18. Sajatovic M, Dawson NV, Perzynski AT, et al. Best practices: optimizing care for people with serious mental illness and comorbid diabetes. *Psychiatric Services (Washington, DC)*. 2011;**62**(9):1001–3.

19. Bauer MS, McBride L. *Structured Group Psychotherapy for Bi-polar Disorder: The Life Goals Program*. New York: Springer; 2003.

20. McKibbin CL, Patterson TL, Norman G, et al. A lifestyle intervention for older schizophrenia patients with diabetes mellitus: a randomized controlled trial. *Schizophrenia Research*. 2006;**86**(1–3):36–44.

21. Sajatovic M, Gunzler DD, Kanuch SW, et al. A 60-week prospective RCT of a self-management intervention for individuals with serious mental illness and diabetes mellitus. *Psychiatric Services (Washington, DC)*. 2017;**68**(9):883–90.

22. Mueser KT, Bartels SJ, Santos M, Pratt SI, Riera EG. Integrated illness management and recovery: a program for integrating physical and psychiatric illness self-management in older persons with severe mental illness. *American Journal of Psychiatric Rehabilitation*. 2012;**15**(2):131–56.

23. Bartels SJ, Pratt SI, Mueser KT, et al. Integrated IMR for psychiatric and general medical illness for adults aged 50 or older with serious mental illness. *Psychiatric Services (Washington, DC)*. 2014;**65**(3):330–7.

24. Mueser KT, Corrigan PW, Hilton DW, et al. Illness management and recovery: a review of the research. *Psychiatric Services (Washington, DC)*. 2002;**53**(10):1272–84.

25. Pratt SI, Van Citters AD, Mueser KT, Bartels SJ. Psychosocial rehabilitation in older adults with serious mental illness: a review of the research literature and recommendations for development of rehabilitative approaches. *American Journal of Psychiatric Rehabilitation*. 2008;**11**(1):7–40.

26. Pratt SI, Bartels SJ, Mueser KT, Forester B. Helping older people experience success: an integrated model of psychosocial rehabilitation and health care management for older adults with serious mental illness. *American Journal of Psychiatric Rehabilitation*. 2008;**11**(1):41–60.

27. Bartels SJ, Pratt SI. Psychosocial rehabilitation and quality of life for older adults with serious mental illness: recent findings and future research directions. *Current Opinion in Psychiatry*. 2009;**22**(4):381–5.

28. Bartels SJ, Forester B, Mueser KT, et al. Enhanced skills training and health care management for older persons with severe mental illness. *Community Mental Health Journal*. 2004;**40**(1):75–90.

29. Patterson TL, McKibbin C, Taylor M, et al. Functional adaptation skills training (FAST): a pilot psychosocial intervention study in middle-aged and older patients with chronic psychotic disorders. *American Journal of Geriatric Psychiatry*. 2003;**11**(1):17–23.

30. McQuaid JR, Granholm E, McClure FS, et al. Development of an integrated cognitive-behavioral and social skills training intervention for older patients with schizophrenia. *Journal of Psychotherapy Practice and Research*. 2000;**9**(3):149–56.

31. Mueser KT, Pratt SI, Bartels SJ, et al. Randomized trial of social rehabilitation and integrated health care for older people with severe mental illness. *Journal of Consulting and Clinical Psychology*. 2010;**78**(4):561–73.

32. Bartels SJ, Pratt SI, Mueser KT, et al. Long-term outcomes of a randomized trial of integrated skills training and preventive healthcare for older adults with serious mental illness. *American Journal of Geriatric Psychiatry*. 2014;**22**(11):1251–61.

33. Vaccaro JV, Liberman RP, Wallace CJ, Blackwell G. Combining social skills training and assertive case management: the social and independent living skills program of the Brentwood Veterans Affairs Medical Center. *New Directions for Mental Health Services*. 1992;(53):33–42.

34. Patterson TL, Mausbach BT, McKibbin C, et al. Functional adaptation skills training (FAST): a randomized trial of a psychosocial intervention for middle-aged and older patients with chronic psychotic disorders. *Schizophrenia Research*. 2006;**86**(1–3):291–9.

35. Patterson TL, Bucardo J, McKibbin CL, et al. Development and pilot testing of a new psychosocial intervention for older Latinos with chronic psychosis. *Schizophrenia Bulletin*. 2005;**31**(4):922–30.

36. Mausbach BT, Bucardo J, Cardenas V, et al. Evaluation of a culturally tailored skills intervention for Latinos with persistent psychotic disorders. *American Journal of Psychiatric Rehabilitation*. 2008;**11**(1):61–75.

37. Beck AT, Rush AJ, Shaw BF, Emery G. *Cognitive Therapy of Depression*. New York: Guilford; 1987.

38. Kingdon D, Turkington D. *Cognititive-Behavioral Therapy of Schizophrenia*. New York: Guilford; 1994.

39. Liberman RP, Van Putten T, Marshall BD, Jr., et al. Optimal drug and behavior therapy for treatment-refractory schizophrenic patients. *American Journal of Psychiatry*. 1994;**151**(5):756–9.

40. Psychiatric Rehabilitation Consultants. Modules in the UCLA social and

independent living skill series. Camarillo, C.A.: Psychiatric Rehabilitation Consultants; 1991.

41. Granholm E, McQuaid JR, McClure FS, et al. A randomized, controlled trial of cognitive behavioral social skills training for middle-aged and older outpatients with chronic schizophrenia. *American Journal of Psychiatry.* 2005;**162**(3):520–9.

42. Laursen TM, Munk-Olsen T, Vestergaard M. Life expectancy and cardiovascular mortality in persons with schizophrenia. *Current Opinion in Psychiatry.* 2012;**25**(2):83–8.

43. Yarborough BJ, Janoff SL, Stevens VJ, Kohler D, Green CA. Delivering a lifestyle and weight loss intervention to individuals in real-world mental health settings: Lessons and opportunities. *Translational Behavioral Medicine.* 2011;**1**(3):406–15.

44. Svetkey LP, Harsha DW, Vollmer WM, et al. Premier: a clinical trial of comprehensive lifestyle modification for blood pressure control: rationale, design and baseline characteristics. *Annals of Epidemiology.* 2003;**13**(6):462–71.

45. Yarborough BJ, Leo MC, Stumbo S, Perrin NA, Green CA. STRIDE: a randomized trial of a lifestyle intervention to promote weight loss among individuals taking antipsychotic medications. *BMC Psychiatry.* 2013;**13**:238.

46. Green CA, Yarborough BJ, Leo MC, et al. The STRIDE weight loss and lifestyle intervention for individuals taking antipsychotic medications: a randomized trial. *American Journal of Psychiatry.* 2015;**172**(1):71–81.

47. Van Citters AD, Pratt SI, Jue K, et al. A pilot evaluation of the In SHAPE individualized health promotion intervention for adults with mental illness. *Community Mental Health Journal.* 2010;**46**(6):540–52.

48. Bartels SJ, Pratt SI, Aschbrenner KA, et al. Clinically significant improved fitness and weight loss among overweight persons with serious mental illness. *Psychiatric Services.* 2013;**64**(8):729–36.

49. Samitz G, Egger M, Zwahlen M. Domains of physical activity and all-cause mortality: systematic review and dose-response meta-analysis of cohort studies. *International Journal of Epidemiology.* 2011;**40**(5):1382–400.

50. Larsson UE, Reynisdottir S. The six-minute walk test in outpatients with obesity: reproducibility and known group validity. *Physiotherapy Research International.* 2008;**13**(2):84–93.

51. Wise RA, Brown CD. Minimal clinically important differences in the six-minute walk test and the incremental shuttle walking test. *Journal of Chronic Obstructive Pulmonary Disease.* 2005;**2**(1):125–9.

52. Rasekaba T, Lee AL, Naughton MT, Williams TJ, Holland AE. The six-minute walk test: a useful metric for the cardiopulmonary patient. *Internal Medicine Journal.* 2009;**39**(8):495–501.

53. Bartels SJ, Pratt SI, Aschbrenner KA, et al. Pragmatic replication trial of health promotion coaching for obesity in serious mental illness and maintenance of outcomes. *American Journal of Psychiatry.* 2015;**172**(4):344–52.

54. Elmer PJ, Obarzanek E, Vollmer WM, et al. Effects of comprehensive lifestyle modification on diet, weight, physical fitness, and blood pressure control: 18-month results of a randomized trial. *Annals of Internal Medicine.* 2006;**144**(7):485–95.

55. Whelton PK, Appel LJ, Espeland MA, et al. Sodium reduction and weight loss in the treatment of hypertension in older persons: a randomized controlled trial of nonpharmacologic interventions in the elderly (TONE). *JAMA.* 1998;**279**(11):839–46.

56. Daumit GL, Dickerson FB, Wang NY, et al. A behavioral weight-loss intervention in persons with serious mental illness. *New England Journal of Medicine.* 2013;**368**(17):1594–602.

57. Casagrande SS, Jerome GJ, Dalcin AT, et al. Randomized trial of achieving healthy lifestyles in psychiatric

rehabilitation: the ACHIEVE trial. *BMC Psychiatry.* 2010;**10**:108.

58. Vazin R, McGinty EE, Dickerson F, et al. Perceptions of strategies for successful weight loss in persons with serious mental illness participating in a behavioral weight loss intervention: a qualitative study. *Psychiatric Rehabilitation Journal.* 2016;**39**(2):137–46.

59. Leutwyler H, Hubbard E, and Dowling G. Adherence to a videogame-based physical activity program for older adults with schizophrenia. *Games for Health Journal.* 2014;3(4):227–233.

60. Leutwyler H, Hubbard E, Cooper B, and Dowling G. The impact of a videogame-based pilot physical activity program in older adults with schizophrenia on subjectively and objectively measured physical activity. *Front Psychiatry.* 2015;**6**:180.

Changing Caregiver Needs with Increasing Age of People with Schizophrenia

Harriet P. Lefley, Ph.D. and Brian R. Ghezelaiagh

People with schizophrenia represent a variant population. At one end of the curve are extremely productive individuals such as John Nash [1] or Elyn Saks [2], who had the strength to overcome their perceived deficits and even make highly important contributions to society. The current emphasis on recovery as a therapeutic goal focuses on autonomy rather than on continuity of oversight by a treatment and caregiving system. It seems clear, however, that numerous individuals with this diagnosis cannot live independently. This chapter deals with the much larger number of persons with schizophrenia who require both continuing psychiatric oversight and some level of caregiving throughout much of their lives.

As people with schizophrenia age, many of their caregivers grow even older in terms of their capacity for fulfilling this need. In this chapter, we deal for the most part with family-member caregivers rather than salaried home help or employees of a care facility. Typically, over the years the caregivers are one or more parents, although, to a lesser degree, they may be spouses, siblings, other relatives, or even close friends. We begin with some beneficial aspects of parallel aging, and then we will move on to those aspects that pose serious threats to the stability of the relationship.

The agreeable patient: the ideal of reciprocity

Despite much research over the years on caregiver burden, we have little knowledge of the burden of dependency on the recipient of the care. Sometimes this is handled by role reversal. In this situation, a person whose schizophrenia has not abated to the point of living independently, and who continues to live at home with caregiver oversight, has developed a functional role in the family economy. In many cases this is a younger person who can help aging parents with driving, shopping, lifting heavy objects, and doing other tasks that require younger bodies. Some symptom-controlled long-term patients are able to provide love and companionship to parents dealing with the trials of their own old age. His or her presence may be especially valuable if the caregiver is now a widowed parent.

These are productive roles that are validly helpful to all parties and to the patient's self-esteem. If they are not already in evidence, patients' helpful contributions to the household can often be established and reinforced in the problem-solving phase of family psychoeducation, as well as in brief family therapy.

The difficult and potentially violent patient

Family dynamics may change substantially as a mentally ill person begins to perceive the growing fragility of the caregivers on whom he or she has learned to depend. Feelings of dependency may themselves provoke a resentment that explodes into violence, particularly if reinforced by paranoid ideation. The dilemmas of living with violence are exemplified in a description of living with an abusive adult child who is mentally ill [3]. The authors' suggested intervention focuses on reinforcing social networks for both the patient and family caregivers, but also emphasizes the rights of the latter to self-protection.

Satisfying caregivers' rights to self-protection may involve actions that are beyond the scope of psychotherapeutic interventions. Typically, violence against an aging caregiver means calling the police. But families who expected their loved one to be taken to a treatment facility have too often found that they were taken to jail, some after being tased or manhandled by untrained officers. Even in the few cities with mental health courts that divert offenders with schizophrenia to the treatment system, this solution is typically for petty misdemeanors or less serious, nonviolent felonies [4]. This is rarely an option for assaults on an aging parent.

Non-assaultive crises

We are all aware of crisis situations generated by psychotic episodes. The patient may pose a danger to him or herself or others with verbal threats, act irrationally in potentially dangerous situations, and obviously require professional interventions that undoubtedly will be rejected. Many caregivers are not aware of alternative resources in times of crisis. This is particularly true for older caregivers who, after many years, may have reached a mutually satisfactory or acceptable accommodation with the behaviors of a family member with schizophrenia, but now find they are unable to handle the load. Much depends now on their knowledge of the resources that are available to them, particularly if they are fortunate enough to live in an area with police units trained to deal with mental illness. But these are still rarely available, and after years of quietly coping with difficult, perhaps even dangerous behaviors, older caregivers may now be too tired to avoid the repetitive need for police interventions. Typically, these have led to too brief, fruitless stays in an emergency room or crisis intervention unit or even in jail. The aftermath is usually ugly: the patient furious at caregivers and unlikely to resume taking medications willingly. In this case, an intervention from a case manager or a long-term personal psychiatrist may be needed to change the family dynamics. In many cases this involves planning that will serve the needs of the aging caregiver and enable the patients' separation from a now decaying and potentially destructive relationship with the family members on whom they have had to depend.

A patient's acceptance of familial caregiving depends of course on his or her prior history with those administering care, and the degree to which the person is willing to accept a subordinate position as grantee. This varies considerably in terms of the patient's prior history, and because family members are often the last resort to provide for individuals unable to support their own needs, interactions over time are likely to reflect earlier relationships.

Parental caregivers

In almost all disorders, when the need for caregiving arises it is primarily women who shoulder the burden. But men suffer too. Ghose and Greenberg [5] compared 95 older (mean age 70 years) married fathers of adult children with schizophrenia with a well-matched comparison group of 95 fathers with no mental illness in the family. Despite their spouses being the major caregivers, fathers of adults with schizophrenia had higher levels of depression, poorer perceived health, lower psychological well-being, and less marital satisfaction. Thus, regardless of the division of responsibilities, there seem to be psychological costs that are are not related to the burdens of caregiving per se.

As they age, parents lose physical strength and their threshold for tolerance of difficult behaviors lowers. But as previously noted, there is also the possibility of greater reliance on the family member with schizophrenia as a source of companionship and household help. In many years working with family support groups, Lefley [6,7] found that an aging family member with schizophrenia may offer needed help with numerous household chores. A younger, stronger person can be greatly beneficial to aging caregivers, and fulfillment of a much-needed role in itself is therapeutic. Most psychoeducational interventions that involve both patient and family typically have a problem-solving component, in which all members participate. The problem is limited to an issue for the entire household (e.g., where to go on summer vacation, whether to paint the house, fix the roof, etc.) and never to the patient's behavior. When patients are able to give an opinion, to formulate their own role in the problem's resolution, this provides benefits for all the members. This exercise can enhance the patient's self-esteem and even change the family dynamic.

In another scenario, aging family caregivers may offer ongoing financial and social support, but not a home. Although there is currently a much-needed focus on reinforcing potential for recovery and independent living, it is clear that many persons with schizophrenia cannot live alone. If they cannot live at home with relatives, they typically reside in an assisted living facility. Here, the family needs ongoing contact with the patient's caregiving staff, and with the treating psychiatrist and social worker if the patient is to make optimal progress. It has been many years since families were deliberately excluded from these interactions, although there are still mental health professionals who subscribe to these essentially countertherapeutic beliefs. It is only recently that Health Insurance Portability and Accountability Act (HIPPAA) rules were changed to facilitate sharing needed information with patients' caregivers.

Some research findings on aging caregivers

A number of studies have been conducted among members of the National Alliance on Mental Illness (NAMI), the major organization for families of people with serious mental illness. Some were oriented toward service needs of aging caregivers, others toward future planning for replacement of aging caregivers after their death. In one study [8] of service use and unmet needs of older persons with severe mental illness, 196 caregivers in 41 states (with a response rate of more than 90% to a mailed questionnaire) reported major unmet service needs related to their own deteriorating health and home situations. Respondents had a mean age of 67 (range 50–88) years; 90% were between 65 and 79 years of age and 10% were 80 years or older. The majority were mothers (79%) and 57% were married. The mentally ill offspring were primarily male (76%) with a mean age of 38 years. Only one-third were involved in outside activities such as day treatment or supported employment. More than half spent their typical days at home relying on their mother for all services and doing little on their own behalf. There was special need for outreach services when the caregivers perceived more age-related changes in themselves and when their offspring typically spent the day at home without outside stimulation. The need for social outlets, particularly for outpatient support groups, was readily apparent, although these are rarely offered in standard clinical settings.

Smith's research on aging caregivers also focused on future planning for their replacement after their death. In the cited study [8], a component on permanency planning was completed by the 196 older caregivers. The survey specifically focused on the extent of residential and financial planning for future care, the desire of other family members to assume caregiving, and the perceived need for the service system to assist in planning. Results indicated that almost half of the respondents had devoted very little effort to where their mentally ill child would live in the future. However, 66% had done some financial planning, primarily through trusts (34%) or money willed to another relative on behalf of the ill offspring (24%). Although the vast majority (76%) said they would like one of their other children to take over caregiving when they died, only 25% thought this might happen.

Additional research on older NAMI caregivers, primarily in two eastern states, was conducted in order to explore their concerns about what would happen to their loved ones after they died [9]. In this study, four focus groups of elderly caregivers were convened to identify problems of planning for future care. A survey instrument derived from these discussions was specifically addressed to older caregivers and appeared in NAMI newsletters in Maryland and Florida. Selection criteria were that respondents be: (a) 65 years or older, and (b) the major caregiver of a person with severe and persistent mental illness. Fixed-choice items related to possible barriers in: (a) the caregivers' personal lives, (b) the attitudes and behaviors of the person with mental illness, and (c) limitations of the service system. The returns yielded 210 usable responses. The majority of caregivers (79%) were mothers, 90% were between 65 and 79 years of age and 10% were 80 years or older. Three-quarters of the relatives with mental illness had a diagnosis of schizophrenia; the remainder were diagnosed with bipolar disorder. The ages of those needing caregiving were as follows: 33% in their thirties, 56% in their forties, and 11% 50 years or older.

Respondents were asked about their planning for the future: 44% reported no planning at all, 38% reported some partially completed planning, and 18% reported a completed plan. Major obstacles were: (a) the caregivers' lack of knowledge about how to plan (50%), (b) the disabled relative's resistance to change (52%), and (c) limited housing resources in the local mental health system (48%). Although 43% found their relative unstable much of the time, an equal number (44%) said their relative refused to use available resources. The option of getting their family member into a program with case management and linked residential services seemed unlikely.

The findings indicated that even with their own aging and prospective disability or death, older parental caregivers have problems making future plans. Although they are more likely to attribute this to their own failings or to the patient's resistance, rather than to deficits in the service system, the system itself has neglected the need for future planning with their patients, both instrumental and psychological, in the event of the death of an aging caregiver. Mental health professionals who serve older patients with schizophrenia would do well to consider how to prepare them for the inevitable loss of an elderly caregiving parent [10].

Sibling caregivers

In the research cited above, most parents assumed that after they died their other children would assume some caregiving responsibilities, but to a much lesser degree. Typically this was limited to occasional visits and some financial help, but did not involve their own homes. The parents were faced with a clear dilemma: although they worried about their ill child, they were also reluctant to inflict that responsibility on the patient's siblings.

Much depends of course on the prior relationship. The literature on family relationships in schizophrenia shows considerable sibling resentment, particularly during the teen years [6]. They were often ashamed of the ill sibling, reluctant to publicize or even acknowledge their relationship, and resentful about the undue attention given by the parents to the ill family member. As children and teenagers they were often afraid to be seen in public with their ill brother or sister. Many siblings later feel guilty about their former attitudes and may try to make up for it in later life. Others retain conflicted or suppressed hostile feelings and may resent taking on a caregiving role, however slight its demands, so the relationship may become tainted by unacknowledged resentment and become countertherapeutic. In workshops on future planning conducted for 400 elderly parents and 60 siblings, the siblings answered a survey regarding their future caregiving expectations, anticipated difficulties, and need for help. Nearly all expected to be involved, but were more likely to provide social and emotional support than the instrumental support provided by their parents. Nearly half indicated that the patient's hostility and lack of cooperation were major barriers to his or her acceptance of effective care [9].

It should be noted that this was a highly motivated participant group eager to learn more about their siblings' illness and how they can help their parents. But much depends upon the specific diagnosis and the former degree of affection. Happily, we find an increasing literature in which now successful adult siblings both acknowledge the relationship and develop mutual roles in fighting societal stigma against mental illness.

Spousal and child caregivers

In schizophrenia the marriage rate is low, and divorce and separation are common among people with schizophrenia who do marry. Even among spouses who evidence love and respect for each other, the burden of sporadic psychosis may become too much too bear, especially if there are children [1]. Spouses who remain, and who assume a caregiving role, may do so for religious reasons, for their own psychological needs, or in many cases, because of their love for the ill spouse. The relationship may become closer, depending on the level of functioning and irrational behaviors. In relation to parental caregiving, however, caregiving by aging spouses of persons with schizophrenia is minimal. Most caregiving literature in later life focuses on the dementias. Caregiving by elderly spouses of schizophrenia patients is undoubtedly minimal in comparison with aging spouses of those with dementias. In the latter case, there are memories of a functioning mate and typically a history of a productive life and reciprocity, of mutual contributions to the other's welfare before behavioral changes occurred. Some individuals with schizophrenia have children. Unlike the attention given to adult children caring for persons with Alzheimer's disease, children caring for their elderly parents with schizophrenia have been neglected by the research and social service communities (see http://schizophrenia.com/family/longbereave.htm).

Services that aid patients and alleviate caregiver burden

We have few services that are specifically oriented toward older patients and fewer still for their aging caregivers. Senior center programs are not typically oriented toward serving aging persons with schizophrenia, and few mental health centers focus on this specific population. With decreasing mental health funding, fewer case managers are available for home visits to offer help, or social workers to serve the special needs of older caregivers. Geriatric psychiatrists serve the patient and may offer help to their caregivers, but this is rarely part of standard practice. Many states have adopted Stein and Test's [11] Program of Assertive Community Treatment (PACT). Their home visits would be a boon for aging caregivers, but the program itself was developed for younger people to learn the skills to manage their own lives.

We have spoken previously of occasional periods of psychotic decompensation that are increasingly harder for aging caregivers to manage. A history of calling the police has usually resulted in worse results than anticipated. Today many states offer a legal mechanism for enforcing treatment, often a last hope for families who can no longer cope.

Assisted outpatient treatment

For patients with a prior history of repeated hospitalizations or arrests, the answer may be Assisted Outpatient Treatment (AOT), also known as "outpatient commitment." The Treatment Advocacy Center (TAC) has advocated for AOT legislation for years. This involves a court mandate for psychiatric treatment, with penalties for noncompliance. AOT commits patients to adhere to treatment plans that have been developed by the patients and their healthcare providers. These plans typically include case management, personal therapy, education, and other rehabilitative tools to promote recovery. In their description, TAC emphasizes that "AOT participants receive due process protections and orders are made only after a hearing before a judge" (www.treatmentadvocacycenter.org/fixing the system/promoting-assisted-outpatient-treatment; accessed October 2018). In the United States, AOT has been widely supported by governmental and professional organizations. As of February 2017, 46 of 50 states and the District of Columbia had enacted laws that authorize the use of AOT.

On the other hand, it must be noted that although AOT has been endorsed by NAMI, the practice has been vigorously condemned by consumer organizations and many of their advocates. The issue of basic civil rights and personal autonomy looms large here. However, the consumer organizations seem largely to represent the population of present or former psychiatric patients who are recovery-oriented, higher-functioning individuals that are not dependent on caregivers. Although NAMI also has a substantial and active consumer membership, it was founded by and remains the major organization for family members of individuals with serious and persistent mental illnesses, especially those with psychotic features. Many of these families have remained lifelong caregivers of dependent, often difficult adults well into older age.

The international picture

Continuity of caregiving for persons with serious mental disorders is both a national and an international problem. In many mental health systems, home caregiving by families is considered a given [12]. In China, for example, co-residence with adult children, particularly for those with a mental illness, is culturally normative. Yet much depends on the services offered by the local mental health system. In a recent comparison of caregivers of family members with schizophrenia in Hong Kong and another major city, Guangzhou, 72.5% of the caregivers were living with the mentally ill family member [13]. But the percentage was 90% in Guangzhou and only 41% in Hong Kong. The authors noted that this was probably due to the difference between the two cities in the availability of psychiatric rehabilitation and community mental health services. Thus, it seems that cultural norms may yield to the availability of alternative resources for care. Further multi-scale research by Zeng et al. [14] indicated that Guangzhou family members experienced significantly more caregiver burden than did those in Hong Kong. Facts influencing their perceived burden included the number of hours spent with the patient, subjective and objective support (including financial assistance), and overall quality of life.

In most of the non-Western world, family members continue to be the primary caregivers of persons with chronic mental illnesses. In India greater than 90% of these individuals live with families. Chadda et al. [15] note that in India there is an increasing trend toward nuclear families and continued poor institutional support for persons with long-term mental illness. This combination makes for increased caregiver burden. Responsibilities include taking care of the patient's day-to-day needs, monitoring mental status, and accessing services, which often are remote. These constant stressors take a toll, and it is suggested that as high as 80% of caregivers experience burnout [15].

In Iran, 65–75% of patients with schizophrenia and other long-term mental illnesses are living with family members. According to von Kardoff et al. [16], these families prefer to keep mentally ill dependents within the family. Yet they struggle with emotional, physical, and financial challenges, obstacles to pursuing leisure activities, social stigma, friction in relationships, and difficulties obtaining governmental support. The author also notes that in spite of strong family ties and feelings of family obligation, mental illness still remains highly taboo in the culture. Because family caregiving remains close to the norm in much of the non-Western world, and because families tend to cluster rather than separate, it may be that the task of aging caregivers is relatively easier when there are others to share and later take over the burden. However, this is a hypothesis that has yet to be explored.

In contrast, in the United States, the survey results of the NAMI studies have been used as a basis for practical planning and family training in the University of Maryland Mental Heath Services Training Collaborative and the Maryland Department of Health and Mental Hygiene. Hatfield wrote an informative publication [17] on planning for the future care for relatives with serious and persistent mental illness. The survey responses of NAMI respondents indicate the fear that many patients who have relied on parental caregiving for years are likely to fight any change. Some may decompensate at the loss not only of a caregiver, but also of known surroundings that comfort them. Maryland's planning document has sections on overcoming reluctance to planning, needs assessments, selecting an advocate or guardian, and preparing the person with mental illness for eventual loss of the caregiver [17].

For parents who have money to leave their children, the PLAN (Planned Lifetime Assistance Program) was developed to provide for their adult children with disabilities after their death or their own inability to care for them. PLAN covers all disabilities. It is essentially a specific future-case plan developed to ensure ongoing case management and security of a disabled loved one. A financial mechanism such as a special needs trust or third-party trust is created to pay for these activities and services. A service provider and/or trustee is identified to guarantee that the plan is implemented. More information may be obtained from NAMI (www.nami.org). However, the local bar association may be the best resource for finding an attorney who specializes in disability law and can set up a special needs trust.

Are we seeing the "aging out" of family caregivers? Some indicators from the United Kingdom

The U.K. has a major organization called the Carers' Trust, which serves the needs of caregivers for persons with serious and long-lasting physical as well as psychiatric conditions. ("Carers," the British term, seems to be more appropriate than "caregivers" when families assume this task.) Although it covers all disabilities, the Carers' Trust has been involved in a special campaign with the Royal College of Psychiatrists. Called Partners in Care, this coalition reflected psychiatrists' efforts both to educate and to become educated themselves about the problems of carers coping with severe and persistent mental illness.

A current study by the Carers' Trust explored specific problems of elderly carers in the United Kingdom. The results of the survey are remarkably similar to those found in the United States studies. According to their report, the last (2011) U.K. census indicated that there were 1.8 million carers aged 60 and over in the U.K., including 151,674 between 80 and 84, and 87,346 aged over 85. Results of a representative focus group sample of 100 elderly carers showed similar problems to those in the U.S.: care coordination, carers' own health issues and need for relief, transport, benefits and finances, planning for the future, and problems finding housing.

This report appeared in a recent issue of *Meriden* [18], the bulletin of the Meriden Family Programme, which is funded by the British government's National Health Service (NHS) to serve the needs of family carers for adult patients with schizophrenia and other major psychiatric disorders. As a component of the NHS, for the past 20 years the Meriden Family Programme has focused on training various mental health disciplines in how to help these family carers. The emphasis is on providing family psychoeducation (FPE) (as opposed to a presumption of the need for psychotherapy) for serious mental illness. FPE is an evidence-based treatment approach to schizophrenia [19,20]. It is based on the premise that family carers need from professionals that which they have long been requesting: education, support, problem-resolution, and illness management techniques.

The Carers' Trust noted a phenomenon already evident in the United States: "People are caring far longer and later in their lives" ([18] p. 19). This phenomenon is apparent in the American NAMI samples and may reflect a historical trend in societal approaches to dealing with serious mental illness. The family caregivers who replaced long-term hospitalization of the now-closed mental institutions may be aging out of their capability for providing care. Yet the promised community residential resources have not been sufficiently provided to meet the need. We already know the outrageous replacement of hospital beds by jail cells. For the more fortunate patients living with relatives, the continuity of family caregiving may be increasingly problematic, especially in cultures where adult children are expected to leave home and take care of their own futures. Although deinstitutionalization undoubtedly has had many salutary effects in demonstrating patients' potential for recovery, we are increasingly seeing the negative effects on those with severe and persistent mental illnesses.

Conclusion

If parental caregivers are aging out in the Western world, and other close relatives are unlikely to assume their tasks, who replaces them? And if government support for the disabled population is subject to political vagaries, how will this be funded? The future financial planning indicated in the NAMI studies is of course only good for a highly limited population: those who can afford it. The world of aging caregivers is culturally and sociologically diverse, and caregivers are not necessarily represented by the primarily middle-class families in NAMI or Mental Health America. Most aging people with schizophrenia are poor. They rarely have a work history sufficient to rely on regular social security, and most must survive on reduced disability income. In the United States, the for-profit network of assisted living facilities where more aging people with schizophrenia are likely to live are usually unstimulating and inadequately supported by the mental health system. At most, patients may see a few visiting psychiatrists or have brief monthly medication evaluations at a mental health center. They also have too few resources for the type of interactive activities that often are available to older retirees.

Family members have in large part been excluded from the treatment system, and their caregiving skills are generally developed with little help from professionals. As the NAMI data show, their relatives with schizophrenia are insufficiently challenged to help with their own care. Many older persons with schizophrenia are unfamiliar with the idea of an interesting life. The later years might be more stimulating if the seeds had been sown early enough in their interactions with mental health professionals – in psychiatric rehabilitation or work development programs, or even in discussion groups, as well as therapy groups [21]. And many would benefit from participation in consumer network activities. These are networks of persons with a diagnosed mental illness who have outside activities and classes as part of the mental health system. These are now available with funding from many state mental health offices of consumer affairs. In the meantime, mental health systems should offer more outreach to aging caregivers of aging patients with schizophrenia, on the same level as caregivers for the dementias. For both populations, the need is great.

References

1. Nasar, S. (1998). *A Beautiful Mind: A Biography of John Forbes Nash*. New York: Simon & Schuster.

2. Saks, E.R. (2007). *The Center Cannot Hold: My Journey Through Madness*. New York: Hyperion.

3. Band-Winterstein, T., Avieli, H., Smeloy, Y. (2015). "He is still my son": aging and living in the shadow of an abusive adult child with mental disorder. In S.R. Maxwell, S.L. Blair (eds.), *Violence and Crime in the Family: Patterns, Causes, and Consequences*. (Contemporary Perspectives in Family Research, Volume 9). Bingley, UK: Emerald Groups Publishing Limited, 155–76.

4. Iglehart, J.K. (2016). Decriminalizing mental illness: the Miami model. *New England Journal of Medicine*, 374, 1701–3.

5. Ghose S., Greenberg, J. (2009). Aging fathers of adult children with schizophrenia: the toll of caregiving on their physical and mental health. *Psychiatric Services*, 60, 982–4.

6. Lefley, H.P. (1996). *Family Caregiving in Mental Illness*. Thousand Oaks, CA: Sage.

7. Lefley, H.P. (2010). Treating difficult cases in a psychoeducational family support group for serious mental illness. *Journal of Family Psychotherapy*, 21, 253–68.

8. Smith, G.C. (2003). Patterns and predictors of service use and unmet needs among aging families of adults with severe mental illness. *Psychiatric Services*, 54, 871–7.

9. Hatfield, A.B., Lefley, H.P. (2000). Helping elderly caregivers plan for the future care of a relative with mental illness. *Psychiatric Rehabilitaion Journal*, 24, 103–7.

10. Lefley, H.P., Hatfield, A.B. (1999). Helping parental caregivers and mental health

consumers cope with parental aging and loss. *Psychiatric Services*, 50, 369–75.

11. Stein, L., Test, M. (1980). Alternative to mental hospital treatment. *Archives of General Psychiatry*, 37, 392–7.

12. Lefley, H.P. (2010) Mental health systems in cross-cultural context. In T.L. Shcheid, T.N. Brown (eds.), *Handbook for the Study of Mental Health: Social Contexts, Theories, and Systems*. 2nd edn. New York: Cambridge University Press, 135–61.

13. Lam, P.C.W., Ng, P., Pan, J., Yung, D.W.K. (2015). Ways of coping of Chinese caregivers for family members with schizophrenia in two metropolitan cities: Guangzhou and Hong Kong, China. *International Journal of Social Psychiatry*, 61, 591–9.

14. Zeng, Y., Zhou, Y., Lin J. (2017). Perceived burden and quality of life in Chinese caregivers of people with serious mental illness: a comparison cross-sectional survey. *Perspectives in Psychiatric Care*, 53, 183–9.

15. Chadda, R.K. (2014). Caring for the family caregivers of persons with mental illness. *Indian Journal of Psychiatry*, 56, 221.

16. Von Kardoff, E., Soltaninejad, A., Kamali, M., Eslami Shahrbabaki, M. (2016). Family caregiver burden in mental illnesses: the case of affective disorders and schizophrenia: a qualitative exploratory study. *Nordic Journal of Psychiatry*, 70, 248–54.

17. Hatfield, A.B. *Planning for the Future Care of Relatives with Mental Illnesses*. Baltimore: Maryland Department of Health and Mental Hygiene.

18. Meriden. (2017). *The Meriden Family Programme. Meriden*, (2017). 4(4), 19.

19. Lefley, H.P. *Family Psychoeducation for Serious Mental Illness*. (Evidence-Based Practice Series: V.1.) New York: Oxford University Press.

20. Dixon, L., McFarlane, W.R., Lefley, H., et al. (2001). Evidence-based practices for services to families of people with psychiatric disabilites. *Psychiatric Services*, 52, 903–10.

21. Lefley, H.P. (2009). A psychoeducational support group for persons with serious mental illness. *Journal for Specialists in Group Work*, 34, 369–81.

16 Personal Accounts of Living with Schizophrenia across a Lifetime: Coping Strategies and Subjective Perspectives

Tova Band-Winterstein, Ph.D., Hila Avieli, Ph.D., and Peli Mushkin

Studies within the medical, psychological, and gerontological traditions have established that aging is not a uniform process, meaning that people tend to age differently, and that within the same individual, different organs and systems change with age at varied rates [1]. This non-uniformity is even more striking in aging individuals with schizophrenia (AIWS). Most studies point out that for these individuals, aging is associated with a moderate improvement in psychotic symptoms, a reduction in psychiatric relapses and better self-management [2]. On the other hand, with age often comes an increase in negative symptoms, resulting in a "flat" affect, a lack of ability to begin and sustain activities, reduced social interactions, and self-neglect [3–6]. However, a recent review provides cumulative data from cross-sectional and longitudinal studies, suggesting that this common notion – of reduced positive symptoms and increased negative symptoms – does not accurately reflect aging with regard to schizophrenia. Therefore, schizophrenia in later life cannot be conceptualized as a quiescent or stable end-state, but rather one of fluctuating symptoms and varying levels of functioning [7]. Thus, the non-unified and ever-changing nature of schizophrenia in later life often leads to certain gaps and a general sense of ambiguity in the growing body of knowledge regarding AIWS. Therefore, the voices of AIWS themselves and their personal experiences during this stage of life may provide a broader perspective of the phenomenon.

Subjective accounts of aging with schizophrenia

There is a growing consensus that to fully appreciate life with schizophrenia, research must go beyond the symptoms and the diagnosis in order to better understand the full spectrum of human experience, including knowledge of the hardships and joys of those who experience it first hand [8,9]. Subjective accounts can provide an in-depth understanding regarding AIWS' insight and conceptualization of their own situation. Studies focusing on personal accounts of AIWS reveal that many are preoccupied with questions regarding the cause of their illness. However, while numerous causal explanations of schizophrenia have been proposed over the years, each inspired by a different academic tradition [10], only a few have presented AIWS' self-etiology of the illness [11–13]. These self-etiologies are usually considerably different from outsiders' explanations. Yet, understanding them is important because they might influence the individual's preferences and expectations regarding the course of the illness or the treatment [14], as well as promote help-seeking behaviors [15] and compliance with the treatment [16]. Another issue that often comes up in subjective accounts as being central to AIWS' lives is day-to-day coping and the development of an overall coping strategy [17]. This issue was addressed by several studies that deliberated between two general coping strategies: *active* or *behavior-focused coping* (e.g., seeking new treatment methods) and *passive* or *avoidant coping* (e.g., ignoring the symptoms) [18–20].

However, subjective accounts of coping reveal a more complex picture. Intertwined with the sense of sadness and loss, AIWS narrate a continued sense of hope and an active search to achieve and maintain the valued social roles of adulthood. These narratives are expressed through a striving to achieve independent living, work in the community, and plan for the future, to ensure they will not be left helpless and alone when their family members can no longer care for them [17,21].

Finally, the attempt to engage in a meaning-making process is common to many aging individuals, including AIWS. Previous studies, taking an objective viewpoint, revealed lifelong deprivation due to poverty, abandonment, and drug use [22], decreased quality of life [23], and social isolation in old age [24]. However, these aspects of schizophrenia, often highlighted by other research traditions, may present a broken and fragmented reality, and poorly reflect the holistic experience of trying to unravel the meaning of living with life-long mental illness. Interviews with AIWS regarding their subjective experience uncover a vast array of retrospective reflections about the meaning of life with schizophrenia, which accumulate over time and shape these individuals' golden years. Some of these elderly individuals depict intense and multidimensional suffering, while others describe an enhanced ability to enjoy life [25,26].

Despite the importance of introducing AIWS' narratives into the research, the inclusion of an insider perspective in the existing literature is scarce [27,28]. Recently, some qualitative studies have focused on AIWS experience, emphasizing various aspects of this phenomenon, including older women's experience of schizophrenia [29], functional abilities [30], homelessness [22], and AIWS' dignity and identity [31].

This chapter will attempt to broaden the perspective on the subjective experience of AIWS, and hopefully provide an added value to the theoretical framework of aging and schizophrenia. Thus, it explores three major issues that continually emerged throughout the AIWS's narratives: Why did this happen to me? How do I cope? What does it all mean for me?

Methodological notes

Schizophrenia and aging are two bodies of knowledge that benefit from the direct accounts of the people experiencing these processes. Therefore, we chose to apply the phenomenological principle that sentiments, responses, and actions are informed by social location [32].

The AIWS participants were purposefully selected by criterion sampling in order to obtain the broadest interpretive information possible from the AIWS [32]. Sampling included 18 participants, 11 men and 7 women, current age over 60, diagnosed with schizophrenia spectrum disorders before the age of 40, living in the community, with adequate verbal, cognitive, and mental state capacities to respond to face-to-face in-depth interviews. The participants' ages ranged from 60 to 69 years, with a mean age of 63. Most of the participants were single or divorced at the time of the interviews and were living in community supported housing, while others were employed in sheltered settings. The final sample size (18 participants) was determined according to Morse's principle of theoretical saturation [33].

Data collection included in-depth interviews and was based on an interview guide [34,35]. The interview guide included four content areas and key subjects. One focused on the participant and his/her family ties in the past and present (sample item: "Tell us about yourself"). The second dealt with everyday life with schizophrenia, in which the participants were asked, for example, to describe their daily life and how it has changed over the years. The third centered on aging with schizophrenia (sample item: "When you think about your age and schizophrenia, what comes to mind?"). The fourth area addressed the topic of well-being, old age, and schizophrenia – a retrospective viewpoint (sample item: "How do you perceive your quality of life at this stage of your life?").

Content analysis of the transcribed interviews was performed by a team of researchers experienced in qualitative methodology. As an initial step, transcripts were read from a phenomenological perspective allowing for an in-depth acquaintance with the text. Second, the data were coded and grouped according to meanings relevant to the study aim, and conceptualized into unique theoretical categories. Third, major themes were organized by means of a transition from the theoretical to the interpretative level. The analysis provided us with new information about AIWS and revealed several key themes underlining the experience of aging with schizophrenia. We have chosen some of these themes and examined them in this chapter generating explanations for their illness, the impact of their illness on their life stories, and making life meaningful with advancing age.

Narrating schizophrenia: "Why did this happen to me?"

After years of living with and experiencing schizophrenia, individuals tend to narrate their life stories in a way that enables them to accept the illness and the way it has shaped their lives. In contrast to the "empirical truth," their experience includes various subjective narratives. The first is narrated as general mantras and popular beliefs, such as:

> It leaves you to your fate, it does not ask you... we believe that you are thrown into the "movie" of your life and it tells you that's how it's going to be, whether you like it or not... Now, I know that this life is all [a matter of] Fate.
>
> from [13] with permission of Taylor & Francis Ltd, www.tandfonline.com

Another narrative refers to the external attribution of superstitions such as:

> I think I've been hexed... I think that's why I'm sick... They put something in my coffee... they gave me an amulet. It lasted for two and a half years... then its power wore off.
>
> from [13] with permission of Taylor & Francis Ltd, www.tandfonline.com

This participant, in this stage of life, seeks a coherent explanation that will assist him to understand the nature of his illness.

Another way of narrating the illness relates to the belief in "reward and punishment":

> I'll tell you the truth, I've sinned... Nothing's gone right for me... I've cursed God and denounced Him. I've sinned against Him, heaven forbid. Now that I am old, I'm sure He'll forgive me one day, so that I can go to Heaven.
>
> from [13] with permission of Taylor & Francis Ltd, www.tandfonline.com

Finally, some narratives are based on actual facts and events that took place during the life course of the individual with schizophrenia. However, the structure of these narratives does not necessarily have a coherent cause and effect, for example:

> So, my wife left me... and she took the kids, and I didn't see them... not since they were 13... I would see them for half an hour and then they'd be gone... difficult, very difficult. I loved them so much... that's why I became sick.
>
> from [13] with permission of Taylor & Francis Ltd, www.tandfonline.com

In line with these illustrations, it seems that AIWS attempt to construct their own self-etiology regarding the illness, in order to make sense and attribute meaning to a lifetime of having to cope with schizophrenia.

Schizophrenia: figure or background and coping with lifelong mental illness

These subjective ways of narrating the illness lead AIWS to develop the two major coping strategies that can best serve their narratives. The first strategy is anchored in a basic assumption that the illness is a central constituent overshadowing life, while the second strategy views the illness as an entity that does not necessarily involve or impact other aspects of one's life story.

"The illness controls me": schizophrenia as the essence of life

Schizophrenia, when perceived as the essence of life, has an all-encompassing hold over one's life, and is subjectively described as an all-consuming factor. In this case, it prevents AIWS from establishing and maintaining social ties, thus strengthening avoidance behaviors:

> I don't have any friends..., at work also, I can't... the illness won't let me... the illness controls me – that's the problem. It controls me, so that I'll be afraid to go to people's houses... I can't be in touch with a man... now there is no option of getting married or even dating. No relationships...

Another way in which schizophrenia becomes a central component in life is clearly illustrated by another participant, who narrates a life that is so intensively focused on the illness that it almost "colors" his entire being.

This is manifested in extreme emotional outbursts and heartrending feelings that leave no emotional resources for anything else:

> It started when I was in the ninth grade, that was the first time, and since then, it has gotten worse and worse. I would sit down and cry, feel horrible... I couldn't go to school; I used to blow up at my mother. I was hospitalized for three months in a psychiatric facility and received treatment. Since then, this has been my life. I get hospitalized every time I don't feel well. It's hard to function like this, hard to work, hard to live like this.

"I'm a strong person...": living life while managing schizophrenia

The second strategy is based on not viewing schizophrenia as a dominant force that impacts and shapes all aspects of life, but rather as a sort of background "noise," which does not prevent AIWS from finding ways of being in the world, despite the illness. This strategy enables the AIWS to reflect upon their lives and appreciate other aspects of it, as illustrated in the following quotes:

> *For an ill person, with all the medication I take, I do a lot with my life. Not everyone gardens twice a week and studies computers, and I'm still going strong... a person must function! I've had hard times before and I overcame them... I have an enormous amount of strength and a strong sense of endurance. If I want help, I help myself; there is no one else to help me... I want to be amongst the living, and this takes effort. This is life and a man should deal with things as they are. Crying or having people feel sorry for me won't help. I don't want to drift away from life. I think of the present and hope for the best. I insist on functioning. If I didn't, I would spend all my life in a hospital.*

In this quote, the participant reflects upon the notion that he needs strength to overcome the hardships of the illness and avoid being an object of others' pity. Another way of gaining control over the illness is illustrated in the following quote:

> *I know what's right and what's wrong when it comes to the illness ... I've been in control of it for a long time now. I've suffered for years. Now I'm in control ... I manage on my own, carry out my daily routines; I even help others to overcome (their difficulties)...*
>
> from [36] with permission of SAGE Publications

It seems that at this specific stage of their life, the AIWS tend to reflect on the role schizophrenia plays in their lives. While some of them emphasize its centrality, others are able to function in spite of it.

Between adversity and personal growth: meaning-making and aging with schizophrenia

Old age retrospectively enables AIWS to try to achieve a sense of closure by bridging the gap between lifelong experiences of adversity and present experiences of growth. In other words, the subjective experience of schizophrenia along the life course is narrated as a multidimensional cumulative form of suffering, consisting of physical and mental agony, and losses regarding several major life domains. On the other hand, old age may also provide a "window of opportunity" for some AIWS to finally live a "normal" life.

Lifelong experiences of adversity

The different dimensions of adversity that emerged from the participants' narratives include: social and familial rejection; the harsh symptoms accompanying schizophrenia, the hardships of hospitalization and the side effects of medication; loss of employment and independent accommodation; and the loss of hope of ever being a partner and a parent. The following phrases and quotes illustrate these diverse forms of adversity:

> *I tried talking to people. Only junkies agreed to accept me. The neighbors cut off all ties with me because I harassed them. They wouldn't open their doors to me. I went over to a payphone and sat there, I slept out in the street; I talked to a lot of people in the streets, and collected cigarette stamps... (Silence) I felt very miserable... who could ever want me? They threw me out like garbage...*
>
> from [26] with permission of Elsevier

While this participant emphasizes the tragic loss of social ties, another participant describes his familial losses:

> *I've been through hell; I swear, I wouldn't wish this on anybody, and always alone, all alone. My mother was here once for a day and then ran off, she told me being with me was torture... I went over to my parents' house once and they threw me out... My mother is 84, I don't acknowledge her as my mother; when she dies, I won't go to her funeral. I got nothing from her, nothing, no money, no nothing, it's like I have a mother, but I don't have a mother...*
>
> from [26] with permission of Elsevier

The third quote illustrates the harsh personal price of losing one's family ties and family life:

> *He found somebody else, because of all the treatment I went through, he couldn't deal with it anymore... I came back home after a month-and-a-half in the hospital, and [he was gone]. He just left without saying a word... I have two kids; my son comes over sometimes, but my daughter isn't in touch. I haven't seen her since the holidays. I gave her trouble then... and she hasn't come over since ...*

All of the participants emphasized feelings of being marginalized, betrayed, and stigmatized by family and friends. They describe complex and fickle social interactions that characterize the nature of their existence. It seems that this subjective voice mirrors the difficulties AIWS confront when they come into contact with society.

In addition to the above, AIWS describe the adversity connected to the illness's symptoms:

> *I always have bad thoughts... especially about her cheating on me; I hear voices... bad things... He tells me bad things that I cannot bear to hear ... All these voices give me a terrible headache... It's not just a headache... It's like a wound in my head...*
>
> from [26] with permission of Elsevier

While this participant describes his positive symptoms, the following quote refers to another set of symptoms that cause severe adversity:

> *I lost weight, I weighed 40 kg. I couldn't eat or sleep... I had horrible visions of myself dying... I used to hide under the beds; I had horrible fears that I was going to die. I wanted very much to commit suicide...I was afraid to fall asleep and not wake up anymore....*

The following quotes emphasize medication side effects:

> *Five mg of Artan in the morning, 11 mg at noon, combined with Assival. It makes me sleepy, it makes me feel weak, and it drives me crazy. But that's what the doctor told me to do... In the morning, I can't get up for work. I barely wake up, and when I do – I'm in a bad mood... I feel empty...*
>
> from [26] with permission of Elsevier

Finally, narrating a long history of hospitalizations is described as a major source of distress:

> *They hospitalized me, by force, four or five times... what can I tell you? They made me feel like a doormat over there. They put me in a closed psychiatric ward in the hospital together with criminals and junkies. They just killed me...*
>
> from [26] with permission of Elsevier

The subjective perspective of schizophrenia is experienced as a type of torture that includes cumulative physical pain and agony, accompanied by feelings of helplessness, worthlessness, and de-humanization. Moreover, the loss of employment and the lack of ability to live an independent lifestyle are perceived negatively by AIWS. They feel as if the illness has "robbed" them of every opportunity to fulfill their professional and personal ideals. As a result, this lack becomes a major source of disappointment, frustration, and suffering:

> I was studying Medicine, but I dropped out when I became ill...now I work four hours a day in sheltered employment...

from [26] with permission of Elsevier

> I failed at everything I tried... I can't be a carpenter because I can't concentrate, I forget everything...
> I wish I was free in my own home ...I don't really feel free living in the hostel...

from [26] with permission of Elsevier

An additional level of hardship is expressed in the recognition that IAWS express regarding their loss of hope at ever being a partner or a parent:

> ... It's sad, very sad; no one should live without love... It's hard, it's annoying that I have no love... .... Here everyone loves me (the staff of the sheltered house). It's love, but not like the love between a husband and a wife. This is the hardest thing for people with schizophrenia, the greatest tragedy...

from [26] with permission of Elsevier

Unfulfilled intimate relationships are exacerbated by the loss of never having experienced parenthood:

> I was pregnant, but I aborted my child. I was 38 years old... I panicked – how was I going to be a mother with my anxieties? My child would probably have been taken away from me... I freaked out and told the doctor that I wanted to have an abortion... I told myself he would have turned out to be mentally ill because of my fears... Now I feel very jealous of healthy people; they get love and marriage and children. Only I am alone...

To sum up our discussion of the difficulties faced by AIWS in their daily lives, the participants have a long list of losses which they mourn. This list begins with the loss of their social life and a general experience of social rejection. Then there are the physical and emotional side effects of the disease, including feelings of shame, embarrassment, and low self-esteem. Another major item on this list is the loss of love, expressed as a central theme, which appears on several levels: the family of origin level, the partnership and intimate relationship level, and the future parental experience level. The notion that the illness has deprived and continues to deprive these AIWS of living and experiencing life fully is expressed by feelings of jealousy, sadness, and a resounding sense of missed opportunity.

Present experiences of growth

Experiencing old age leads to new and unique reflection among AIWS regarding life and its meaning. Some of the participants perceived this current chapter in their lives as a window of opportunity – a way to experience life as it is experienced by healthy people. This is described by viewing old age as a positive period, which can provide AIWS with a new quality of life and generate fresh self-perceptions – as individuals and valuable members of the mainstream community. This perception was expressed through the following topics: A balanced course of the illness, as a basis for quality of life in old age; Self-fulfillment as promoting quality of life; Experiencing a sense of belonging; and Aging as an opportunity for normalization.

A more balanced and manageable course of the illness in old age was described by some of the participants. Relying on drugs is a normative phenomenon that characterizes many aging people. Thus, in old age, this common habit of taking medication suddenly makes AIWS feel they are part of a large group of people living with chronic conditions, which can be endured like any other illness. At this point in their lives, participants reported being aware of the specific symptoms of their illness, but seemed confident that they could control the symptoms by using medication, just like any other patient with a chronic illness. Such meaning-making provides a sense of normalization for the AIWS:

> It's not that bad. You live with it, like diabetes, like any other illness ... the pills are like crutches, they hold you up ... some people have diabetes, others have high cholesterol, high blood pressure, and just like everyone else, we have our pills... sometimes I have annoying thoughts, especially at night; I take my pills and they go away. I take Klonex, SeroquSat and Clopicsol [to alleviate] my fears; they are like glasses or crutches for me ... I love the pills ... they are very helpful...

> from [36] with permission of SAGE Publications

Regarding quality of life in old age, the participants described the life domains through which they promote their well-being. Some have achieved self-realization and self-fulfillment through occupation and self-expression, others through creativity and artwork. The participants are able to rejuvenate skills that were lost during the acute phases of their illness. In some cases, this "renaissance" may even be recognized and admired by themselves and others.

> Sometimes I go to painting class and other times I go to music class... yes, I'm an artist, the artist in my family. Next month, I'm going to have my own exhibition at the museum... I'm already handing out invitations. I've been waiting for five months to have this exhibition, I have about 50 paintings already... I've been painting for two years now and they treat me well over there... the art teacher talks about my work quite a bit, and the girl in the reception is nice to me... I'm happy; I like it there

> from [36] with permission of SAGE Publications

The following quote demonstrates the subjective experience of being a central figure in hostel life, accompanied by feelings of self-efficacy and self-confidence. In this stage of life, some participants find themselves in positions where they are able to share their life experience and wisdom, by acting as mentors to others living with schizophrenia. Acquiring a sense of social status is both rewarding and satisfying, as illustrated in this quote:

> I'm the "on call" person here at the hostel and the guys here really love me. They come around to sit and have coffee with me; they come from all the different apartments in the hostel just to sit here in the garden with me. A guy who I met a while ago told me he didn't want to go to a hostel, so I invited him to come here, to my hostel. I told him it was nice here and he would get good food. Now he tells me he is here because of me. "You are my father here in the hostel" he tells me (laughs)...

Experiencing a sense of belonging is another aspect of personal growth in the lives of the AIWS. After years of hospitalization and the everyday reality of the illness creating a sense of distance and alienation from their families of origin, now they find comfort in living in the family-like environment of a hostel or an assisted living residence, as an alternative to a genuine family life. This format allows for a feeling of safety and belonging, on the one hand, and of personal space, on the other:

> I get up, I drink my coffee, I go to work. I come home beat, watch TV, eat and read the Bible. I listen to radio programs with my roommate. Each one of us has her own thing – one likes to cook, the other does the laundry, just like in an ordinary family. Once I get home to the apartment, I just want to stay in...

Comparing a deterministic perspective of being a chronic patient with a mental disorder with the actual subjective experiences of "normality" in AIWS' narratives reveals that aging is experienced as a kind of miracle – the miracle of reaching a ripe, old age against all odds. For these participants, reaching old age itself is both a victory and a life achievement. Whereas normative people who reach old age tend to emphasize its disadvantages, the study participants welcomed aging as a sign of normality. This enabled them to embrace and enjoy old age:

> I suffered physically and mentally from hardcore schizophrenia – and now I'm strong. I'm a lucky man; lucky to be alive, lucky I'm not dead, it's so good to live ... Thank God, many die at younger ages and I have lived to be an old man. It's good to be alive. Yes, I'm happy to get old, I'm not afraid of it... I didn't believe I would live to see this age. It's a miracle. Despite everything that's happened to me, I've reached this age...
>
> from [36] with permission of SAGE Publications

Aging individuals with schizophrenia: searching for a voice

The experience of living and aging with schizophrenia provides an "insider" perspective that is not necessarily compatible with the "outside" views about schizophrenia. In this chapter, we have tried to present personal accounts of living with schizophrenia across a lifetime through biography, life changes, and subjectivity, including a sense of recovery and growth, as well as adversity. This heterogeneous picture has enabled us to depict AIWS' everyday life at this stage, which is not possible using traditional quantitative methods. This echoes Heidegger's view of the phenomenological perspective that provides us with the "sense of being there" based on "the things themselves" [37]. Narrating the causes of the illness, coping strategies, and the subjective perspectives of personal growth and endurance [13,30] corresponds with the recovery model of mental illness [38]. The recovery model states that the meaning-making process and self-advocacy, which are perceived as important in promoting AIWS' quality of life, are also significant in the recovery process [39]. This approach also focuses on the lived experiences and insights of people with mental illness, stressing the importance of personal identities beyond the constraints imposed by psychiatric diagnosis [40].

The literature suggests that people tend to seek an "identity" for their illness [41,42]. When the identity suggested by the medical establishment does not resonate well with their subjective experiences, they continue to seek "alternative identities," which they perceive as more compelling [43]. In other words, the "logical truth" – based on consistent and coherent correlations between cause and effect [43] and which are embedded in the psychiatric regime – is not always compatible with the "metaphysical truth" of AIWS, which reflects various subjective narratives [44].

While old age is sometimes described as a period of hardship and decline, due to physiological, functional, and social changes, for AIWS this stage of life provides a sense of normality, as old age brings about a more balanced illness management regime. Moreover, we found that reaching old age is perceived by AIWS as a sort of "miracle," as this is the first generation of individuals with schizophrenia that actually enjoys longevity similar to the general population. For some of these AIWS, the notion of old age provides an opportunity to view life as an integrated whole, comprised of successfully enduring the many adversities, whilst also enjoying a stage of late blooming. Being able to reflect, look back upon life's major events and trajectories, and reevaluate the meaning attributed to these events [45] is all part of the natural process of "life review" [46,47].

"Life review" refers to the attempt made by aging people to organize their lives according to certain consecutive themes, enabling them to resolve conflicts, deal with the notion of death, and create a better understanding of past events, by emphasizing some events and blurring the meaning of others. Life review has become increasingly common, particularly with elderly persons, as a therapeutic method of reestablishing meaning and promoting self-worth [48]. It seems that AIWS look back on their lives and achievements within the framework of a society that sanctifies health, productivity, and independence and in which stigmatization and social rejection is the prevailing norm regarding adults with disabilities, such as a mental disorder [49]. In this context, they attempt to devote this stage of their lives to reconstructing a life story that may lead to a more peaceful sense of closure.

Note

Quotations not assigned to any reference are from interviews conducted by the chapter's authors and have not previously been published.

References

1. P.B. Baltes and M.M. Baltes. Psychological perspectives on successful aging: the model of selective optimization with compensation. In *Successful Aging: Perspectives from the Behavioral Sciences*, ed. P.B. Baltes and M.M. Baltes, Cambridge, UK: Cambridge University Press, 1990: 1–34.

2. D.V. Jeste, C.A. Depp, and I.V. Vahia. Successful cognitive and emotional aging. *World Psychiatry* 2010; 9(2): 78–84.

3. C.I. Cohen. Outcome of schizophrenia into later life: an overview. *Gerontologist* 1990; 30: 790–7.

4. S. Karim, R. Overshott, and A. Burns. Older people with chronic schizophrenia. *Aging and Mental Health* 2005; 9(4): 315–24.

5. T.H. McGlashan and J.O. Johannessen. Early detection and intervention with schizophrenia: rationale. *Schizophrenia Bulletin* 1996; 22(2): 201–22.

6. J. Bobes, C. Arango, M. Garcia-Garcia, et al. Prevalence of negative symptoms in outpatients with schizophrenia spectrum disorders treated with antipsychotics in routine clinical practice: findings from the CLAMORS study. *Journal of Clinical Psychiatry* 2010; 71(3): 280.

7. C.I. Cohen, P.D. Meesters, and J. Zhao. New perspectives on schizophrenia in later life: implications for treatment, policy, and research. *Lancet Psychiatry* 2015; 2(4): 340–50.

8. E.H. Flanagan, L. Davidson, and J. S. Strauss. Issues for DSM-V: incorporating

patients' subjective experiences. *American Journal of Psychiatry* 2007; **164**(3): 391–2.

9.   J.S. Strauss. Prognosis in schizophrenia and the role of subjectivity. *Schizophrenia Bulletin* 2008; **34**(2): 201–3.

10. E. Walker, L. Kestler, A. Bollini, et al. Schizophrenia: etiology and course. *Annual Review of Psychology* 2003; **55**: 401–30.

11. B. Williams and D. Healy. Perceptions of illness causation among new referrals to a community mental health team: "explanatory model" or "exploratory map"? *Social Science and Medicine* 2001; **53**: 465–76.

12. A.E.Z. Baker and N.G. Procter. A qualitative inquiry into consumer beliefs about the causes of mental illness. *Journal of Psychiatric and Mental Health Nursing* 2013; **20**(5): 442–7.

13. T. Araten-Bergman, H. Avieli, P. Mushkin, et al. How aging individuals with schizophrenia experience the self-etiology of their illness: a reflective lifeworld research approach. *Aging and Mental Health* 2016; **20**(11): 1147–56.

14. S.R. Khalsa, K.S. McCarthy, B.A. Sharpless, et al. Beliefs about the causes of depression and treatment preferences. *Journal of Clinical Psychology* 2011; **67**(6): 539–49.

15. S. Sheikh and A. Furnham. A cross-cultural study of mental health beliefs and attitudes towards seeking professional help. *Social Psychiatry and Psychiatric Epidemiology* 2000; **35**(7): 326–34.

16. K. Bhui and D. Bhugra. Explanatory models for mental distress: implications for clinical practice research. *British Journal of Psychiatry* 2002; **181**: 6–7.

17. C.H. Stein and V.A. Wemmerus. Searching for a normal life: personal accounts of adults with schizophrenia, their parents and well-siblings. *American Journal of Community Psychology* 2001; **29**(5): 725–46.

18. N.H. Solano and S.K. Whitbourne, Coping with schizophrenia: patterns in later adulthood. *International Journal of Aging and Human Development* 2001; **53**(1): 1–10.

19. C. Barrowclough, K.K.L. Berry, E.E.J. Byrne, and N. Purandare. Coping processes in older people with schizophrenia: an investigation of appraisals, coping and social support in patients and non-clinical controls. *Social Psychiatry and Psychiatric Epidemiology* 2006; **41**(4): 280–4.

20. C.I. Cohen, S.K. Hassamal, and N. Begum. General coping strategies and their impact on quality of life in older adults with schizophrenia. *Schizophrenia Research* 2011; **127**(1): 223–8.

21. L.P. Ogden. "My Life as it is has Value": A Narrative Approach to Understanding Life Course Experiences of Older Adults with Schizophrenia. Doctoral thesis, Columbia University, 2012.

22. T. Shibusawa and D. Padgett. The experiences of "aging" among formerly homeless adults with chronic mental illness: a qualitative study. *Journal of Aging Studies* 2009; **23**: 188–96.

23. S.J. Bartels and S. Pratt. Psychosocial rehabilitation and quality of life for older adults with serious mental illness: recent findings and future research directions. *Current Opinion in Psychiatry* 2009; **22**: 381–5.

24. L. Magliano, A. Fiorillo, C. Malangone, et al. Social network in long-term diseases: a comparative study in relatives of persons with schizophrenia and physical illnesses versus a sample from the general population. *Social Science and Medicine* 2006; **62**(6): 1392–402.

25. B.W. Palmer, A.S. Martin, C.A. Depp, et al. Wellness within illness: happiness in schizophrenia. *Schizophrenia Research* 2014; **159**(1): 151–6.

26. H. Avieli, P. Mushkin, T. Araten-Bergman, et al. Aging with schizophrenia: a lifelong experience of multidimensional losses and suffering. *Archives of Psychiatric Nursing* 2016; **30**(2): 230–6.

27. E.B. Larsen and J. Gerlach. Subjective experience of treatment, side-effects,

mental state and quality of life in chronic schizophrenic out-patients treated with depot neuroleptics. *Acta Psychiatrica Scandinavica* 1996; **93**(5): 381–8.

28. G. Higginbottom and P. Liamputtong (eds.) *Participatory Qualitative Research Methodologies in Health.* Thousand Oaks, CA: Sage, 2015.

29. W. Pentland, G. Miscio, S. Eastabrook, et al. Aging women with schizophrenia. *Psychiatric Rehabilitation Journal* 2003; **26**: 290–302.

30. S. Shepherd, C.A. Depp, G. Harris, et al. Perspectives on schizophrenia over the lifespan: a qualitative study. *Schizophrenia Bulletin* 2012; **38**: 295–303.

31. G. Martinsson, I. Fagerberg, C. Lindholm, et al. Struggling for existence: life situation experiences of older persons with mental disorders. *International Journal of Qualitative Studies on Health and Well-being* 2012; **7**(1): 18422.

32. M.Q. Patton. *Qualitative Research and Evaluation Methods*, 3rd edn. Thousand Oaks, CA: Sage, 2002.

33. J.M. Morse. Determining sample size. *Qualitative Health Research* 2000; **10**: 3–5.

34. S. Kvale. The 1,000-page question. *Qualitative Inquiry* 1996; **2**(3): 275–84.

35. D.K. Padgett. *Qualitative Methods in Social Work Research*, Thousand Oaks, CA: Sage Publications, 2016.

36. P. Mushkin, T. Band-Winterstein, and H. Avieli. "Like every normal person": like every normal person?! The paradoxical effect of aging with schizophrenia. *Qualitative Health Research* 2018; **28**(6): 977–86.

37. M. Heidegger. What is metaphysics? *Basic Writings*, New York, NY: Routledge, 1993: 89–110.

38. K.S. Jacob. Insight in psychosis: an independent predictor of outcome or an explanatory model of illness? *Asian Journal of Psychiatry* 2014; **11**: 65–71.

39. M. Leamy, V. Bird, C. Le Boutillier, et al. Conceptual framework for personal recovery in mental health: systematic review and narrative synthesis. *British Journal of Psychiatry* 2011; **199**(6): 445–52.

40. R. Andresen, L G. Oades, and P. Caputi. *Psychological Recovery: Beyond Mental Illness.* Chichester, UK: John Wiley & Sons, 2011.

41. H. Leventhal and D. Nerenz. The assessment of illness cognition. In *Measurement Strategies in Health Psychology*, ed. P. Karoly. New York: John Wiley, 1985.

42. D.A. Karp. Illness ambiguity and the search for meaning. *Journal of Contemporary Ethnography* 1992; **21**(2): 139–70.

43. Y.S. Lincoln and E.G. Guba. *Naturalistic Inquiry*, Thousand Oaks, CA: Sage, 1985.

44. F. Correia and B. Schnieder (eds.) *Metaphysical Grounding: Understanding the Structure of Reality.* Cambridge, UK: Cambridge University Press, 2012.

45. G. T. Reker, J. Birren, and C. Svensson. Restoring, maintaining, and enhancing personal meaning in life through autobiographical methods. In *The Human Quest for Meaning: Theories, Research, and Applications.* New York, NY: Routledge, 2013: 383–408.

46. M. Beaver. Life review/reminiscent therapy. In *Serving the Elderly*, ed P. Kim. New York, NY: Aldine DeGruyter, 1991: 67–88.

47. R.N. Butler. The life review: an interpretation of reminiscence in the aged. In *New Thoughts on Old Age*. Berlin Heidelberg: Springer, 196: 265–80.

48. J.E. Birren and K.N. Cochran. *Telling the Stories of Life through Guided Autobiography Groups.* Baltimore, MD: Taylor & Francis, 2001.

49. M. Oliver and C. Barnes. *Disabled People and Social Policy: From Exclusion to Inclusion.* London, UK: Addison Wesley Longman, 1998.

The Care of Older Adults with Schizophrenia in Developing Countries

17

Rujvi Kamat, Ph.D., and Samir T. Mukherjee, M.D.

Introduction

Prevalence estimates of schizophrenia from studies in developing countries vary from a low of 0.07 per thousand reported in Vietnam to a high of 5.7 per thousand in Swaziland [1]. As life expectancy has increased globally, the global burden of severe mental illness has also increased. A disproportionate burden of geriatric mental illness is borne by the developing world. World Health Organization estimates suggest that by 2025, 75% of the world's older adult population will live in developing countries [2]. Recent estimates suggest that 10 million older adults are expected to be living with schizophrenia by 2050 [3]. Compared to the general population, as people with schizophrenia age, they suffer from increased and premature medical comorbidity and mortality [4]. Older adults with schizophrenia are at greater risk for poor physical outcomes and may have premorbid mild cognitive impairment that persists throughout life. Taken together, there are growing data to suggest that this segment of the population has unique trajectories for aging and psychiatric illness. This is particularly true for older adults with schizophrenia in developing countries.

In this chapter we will address the following questions:

1. What is the global burden of schizophrenia in older adults?
2. What are the specific challenges and priorities in improving schizophrenia-related services for older adults in developing countries?
3. Globally, how do folk and family-based treatments and allopathic medical services compete and coexist?
4. How can novel approaches to leverage information and computer technologies be introduced and used to serve this population in a culturally sensitive manner?

Schizophrenia across cultures

Schizophrenia is a global disorder; estimates suggest that the prevalence per 1000 persons is 3.05 in the least developed countries and 5.7 in emerging-economy countries. Developed countries are estimated to have a prevalence of 5.8 per 1000 persons [5]. Although it is present in every country, the symptoms and presentation are conceptualized differently across cultures. There have been numerous cultural-comparative studies that have examined differences in positive and negative symptoms of schizophrenia across societies. For instance, visual and tactile hallucinations are reportedly more common in patients from Africa and the Near East [6] compared to patients in European regions. Bauer et al. [6]

posited that the higher prevalence of visual hallucinations in patients with schizophrenia in non-Western societies might be related to the cognitive styles and perceived etiology of the illness. In non-Western cultures, somatic, or nutritive factors may be thought to cause the symptoms, whereas in Western societies, the symptom onset is thought to be related to elevated emotional stress. There is some evidence to suggest that negative symptoms are experienced similarly across cultures, but their impact on functioning may depend on the demands placed by the cultural context within which the patient lives [7].

In nearly every society, regardless of theories that the population holds about the etiology, symptoms, or consequences of schizophrenia, the disorder is highly stigmatized. In some societies, "madness" is thought to be contagious or passed through a family. The patient and family may be shunned by their community. In some cultures, patients may be regarded as possessed or ill, but still cared for and included in community activities. Stigma may lead to isolation and neglect. For instance, studies from India have frequently reported that stigma might affect women more than men, and that such stigma serves as a profound barrier to seeking care in this population.

A review of the literature regarding schizophrenia across cultures suggests that stigma and the competing and conflicting explanatory models of mental illness contribute to the course of the illness as well as the extent to which treatments are used by the patient [8]. Some authors have suggested that health-seeking behavior may also be affected by other factors such as religious beliefs, mind–body distinction, and tendency for somatization [9–11]. Individuals with severe mental illness in Asia, for instance, have greater levels of family involvement that is persistent and intense [12]. For individuals and families dealing with schizophrenia, differing explanations for their distress contribute to the conflict experienced in the help-seeking stage of the illness [13]. Typically, individuals in these societies seek help from traditional healers prior to entering the modern medicine system [14]. When patients' social and psychiatric functioning improves in response to treatment, there appears to be a change in the community's perception of schizophrenia from a non-medical/mystical etiology to a medical etiology [8].

Schizophrenia in older adults

Assuming a 0.5% prevalence of schizophrenia in persons over the age of 60, approximately 10 million older adults are expected to be living with schizophrenia by 2050 [3]. The greatest burden of care for older adults with schizophrenia will likely be borne by developing countries, where the increase in life-span and population size is most prominent. As these countries become increasingly urbanized, there is a change in social structures and family dynamics that leaves older adults (especially those with a severe mental illness) at risk for isolation and abandonment [15,16].

As a group, older schizophrenia patients include individuals who have had the disorder for most of their lives, as well as those whose onset of the illness was later in life. The late-onset group is thought to include individuals with onset between the ages of 40 and 60 years, and the very-late-onset group comprises individuals who have psychotic symptoms that begin after the age of 60. In older adults, making a diagnosis of late-onset schizophrenia can be challenging, given the various other etiologies that must be ruled out. The onset of hallucinations and delusions in seniors may be associated with mood disorders, polypharmacy, medical disorders, dementia, or sensory deficits [3]. In emerging communities, a similar split between early, late, and very-late onset is expected; however, data regarding the actual rates and course in these settings are yet to be gathered systematically.

Aging and schizophrenia together raise the concern of increased risk for disability. Patients with schizophrenia have been shown to have higher morbidity and mortality relative to the general population. The accelerated aging observed in individuals with schizophrenia is thought to be related to various biological factors (e.g., inflammation, oxidative stress) [17]. Other comorbidities include congestive heart failure, chronic obstructive pulmonary disease, and hypothyroidism [18]. Such comorbidities are of particular concern in resource-limited settings, where patients with these medical conditions tend to have inadequate access to treatment. Older adults with schizophrenia living in these settings may be at higher risk for undetected and/or inadequately managed medical diseases that consequently worsens their prognosis [19]. Existing data regarding the interplay between aging and schizophrenia, as well as schizophrenia and culture, serve to highlight the need to carefully understand the needs of older adults with schizophrenia in developing countries so that they can be provided with appropriate and optimal care.

Caring for older adults with schizophrenia

The course of schizophrenia across the lifespan is thought to have three components. Early in the course of the illness, there appears to be a deterioration in symptoms, then, as an individual ages, there appears to be a stabilization of symptoms. This is followed by the subsequent onset of a phase of gradual improvement in older adults (e.g., [20]), although many people continue to have fluctuations in symptoms [3]. Other studies suggest that chronically institutionalized patients with schizophrenia do not necessarily show this plateauing and improvement; in fact, there is a possibility of clinical deterioration in very elderly patients [21].

The ideal life-trajectory for older schizophrenia patients can be viewed as a process during which patients transition from diminished psychopathology and functional deficits, to community integration, and finally to successful aging characterized by wellbeing and positive health [3]. In attaining these ideal life-trajectory outcomes, the effective treatment of older schizophrenia patients is a critical component; unfortunately, for a variety of reasons, older patients in developing countries often lack the treatment they need. A 2001 Institute of Medicine report found that two-thirds of people with schizophrenia in developing countries were not receiving any treatment. For example, in China, many patients with severe mental disorders go untreated and rates of institutionalization are relatively low [22]. In rural Chinese communities, the families of older adults with schizophrenia bear the responsibility of caring for the patient. Although the patients may have some degree of integration into the community, their limited (if any) access to treatment may place them at a disadvantage with regard to effective symptom reduction. Inadequate access or utilization of mental health treatments has a detrimental effect on positive health outcomes (e.g., wellbeing, life satisfaction) in this cohort.

Seniors with schizophrenia in developing countries have needs and priorities that are similar to those of elderly patients in other societies. Caring for older adults with schizophrenia requires attention to both the physical and psychiatric needs of the patient. Efforts to integrate primary care and psychiatry services by improving communication between physicians and mental health teams have demonstrated promising beneficial outcomes for patients, as well as healthcare systems. There is a clear benefit to providing comprehensive medical and psychiatric care to older adults with schizophrenia, but the costs for caring for this subset of older adults are often much higher than those for other elderly persons (e.g., individuals with dementia, depression, medical illnesses). The cost of such care places a significant burden on developing countries, where historically, greater monetary and infrastructure resources have been devoted to other healthcare goals, such as improving infant and maternal health outcomes [23].

While the implementation of collaborative strategies between psychiatry and primary care is useful across the spectrum of individuals with schizophrenia, older adults have specific needs that may be best met by professionals with training in geriatric medicine and psychiatry. For instance, compared to younger individuals, older adults are more vulnerable to the adverse side effects of medication, an issue of particular relevance in the management of schizophrenia. There are growing data to suggest that older schizophrenia patients may benefit more from targeted non-pharmacological interventions such as cognitive remediation therapy, social skills training, and cognitive behavioral therapy for psychosis or mood disorders (see [3] for review). Thus, the care of seniors with schizophrenia requires a multidimensional approach that blends collaborative care and case management strategies.

In low-income countries, seniors with schizophrenia face various sociocultural, financial, and systemic barriers to the specialized, multifaceted care they need: (1) their relatives may have a poor understanding of their symptoms and comorbid conditions and may only seek intervention when symptoms reach a high severity level, (2) family members may inaccurately believe that symptoms in older individuals will not respond to treatment, (3) limited financial resources may restrict access to care, and (4) there exists a dearth of adequately trained mental health professionals (e.g., [8,24]).

The shortage of adequately trained mental health providers is a critical issue. In many parts of the world, it is estimated that there is less than one qualified mental health professional for half to a million people (and by extension up to 5000 individuals with schizophrenia) [8]. Consequently, individuals with schizophrenia are rather unlikely to receive formal care. This problem is magnified for older schizophrenia patients who require close monitoring of not only their psychiatric symptoms but their often complex medical comorbidities as well.

Cross-cultural differences in treatment of schizophrenia

Numerous studies to date have demonstrated that multiple and contradictory models of illness exist across different cultures. In non-Western cultures, non-medical beliefs (e.g., punishment by God, karma, evil spirits) coexist with biomedical concepts of disease, with chronic diseases being more likely to be attributed to non-medical causes [25]. Patients and caregivers in these pluralistic societies may use these contradictory models simultaneously with the possible intention of coping with different facets of the illness.

As mandated by the World Health Organization (WHO), all member countries conform to a standardized set of curative, preventative, and epidemiological practices, which are based on allopathic systems of care. In developing countries, this model is referred to as "modern" medicine. However, in regions such as India, China, the Middle East, and Africa, the traditional systems of medicine exist in parallel with allopathic or modern medicine [26]. In traditional medicine, mental illnesses are often conceptualized in the context of mystical or religious beliefs (e.g., punishment by God, the result of karma or evil spirits, or a reflection of psychic imbalance in the body). Treatments in the traditional healthcare system tend to reflect a combination of religious practices, mysticism, and rational healing [26]. Traditional healers may utilize rituals and/or herbal remedies to target the culturally accepted cause of the psychiatric symptoms.

In contrast to the diversity of traditional care approaches across cultures, the practice of contemporary psychiatry does not vary: psychiatrists trained in allopathic medicine utilize similar psychopharmacological approaches, regardless of the prevailing beliefs regarding the etiology of psychiatric distress. However, psychiatrists in developing countries do experience unique challenges that come with practicing in pluralistic societies. For example, they must compete with faith and traditional healers, as well as serve the role of educating patients and family members regarding the nature of the illness and its biological mechanisms (and do so in the context of the cultural norms). Psychiatrists in the developing world also work at the frontline of cultural awareness and acceptance of mental illnesses such as schizophrenia. Across cultures, reports suggest that many patients, despite their traditional beliefs regarding the etiology of schizophrenia, are willing to take antipsychotic medication; this serves to highlight the complexity of providing psychiatric care in these pluralistic societies.

There have been a growing number of studies of the outcomes associated with traditional systems of care versus allopathic treatments in schizophrenia. One review examined the outcomes associated with Ayurvedic medicine (a traditional, holistic Indian medical system) versus antipsychotic medications for schizophrenia. The authors reported equivocal results for the use of Ayurvedic herbal remedies alone, but noted that these treatments may be used as adjuncts to antipsychotic medication [27]. Despite the lack of definitive evidence in support of the use of traditional remedies in treating schizophrenia, it should be noted that many non-Western systems of medicine emphasize the importance of emotional and mental wellbeing, a focus that until recently has been underappreciated in Western psychiatric practice. Awareness and appreciation by psychiatrists of the non-medical illness conceptualizations of their patients may yield positive patient outcomes. Thus, there appears to be a need to blend the allopathic and traditional models.

Globally, there is a marked diversity in socioeconomic resources and psychosocial networks; thus it has been challenging to create a model of psychiatric care that can be implemented universally. The combination of traditional and allopathic care models may be attained through a decentralized system of mental healthcare focused on community-based outreach programs. For example, in India, health workers identify patients with mental illness and refer them to primary care centers where they are evaluated by medical professionals and if needed, referred for specialized psychiatric care. This model has been shown to reduce symptoms of psychosis, family burden, and disability [28]. Additionally, the outreach-worker model also appears to aid in identifying untreated schizophrenia, while ensuring medication compliance. Although not yet rigorously investigated, such models may be particularly beneficial for older adults with schizophrenia who may have physical comorbidities that prevent them from traveling great distances to seek care for their psychiatric symptoms. Overall, such community-based models appear to be an effective tool for improving the quality and extent of care available to individuals with schizophrenia in rural communities. Outreach workers also help with educating patients and family members regarding the nature of schizophrenia and available resources to treat the disorder. By establishing close ties with the community, mental health workers may help to customize care in the context of prevalent sociocultural beliefs and assist with reducing stigma associated with schizophrenia [8]. Outreach workers may serve to promote communication between traditional and modern healthcare services, whose coexistence is often marked by distrust and hostility. Of course, efforts to care for individuals with schizophrenia in developing countries cannot end with the outreach worker. Once patients are identified, a skilled health practitioner may make the diagnosis and initiate drug treatment, while attending to the physical health needs of the individual. Inpatient units for short-term care of patients with acute psychosis are also needed [8]. For seniors especially, the presence of geriatric specialists within these inpatient units would represent the ideal care model.

Innovative technologies to serve older adults with schizophrenia

There is a global shortage of medical providers with a specialization in geriatric psychiatry. This dearth of trained geropsychiatrists is particularly of concern in developing countries where there are already multiple barriers facing older patients with regard to accessing appropriate psychiatric care. In the Western world, there has been an increasing interest in developing and implementing innovative strategies that harness technology to foster communication between patients and their providers. Through information communication technology (ICT), telecommunication and internet-based systems can be used to coordinate care and provide mental healthcare to patients who live in remote regions and are unable to leave their homes. Adoption of technology by older adults is still limited, but they tend to accept familiar technologies such as phones that they perceive to be useful and easy to operate. There is growing interest in investigating this modality in seniors with schizophrenia. For instance, in a group of patients with schizophrenia and their caregivers, Rotondi et al. [29] demonstrated the beneficial effects on stress and social support of a telehealth-based psychosocial intervention. As wireless devices and the accompanying infrastructure become more pervasive and better equipped to monitor and assess psychiatric symptomatology, they may be an increasingly important component in improving outcomes for patients with schizophrenia across the lifespan.

In developing countries, mobile phone technology is a particularly promising tool to connect medical providers and patients. Globally, mobile telephone subscriptions have far outpaced the demand for fixed or landline telephones. Cellular technologies in emerging countries are relatively cheap and are available to not only financially secure individuals, but also typically marginalized sections of society such as the poor and the uneducated. Emerging data from resource-limited settings suggest that people across social strata have been able to access this technology and use it to disseminate information and develop innovative strategies [30]. Cell-phone-based interventions have been used to provide patients with appointment or medication reminders, tools to manage and monitor their disease, and symptom education. Across populations, these ICT interventions have shown improvements in medication compliance, disease outcome, and sustained involvement in healthcare. The high penetration of mobile phone technology in resource-limited settings, the acceptance of cell phones by older adults, and existing data supporting their role in enhancing the standard of care suggest that this is a useful tool that geriatric psychiatry providers can harness in developing countries.

In particular, interventions relying on mobile phones may be suitable for older adults with schizophrenia who have limited mobility due to physical limitations or live in rural areas and don't have access to providers based in larger cities.

When applying ICT-based interventions in populations of older schizophrenia patients in developing countries, particular attention must be paid to adapting the strategies to fit the local cultural context. Seniors in different parts of the world may have varying levels of familiarity with technology and, prior to deploying ICT-based interventions, they may need targeted training sessions to use the devices. Studies examining intention and adoption of technology in older adults in other cultures have reported unique patterns of predictors. For example, Pan and Jordan-Marsh [31] found that among Chinese older adults, perceived ease of use was a strong predictor of Internet use intention. In their study, factors such as perceived ease of use and whether or not technology use was the norm also influenced adoption of technology. These data suggest that when developing new technologies for seniors in different cultures, their expectations for the technology and their perceptions regarding the norms and user-friendliness certainly warrant consideration.

Seniors in developing countries, let alone those with mental illnesses, are seldom the target consumers for global ICT developers; these technologies are typically developed in Western countries and imported to the developing regions. Governmental and nongovernmental organizations in these countries need to be involved in providing older adults with the technologies and the training to utilize the devices. Incentives for local, culturally sensitive ICT interventions that take into account norms of communication would also help to increase the acceptability and use of these strategies.

Future directions for research in aging and schizophrenia in developing countries

The global demographics of older people with schizophrenia have been shifting with regard to their absolute numbers in developing countries. Given the socioeconomic and cultural diversity in different parts of the world, the models of caring for seniors with schizophrenia that were developed in Western societies cannot be directly transferred into other settings. Thus, there is a need to continue researching suitable diagnostic approaches, sociocultural and biological predictors of disease outcomes, and strategies to improve access to interventions for older schizophrenia patients in developing countries. Specifically, there is a need to support research by investigators from the same cultural background as the target population. Such researchers may have a better appreciation of the cultural nuances at play and may leverage these insights into designing studies that are optimally suited to tease apart the illness, environmental factors, and cultural variables involved in a more reliable manner.

Attention must be paid to the disputed finding that individuals with schizophrenia in developing countries have better outcomes. Three studies, the International Pilot Study of Schizophrenia (IPSS), the Determinants of Outcome of Severe Mental Disorder (DOSMeD), and the International Study of Schizophrenia (ISoS), reported that individuals with schizophrenia in non-industrialized communities had a better prognosis. Proposed factors underlying this discrepancy include the nature of family support and styles of interaction, as well as the extent of industrialization and urbanization [32]. On the other hand, there is emerging evidence suggesting that patients in developing countries have increasing levels of disability and experience no remission in their psychiatric symptoms (see [32] for a review). Methodological limitations across studies have contributed to the inconclusive data regarding schizophrenia outcomes in developing countries. There continues to be a pressing need to systematically characterize the extent of disability and psychiatric burden experienced by older schizophrenia patients in developing countries, as they are at significant risk of being marginalized.

Individuals across cultures experience aging in markedly different ways, and the process of aging in different communities may be associated with differing predictors and outcomes. For instance, in collectivistic cultures often found in developing countries, the experience of aging may not be associated with isolation and a sense of a lack of purpose that is often reported in individualistic, Western societies. On the other hand, limited healthcare resources may render individuals in developing parts of the world more vulnerable to preventable medical comorbidities (e.g., diabetes, cardiovascular disease, impaired sensory functioning) associated with aging as compared to their counterparts in resource-rich settings. The complex interactions between these factors and their relative contributions to the trajectory of aging across the world are yet to be fully characterized. Extending this to the realm of schizophrenia, it remains to be seen whether the culture-specific patterns of aging influence the course of this illness across the world. Given the growing focus on positive psychiatry, issues related to the predictors and prevalence of successful aging in older schizophrenia patients are also worthy of close study.

Finally, there is a need to investigate, develop, and deploy community-based resources and interventions to address the needs of older adults with schizophrenia in developing countries. Social and economic policy changes may serve to address this. At the governmental and non-governmental levels, issues of particular relevance to older psychiatric patients such as healthcare, housing, income security, and long-term care will need to be addressed. Developing countries may need assistance in meeting the mental healthcare needs of their seniors. This may be accomplished through strategies to subsidize psychopharmacological medications and by providing geriatrics-focused training to mental health providers to assist in identifying and treating older patients. Additionally, providing grants, access to foreign collaboration, and resources for local researchers to develop and implement interventions targeted to the needs of seniors with schizophrenia in their communities will benefit developing countries. Such efforts will require motivation and investment from all stakeholders, but have the potential to benefit individuals who would otherwise remain chronically underserved.

Conclusions

In summary, the projected estimates of the number of older schizophrenia patients globally have important implications for the care of these individuals, as well for as health policy and research. Developing countries already bear a significant burden in terms of caring for older adults with schizophrenia; by 2050, over 10 million older adults will be living with schizophrenia and a large proportion of these individuals will be living in emerging economies. While patients across the world share similar priorities of optimal symptom management, reduced disability, community integration, and high quality of life, the cultural and socioeconomic realities vary widely. As a group, older adults with schizophrenia in developing countries face unique challenges in receiving the care they need due to issues such as stigma, lack of access, and limited availability of geriatric specialists.

Cultural norms also influence the types of interventions sought, with traditional approaches often competing with allopathic interventions. Providers practicing allopathic medicine can successfully treat patients, but they may be hampered by the need to care for large numbers of elders. To mitigate the strain on the relatively small number of mental health providers, we must turn to novel interventional tools. There is promising evidence supporting the use of technological approaches such as cell phones and Internet-based services. These innovative technologies are being investigated with the hope of using them to reach marginalized communities and maintain contact with patients in resource-limited settings. There is a pressing need to integrate cultural, educational, and technological strategies in caring for older adults with schizophrenia. By working towards changing cultural attitudes and stigma associated with this illness, providing geriatrics-focused education for mental health providers, and developing culturally sensitive, senior-friendly technologies, we have the potential to promote the wellbeing of elderly schizophrenia patients on a global scale.

References

1. Nuevo R, Chatterji S, Verdes E, et al. The continuum of psychotic symptoms in the general population: a cross-national study. *Schizophrenia Bulletin.* 2010;38:475–85.

2. World Health Organization. *World Health Statistics 2009.* World Health Organization; 2009.

3. Cohen CI, Meesters PD, Zhao J. New perspectives on schizophrenia in later life: implications for treatment, policy, and research. *Lancet Psychiatry.* 2015;2:340–50.

4. Jeste DV, Wolkowitz OM, Palmer BW. Divergent trajectories of physical, cognitive, and psychosocial aging in schizophrenia. *Schizophrenia Bulletin.* 2011;37:451–5.

5. Saha S, Chant D, Welham J, McGrath J. A systematic review of the prevalence of schizophrenia. *PLoS Medicine.* 2005;2:e141.

6. Bauer SM, Schanda H, Karakula H, et al. Culture and the prevalence of hallucinations in schizophrenia. *Comprehensive Psychiatry.* 2011;52:319–25.

7. Myers NL. Update: schizophrenia across cultures. *Current Psychiatry Reports.* 2011;13:305–11.

8. Patel V, Farooq S, Thara R. What is the best approach to treating schizophrenia in developing countries? *PLoS Medicine.* 2007;4:e159.

9. Lauber C, Rössler W. Stigma towards people with mental illness in developing countries in Asia. *International Review of Psychiatry.* 2007;19:157–78.

10. Ng CH. The stigma of mental illness in Asian cultures. *Australian and New Zealand Journal of Psychiatry.* 1997;31:382–90.

11. Yip K-S. Taoism and its impact on mental health of the Chinese communities. *International Journal of Social Psychiatry.* 2004;50:25–42.

12. Lin K-M, Inui TS, Kleinman AM, Womack WM. Sociocultural determinants of the help-seeking behavior of patients with mental illness. *The Journal of Nervous and Mental Disease.* 1982;170:78–85.

13. Campion J, Bhugra D. Experiences of religious healing in psychiatric patients in South India. *Social Psychiatry and Psychiatric Epidemiology.* 1997;32:215–21.

14. Al-Krenawi A, Graham JR, Dean YZ, Eltaiba N. Cross-national study of attitudes towards seeking professional help: Jordan, United Arab Emirates (UAE) and Arabs in Israel. *International Journal of Social Psychiatry.* 2004;50:102–14.

15. Hooyman N, Kiyak HA. *Social Gerontology: A Multidisciplinary Perspective,* 9th edn. Boston, MA: Allyn & Bacon; 2011.

16. Levkoff SE, Macarthur IW, Bucknall J. Elderly mental health in the developing world. *Social Science and Medicine.* 1995;41:983–1003.

17. Kirkpatrick B, Messias E, Harvey PD, Fernandez-Egea E, Bowie CR. Is schizophrenia a syndrome of accelerated aging? *Schizophrenia Bulletin.* 2007;34:1024–32.

18. Hendrie HC, Tu W, Tabbey R, et al. Health outcomes and cost of care among older adults with schizophrenia: a 10-year study using medical records across the continuum of care. *American Journal of Geriatric Psychiatry.* 2014;22:427–36.

19. Vahia IV, Diwan S, Bankole AO, et al. Adequacy of medical treatment among older persons with schizophrenia. *Psychiatric Services.* 2008;59:853–9.

20. Jeste D, Twamley E, Eyler Zorrilla L, et al. Aging and outcome in schizophrenia. *Acta Psychiatrica Scandinavica.* 2003;107:336–43.

21. Putnam KM, Harvey PD, Parrella M, et al. Symptom stability in geriatric chronic schizophrenic inpatients: a one-year follow-up study. *Biological Psychiatry.* 1996;39:92–9.

22. Ran M, Xiang M, Huang M, Shan Y. Natural course of schizophrenia: 2-year follow-up study in a rural Chinese community. *British Journal of Psychiatry.* 2001;178:154–8.

23. Subedi S, Tausig M, Subedi J, Broughton C, Williams-Blangero S. Mental illness and disability among elders in developing countries: the case of Nepal. *Journal of Aging and Health.* 2004;16:71–87.

24. Ran M-S, Xiang M-Z, Conwell Y, et al. Comparison of characteristics between geriatric and younger subjects with schizophrenia in community. *Journal of Psychiatric Research.* 2004;38:417–24.

25. Johnson S, Sathyaseelan M, Charles H, Jeyaseelan V, Jacob KS. Insight, psychopathology, explanatory models and outcome of schizophrenia in India: a prospective 5-year cohort study. *BMC Psychiatry.* 2012;12:159.

26. Vahia IV, Vahia VN. Schizophrenia in developing countries. In *Clinical Handbook of Schizophrenia*, ed. KT Mueser, DV Jeste. New York: Guilford Press; 2008: 549–58.

27. Agarwal V, Abhijnhan A, Raviraj P. Ayurvedic medicine for schizophrenia. *Cochrane Database of Systematic Reviews.* 2007;(4):CD006867.

28. Chatterjee S, Naik S, Dabholkar H, et al. Trials of interventions for people with psychosis. In *Global Mental Health Trials*, ed. G Thornicroft, V Patel. London: Oxford University Press, 2014: 141–59.

29. Rotondi A, Haas G, Anderson C, et al. A clinical trial to test the feasibility of a telehealth psychoeducational intervention for persons with schizophrenia and their families: intervention and 3-month findings. *Rehabilitation Psychology.* 2005;50:325.

30. Kaplan WA. Can the ubiquitous power of mobile phones be used to improve health outcomes in developing countries? *Globalization and Health.* 2006;2:9.

31. Pan S, Jordan-Marsh M. Internet use intention and adoption among Chinese older adults: from the expanded technology acceptance model perspective. *Computers in Human Behavior.* 2010;26:1111–19.

32. Patel V, Cohen A, Thara R, Gureje O. Is the outcome of schizophrenia really better in developing countries? *Revista Brasileira de Psiquiatria.* 2006;28:149–52.

Chapter

18

Schizophrenia in Later Life: Public Policy Issues in the United States

Michael B. Friedman, M.S.W., Lisa Furst, M.S.W., M.P.H., Paul S. Nestadt, M.D., Kimberly A. Williams, M.S.W., and Lina Rodriguez, M.S.W.

Without doubt, life for older adults with schizophrenia and other long-term psychotic disorders is better now than it was in the days when hundreds of thousands of old people were warehoused in state asylums. But even more than half a century after the shift from an institution-based to a community-based mental health system, this population still faces many serious problems.

This chapter is based on the premise that significant changes in mental health policy could result in improvements in the lives of older people (55+) with schizophrenia and other long-term psychotic disorders. These disorders typically have a terrible impact on both length and quality of life. People with schizophrenia and other long-term psychotic disorders die 10–20 years younger than the general population [1]. They are likely to be disabled and to rely on public financial assistance [2] to live in the community. They are more likely to be homeless [3] or to have unstable housing [4]. Although widely feared, they are in fact more likely to be victims rather than perpetrators of violence [5], except violence towards themselves. They are far more likely to complete suicide than the general population [6,7]. In addition, they are unlikely to be welcomed in mainstream society, and this affects access to housing and good healthcare, job prospects, family and social life, recreational opportunities, access to houses of worship, and more.

Although the psychological condition of people with schizophrenia tends to improve over time [8], additional problems are likely to emerge as they grow older. They may be at a higher risk than other older adults for chronic physical conditions such as diabetes, cardiac conditions, and respiratory problems, among others [1,9]. They may also be at slightly higher risk of developing dementia [10]. In addition, they are more likely to suffer the residual effects of hard lives that often include periods of homelessness and substance abuse.

As they age, older adults living with long-term psychotic disorders are less likely to get competent psychiatric treatment, in part because there is a tremendous shortage of geriatric psychiatrists and other mental health professionals, and in part because the side-effects and increased risk of premature disability and death associated with anti-psychotic medications make them more difficult to manage for older adults than for younger [11]. In addition, psychosocial supports for people with schizophrenia are generally designed for younger adults and often not adjusted for older adults. For example, rehabilitation programs focus heavily on vocational goals rather than goals more appropriate to older adults, such as socialization and recreation.

Most importantly, special housing programs for people with serious mental illness, which are in short supply for younger populations, rarely have the capacity to care for people with co-occurring serious, long-term, physical and behavioral conditions. As a result, older adults with serious long-term psychiatric disabilities often live in facilities not suited to their needs, including nursing homes, adult homes, and various supportive housing programs designed for younger, physically healthier populations.

In addition, some older adults with psychiatric disabilities live with parents, who are likely to be very old [12] and who may be increasingly disabled themselves, or with other family caregivers, all of whom are hard pressed to provide needed care and who often need considerable support themselves.

Despite all these challenges, people with schizophrenia who survive into old age can lead lives that they find satisfying and meaningful. A diagnosis of schizophrenia or other long-term psychotic disorder need not doom individuals to terrible lives. The quality of individuals' lives can be better or worse, and which it is depends to a considerable extent not only on the treatment and care that they get, but also on the conditions in which they live.

Public policy matters to this, and in this chapter we will explore how changes in public policy could help people with schizophrenia or other psychotic conditions to lead tolerable lives in old age.

In the sections that follow, we will discuss policy implications related to:

- The mortality gap
- Income supports
- Housing needs
- Treatment issues
- Psychosocial interventions
- Systems coordination and leadership
- Workforce issues
- Research needs.

The mortality gap

As we noted earlier, people with serious long-term mental illness die 10–20 years younger than the general population [1]. This suggests that the life expectancy of this population in the United States is between 60 and 70 years. In our view, increasing life expectancy to about 80 years should be a major goal of geriatric mental health.

Why is life expectancy so low for people with serious long-term mental illness?

The primary causes of death for this population are – as they are for others – physical diseases [9,13], especially cardiac conditions, cancer, respiratory diseases, and diabetes. But the differences in rates of death are associated not only with greater prevalence of physical illnesses but also with suicide [1].

Increased risks of physical illness undoubtedly reflect high rates of smoking [14,15] and obesity [16] among this population. Obesity can be a consequence of poor nutrition and lack of exercise, but also of some anti-psychotic medications. This leads to much speculation that taking these drugs to ameliorate psychotic symptoms may contribute to lower life expectancy [12]. However, there is at least one study that concludes that consistently taking second generation anti-psychotic medications prescribed properly and in safe doses actually prolongs life because it contributes to other improvements in how people live [17].

It also seems likely that the higher death rate of people with serious, long-term mental disorders is related to high rates of substance abuse and to the consequences of significant periods of life on the streets [18], where living conditions are harsh and dangerous. People who are homeless and living with mental illness frequently suffer from physical health conditions that can become extremely serious if not treated early on [19]. They are also frequent victims of physical and sexual assault [20], which can result in long-lasting physical and psychological damage. In addition, they have high rates of sexually transmitted diseases [21] including being HIV+, the transmission of which is related to a combination of factors, including unsafe sexual behavior, sexual assault, and substance abuse.

It is also clear that people with serious, long-term mental disorders are less likely to get good primary healthcare [22] and, when care is available, they are more likely than their age peers to be inadequately treated. In part this reflects the reluctance of some people with serious, long-term mental disorders to seek healthcare, but it also reflects the reluctance of many primary care and specialty providers to serve this population.

What can be done to reduce the mortality gap?

Most efforts currently focus on improving access to high-quality healthcare, promoting integration of physical and behavioral healthcare [23], and the development of "wellness" initiatives that focus on smoking cessation, stress reduction, improved nutrition, exercise, and weight control [24].

In addition, it is important to develop effective measures to prevent suicide. Older adults with schizophrenia attempt suicide more often than the general population [25], although suicide among people with schizophrenia is most likely to take place shortly after the first psychotic break, when many people experience a sense of hopelessness about ever achieving the promise that they had before they became psychotic [26,27]. To what extent this might apply to first breaks in middle age and older age (late-onset schizophrenia) is unknown. In addition, there is widespread belief that screening for suicide risk in primary care might avert some suicides (even though there is little evidence to support this [28]) and that measures such as safety plans [29] for those who acknowledge suicide ideation can be helpful. Access to good psychiatric treatment also may reduce the incidence of suicide [30].

It also seems likely that limiting access to the means of suicide, particularly to guns, could reduce the rate of suicide in the United States [31]. Guns are the most lethal means of attempting suicide, and as such are the most common method for suicide completion, particularly among older Americans [32].

Public policy implications of the mortality gap

What policy changes are needed to increase life expectancy of people with schizophrenia and other psychotic conditions?

- Improved access to quality healthcare
- Greater integration of physical and behavioral healthcare services
- Improved integration of mental health and substance abuse treatment
- Greater attention to the risk of suicide among older primary care patients living with psychotic disorders
- Improved mental health and substance abuse treatment, with particular attention to clinically appropriate use of anti-psychotic medications

- Improved intervention during and after a person's first psychotic break with particular attention to the prevention of suicide
- More "wellness" programs to reduce morbidity and mortality associated with physical health problems
- More extensive efforts to reduce homelessness
- Attention to the risk associated with access to firearms for people with serious mental disorders
- Redesign of the Medicare and Medicaid programs to facilitate funding of the measures noted above.

Income supports

Public income supports – Social Security Disability Insurance (SSDI), Supplemental Security Income (SSI), Social Security Retirement Benefits, and the Supplemental Nutrition Assistance Program (SNAP), otherwise known as "food stamps" – are what make it possible for unemployed people with psychiatric disabilities to live in the community.

In general, income supports provide a subsistence level of support, which may or may not be adequate to cover housing costs that in many parts of the country go up much faster than the annual cost of living adjustment [33]. This makes maintaining stable housing in the community difficult for many people with long-term psychiatric disabilities and undoubtedly contributes to homelessness.

Income supports are also used to pay for various forms of residential care, including: (1) community residences, (2) supportive housing, (3) senior housing, (4) assisted living, and (5) nursing homes.

Unfortunately, income supports are in jeopardy in the long term. Social Security Disability and Retirement benefits are funded out of the Social Security Trust Fund, and, as of this writing, the disability portion of the Trust Fund is projected to be depleted in 2034 [34]. In addition, SSI, SNAP, and general welfare benefits are always subject to the vicissitudes of politics.

Public policy implications of reliance on income supports

It is widely agreed that it is critical to modify America's current Social Security system to make it financially viable for the foreseeable future. But conservatives generally argue for reducing benefits by, for example, raising the retirement age or toughening standards of disability, while liberals generally argue for increasing income to the fund by, for example, raising the cap on taxable income. Both approaches may be necessary to preserve the fund, but compromise is politically difficult given the ideological divide in the United States today.

In addition, it is a problem that income supports are generally not adjusted for local housing costs. A change in this regard could make it more possible for people living with long-term psychiatric disabilities to maintain safe and stable housing.

Housing and residential care

Stable, safe, and appropriate housing and high-quality residential care are critical for older adults living with schizophrenia or other psychotic conditions, but they are difficult to obtain.

This is an extremely complex matter because older adults with severe, long-term psychiatric disabilities live in many different settings. Some live independently. Some live with caregiving family or friends. Some get formal residential care in senior housing, supportive housing, community residences, assisted living, adult homes, nursing homes, or homeless shelters. Some are literally homeless and live "on the streets." And some are incarcerated in jails or prisons.

Independent living

People with serious, long-term mental disorders encounter several difficulties living independently. First, it is a struggle to pay the rent when cost of living adjustments to public assistance do not keep pace with rising housing costs. Those with housing subsidies, such as Section 8, that cover rents that are over 30–40% of income [35], are protected from this, but relatively few people have such subsidies. Second, people can lose their housing if they have extended hospitalizations. Third, in-home services such as home healthcare and psychiatric services that may be necessary to be able to remain at home are often not available. Fourth, and very importantly, living independently can result in social isolation that contributes to – or is a consequence of – increasing levels of depression.

Living with family

People with serious, long-term mental disorders who live with caregiving family and friends also may encounter difficulties remaining at home. Caregivers typically experience great stress, resulting in high rates of physical and mental disorders, and increased placement of disabled family members in residential care [36]. In addition, as caregivers age, they are more likely to become disabled themselves or to die, leaving the person who requires help to remain in the community without the needed care. Unfortunately, Adult Protective Services, which are supposed to step in when adults cannot live safely in the community, are of notoriously uneven quality and are hampered by the lack of appropriate alternatives.

Living in supportive settings

Older adults with serious, long-term mental disorders who live in settings that provide support or care often do not get services that they need.

Community residences and other specialized mental health housing programs are generally designed for younger adults who are physically healthy. Those who have co-occurring disorders often cannot get admitted to these facilities or, if they do, cannot get appropriate medical care [37]. This is particularly true for those who develop dementia.

Those who live in other residential care facilities such as assisted living, senior housing, supportive housing, homeless shelters, and nursing homes generally cannot get appropriate treatment for mental or substance use disorders even when they can get decent physical healthcare or care for dementia.

Living in jails or prisons

The number and proportion of older adults in jails and prisons in the United States is rising rapidly and will continue to grow as the elder boom gathers force [38]. Although estimates regarding mental illness among incarcerated older adults vary, the rate is clearly much higher than in the general population [39]. Needless to say, they generally fare very badly.

Whether older adults with severe mental disorders and/or dementia who are not dangerous to others should serve their full terms in prisons is controversial. Those who believe that the purpose of imprisonment is punishment generally oppose early release. Those who believe that the purpose is rehabilitation and public safety generally support early release [40].

Public policy implications of residential issues problems

Public policy changes are needed to:

- Provide protection from eviction due to unaffordable rent increases or extended stays out of the home due to hospitalization or imprisonment
- Provide funding for renovations that are needed to live safely at home
- Modify Medicaid and Medicare to fund in-home health and mental health services
- Provide access to activities that counter social isolation including those in senior centers, social adult day care, medical day care, psychiatric rehabilitation, day treatment, and partial hospitalization
- Provide support for family caregivers including respite, counseling, support groups and tax relief
- Develop residential care alternatives that provide as much freedom and access to the community as possible while still providing appropriate care and treatment for people with co-occurring physical and behavioral disorders*
- Avoid incarceration in, or provide early release from, jails and prisons for older adults with severe, long-term behavioral disorders who are not currently a danger to society.

Treatment issues

Most accounts of the needs of older (and younger) adults with schizophrenia or other psychotic conditions focus on psychiatric treatment and then note ancillary, useful interventions such as rehabilitation. Our view is that people with schizophrenia and other psychotic conditions need a comprehensive array of interventions including inpatient and outpatient treatment, but also including housing, income supports, rehabilitation, other community supports, physical healthcare, and case management.

This section of the chapter focuses on clinical treatment.

What forms of treatment help?

In this day and age of community-based mental health policy, outpatient treatment is primary. Inpatient treatment is regarded as a treatment of last resort and, when at all possible, it is provided in local, general hospitals rather than in state or private psychiatric hospitals. The treatment goal usually is to stabilize an acute psychotic flare-up, while keeping the person as close to his or her community and family as possible.

This stance about inpatient treatment is controversial, with some advocating for a return to increased use of long-term hospitalization so as to reduce the number of people with serious, long-term mental illness who are homeless or who have been

---

* The current public policy assumption that it is preferable for people with disabilities to live independently if at all possible needs to be examined in light of the risks of social isolation.

transinstitutionalized to adult homes, nursing homes, or prisons [41]. Advocates for community-based treatment argue in response that if there were enough outpatient treatment and housing for people with serious mental illness, there would be little need for long-term inpatient care [42].

Unfortunately, however, there is not enough outpatient treatment. Geriatric psychiatrists, psychologists, social workers, and nurses are in short supply, and there are very few outpatient programs that have staff who are clinically competent to serve older adults with mental and/or substance use disorders [43]. As a result, treatment for behavioral disorders increasingly falls to primary care providers, who are usually ill-prepared for the job.

It is important to be clear that good treatment includes both anti-psychotic medications and psychotherapy [44], and that both require special skills for working with older adults. Prescribing anti-psychotic medications for older adults is exceedingly difficult because they require lower than usual doses to get a therapeutic effect and to avoid risky side-effects, such as reduced ability to concentrate, greater confusion, loss of energy, fatigue, and heightened risk of cardiac conditions and of falls, which are the largest cause of premature disability and death in older adults. Prescribers became even more wary of recommending these medications in 2008, when the FDA extended a black-box warning regarding the risk of sudden death in elderly dementia patients to all anti-psychotic medications [45]. Psychotherapy also requires special skills for older adults and, of course, more time than primary care providers have available.

The solution currently being developed is integrated physical and behavioral healthcare. There are several evidence-based models of integrated care [46]. Primary healthcare settings can routinely screen for mental and substance use disorders, provide care coordination and care management, and/or include behavioral health providers at their sites. Mental health and substance abuse centers can include physical healthcare at their sites, and Medicare and Medicaid are now promoting the use of complex, integrated managed care structures such as "health homes" and "accountable care organizations," through which care managers help patients with serious, complex conditions to get the help they need from a variety of community-based providers.

Barriers to effective treatment

In addition to limited capacity, uneven clinical competence, and the slow growth of integrated care, treatment for older adults with psychotic disorders suffers from insufficient research to develop evidence-based treatment methods. Clinical research often does not include older adults at all, and, when it does, it often rules out older adults with co-occurring physical disorders [43]. This vastly limits knowledge about effective treatment for actual older adults with behavioral disorders, most of whom have co-occurring disorders.

The quality of clinical services for older adults is also compromised because of limited cultural competence, especially the lack of bilingual providers. This will be an increasing problem in the future as so-called "minority" populations become the majority of Americans.

In addition, many older adults with schizophrenia do not get treatment at all. Low utilization is due partly to service shortages, but it is also due to problems of access. For example, many older adults have limited mobility and need either in-home treatment or good transportation, both of which are hard to obtain. But low utilization is also due to either ignorance about or reluctance to use mental health services, loosely referred to as "stigma." It is important to distinguish between ignorance about mental illness, the possible effectiveness of treatment, and where to get it on the one hand and shame or embarrassment about using mental health services on the other. Public education campaigns, which are commonly recommended, are more likely to help with issues of ignorance than issues of shame [47].

Providers

The public mental health system consists of a variety of providers, including: (1) general hospitals, (2) community mental health and health organizations, (3) drug abuse treatment organizations, (4) state psychiatric centers, (5) the Veterans' Administration (VA), and (6) private organizations and practitioners that accept Medicare and Medicaid or that work in partnerships with non-clinical providers, especially nursing homes. All providers encounter problems related to capacity, funding, and regulation.

Funding of treatment

Inadequate funding is often cited as a major barrier to treatment. Problems include lack of coverage, lack of parity, and failure to cover non-traditional interventions such as care management, outreach and engagement, and offsite services [48].

Coverage issues are less significant for people with schizophrenia and other long-term psychotic conditions who live in the community than for other people with mental or substance use disorders. Even before the passage of the Affordable Care Act (ACA), only 7% of this population were uncovered by the government health insurance. The vast majority (93%) were covered by Medicaid or Medicare (85%), and/or the VA (7%) [49]. It seems safe to assume that some who were not covered in 2010 gained coverage through the health exchanges or expanded Medicaid under the ACA. However, mostly this coverage is for medication, office-based psychotherapy, and day treatment [50]. Other forms of intervention, such as housing and case management, remain difficult to fund through Medicaid or Medicare.

Policy implications of problems related to treatment

Policy changes needed to deal with low utilization and uneven quality of treatment services for people with schizophrenia or other long-term psychotic conditions include:

- Resolution of the debate about the need for increased inpatient services
- Expanded outpatient treatment
- Building a larger clinically and culturally competent workforce
- Improved quality of care through:
  - Enhanced clinical and cultural competence of primary care and behavioral health providers
  - Increased integration of physical and behavioral health services
  - Regulatory controls, advisories, oversight, and education regarding appropriate use of anti-psychotic medications for older adults
  - Evaluation of health homes and accountable care organizations and the like
  - Enhanced clinical research regarding older adults and translation of research into practice
- Funding for outreach and engagement, for off-site/in-home services, and transportation

- Funding for care co-ordination and care management services in outpatient physical and mental health programs
- Full implementation of parity requirements
- Enhanced public education and anti-stigma campaigns.

Psychosocial interventions

In addition to treatment, psychosocial interventions are of vital importance to the survival and quality of life of older adults with schizophrenia and other long-term psychotic conditions. As previously discussed, housing is most important. Other psychosocial interventions include recovery-oriented psychiatric and substance abuse rehabilitation, case/care management, assertive community treatment, programs to counter inactivity and social isolation, peer support and advocacy, wellness programs, including anti-smoking and weight management, access to mainstream social, recreational, and religious opportunities, and family support. The most recent Patient Outcomes Research Team (PORT) findings also recommend supported employment – which is applicable to some, but far from all, older adults – skills training, and token economies for those in long-term hospital or residential care [44].

Recovery-oriented rehabilitation

Various studies indicate that full recovery from schizophrenia, i.e., long-term remission of symptoms, is rare [8,10]. Despite this fact, a belief in recovery has become a powerful component of psychiatric and substance abuse rehabilitation. The concept, however, has been redefined. It no longer means "cured." Instead, it means that it is possible for people with severe mental and/or substance abuse disorders to lead lives that they find satisfying and meaningful despite continuing to have the disorder [51], which can include continuing to have prominent symptoms such as hallucinations and delusions.

Psychiatric rehabilitation has a number of key components: skills development, ongoing support, and environmental modifications, all of which contribute to creating places of belonging and access to mainstream opportunities.

There are many different models of psychiatric rehabilitation, some of which are reimbursable by Medicaid and some of which are not. Most emphasize vocational rehabilitation, which may or may not be relevant to older adults with schizophrenia.

Outreach and assertive community treatment

Many people with schizophrenia and other long-term psychotic conditions, particularly those who have had bad experiences with the mental health system or who abuse substances, are extremely reluctant to go to formal mental health settings for treatment. For this subpopulation, outreach and engagement efforts are critical. Assertive community treatment, which includes a broad range of treatment, rehabilitation, medical services, and dedicated case management, is a proven method for engaging people who otherwise reject care [52].

Access to mainstream society

Older adults with schizophrenia and other long-term psychotic conditions are not readily accepted in mainstream society, especially when their dress and demeanor make it apparent that they have a serious behavioral problem. It is therefore important to help people to develop appropriate social skills, but it is also important to try to build community acceptance. For example, supported employment programs work not only to prepare people for jobs, but to find employers who are willing to make appropriate accommodations. Building acceptance at houses of worship is particularly important because spiritual experience and participation in a religion is exceedingly important to many people with serious mental illness, just as it is to people who are not mentally ill [53].

Despite efforts over many years to outlaw discrimination in housing, work, and access to public places, people with severe and persistent mental illness frequently continue to feel unwanted and then withdraw or turn to organized programs.

Programs to counter isolation and inactivity

There are a number of different kinds of programs that address isolation and inactivity. Many psychiatric rehabilitation programs provide places where clients can go for social interaction and activities. Clubhouses, for example, provide lifetime membership and opportunities for volunteer work and socialization [54]. Alternatively, there are psychiatric day treatment programs that also offer opportunities for socialization and activity in the guise of group therapeutic activities.

Outside of the mental health system, older people with psychiatric disabilities may be served in adult medical day care programs, which are primarily designed for people with dementia and/or physical disabilities. But placid older adults with serious and persistent mental illness often fit into these programs and can be attractive to the programs because they are all Medicaid eligible. These programs also provide medical services that can be beneficial to people with co-occurring physical and mental disorders.

Drift from the mental health system to long-term care

There is a kind of drift from the mental health system to the long-term care system for many older adults with serious and persistent mental disorders. This drift also occurs with residential care as people move from community residences, supportive housing, and the like to nursing homes.

While in the abstract it may make sense for people to move from one system to another and one program to another, in fact it means fracturing relationships that often have lasted for years and are central to the lives of the people being shifted to new programs. This is particularly troubling when it happens towards the end of life, when program staff and clients may be the only important relationships and they may not be able to visit and spend time with their friend as he or she is dying.

In addition, long-term care programs are generally not competent treatment providers for schizophrenia and other long-term psychotic conditions. Nursing homes, for example, which are primarily funded by Medicaid, are not adequately reimbursed to cover mental health treatment as a core service. Instead, they generally have arrangements with mental health providers (individuals or groups) in private practice that bill separately for the services they provide. While some of these groups are quite good, others are reputed to do little more than prescribe medications of questionable value and to have brief contact with patients [55,56].

Wellness programs

Poor health is a major reason for the low life expectancy of people with schizophrenia and other long-term psychotic conditions. Smoking, obesity, and poor physical conditioning are among the major reasons for poor health and drive up the costs of care. For this reason, wellness initiatives that emphasize smoking cessation, nutrition, and exercise have been expanding. Some of these programs are organized at local community centers, which helps to connect people who often are isolated with the mainstream. Whether wellness programs are readily available for those who also have physical limitations is an open question.

Case/care management

Since the late 1970s, when public policy regarding people with serious and persistent mental illness began to emphasize comprehensive community mental health systems with a broad range of community supports as the antidote to the shortfalls of deinstitutionalization, case management has been seen as the connective tissue of the mental health system. Case managers have direct relationships with clients who move among a variety of service programs and who occasionally become disconnected from service. The job of case managers is to keep them in appropriate services and to be available to provide support, especially in times of crisis.

Case management (sometimes called "care" management) is also at the core of various managed care initiatives, such as "health homes," that have emerged for people with co-occurring serious, long-term behavioral and physical health disorders [57–59]. This is the population most likely to experience frequent and very costly crises.

Another form of care management has proven very effective in primary care practices for patients who have been diagnosed with mental disorders and been prescribed medication. Care managers provide follow-up care that includes helping patients to adhere to treatment plans. In some cases, these care managers also provide problem-solving therapy, which is particularly effective for dealing with depression [60].

Family support

Many people with schizophrenia and other long-term psychotic disorders live with family members or friends who serve as their primary caregivers. Serving as a caregiver is, as previously noted, extremely demanding and stressful. Many people burn out and arrange placement out of the home – often in institutional settings such as nursing homes. Research regarding family support for caregivers of family members with dementia [61] indicates that providing family support services, such as crisis intervention, support groups, and counseling at convenient times and places results in reduced depression, anxiety, and physical disorders and delayed placement out of the home by as much as 18 months. Other family support measures include respite – both for a night out and for vacations – and tax relief to help cover the costs of having a disabled person live at home.

Policy implications of the value of psychosocial interventions

Needed policy changes include:
- Shifting Medicare and Medicaid from a medical-only model for funding to include funding to support rehabilitation and recovery models of intervention
- Regulatory changes to support outreach and engagement
- Medicaid and Medicare funding for wellness initiatives and family support
- Tax relief for families who provide care for disabled family members

- Avoiding the disruption that occurs with the shift from the mental health system to the long-term care system due to medical complications by:
  - building capacity to manage physical health issues into mental health programs and vice versa
  - providing continuity of relationships, especially as death approaches
- Continuing and increasing the fight against stigma and discrimination through advocacy, political action, and litigation.

Coordination of systems and leadership

A recent Government Accountability Office report noted that there are over 100 poorly co-ordinated federal agencies and programs dealing with behavioral health issues [62]. These include the National Institutes of Mental Health (NIMH), Drug Abuse (NIDA), and Alcohol Abuse (NIAAA), as well as the Substance Abuse and Mental Health Services Administration (SAMHSA), The Health Resources Services Administration (HRSA), The Agency on Healthcare Research and Quality (AHRQ), the Administration for Community Living (ACL), the Social Security Department, the Centers for Medicare and Medicaid (CMS), The Centers for Disease Control (CDC), The Department of Housing and Urban Development (HUD), Department of Justice, and more.

Because of concerns about poor coordination among these agencies, the 21st Century Cures Act of 2016 includes a provision to create an Assistant Secretary of the Department of Health and Human Services who heads SAMHSA and oversees and coordinates the efforts of the various federal agencies and programs dealing with behavioral health [63].

There is similar fragmentation at the state level, even though in many states the department that handles behavioral health is part of a larger department of health. Despite that, there are frequent failures of communication and coordination, as well as disputes between behavioral health leadership and leadership of state Medicaid agencies, public health leadership, and staff in Governors' offices, especially budget staff.

In addition, geriatric behavioral health tends to be at best an afterthought in federal and state agencies that address behavioral health.

Public policy implications of issues of coordination and leadership

Clearly, there is a need to raise the visibility and priority of geriatric behavioral health in relevant federal and state agencies. Appointing a lead in each relevant agency at a high enough level to have some clout could help geriatric mental health emerge from the shadow of other priorities and interests. In addition, at the federal level it might be helpful to have a Deputy Assistant Secretary for Geriatric Behavioral Health in the new Office of the Assistant Secretary.

Workforce challenges

Fundamental to developing an adequate system of care for older adults with schizophrenia and other long-term psychotic conditions is addressing the inadequate size and competence of the current workforce. There are far too few geriatric psychiatrists, psychologists, social workers, and nurses, and this situation is not likely to improve in the foreseeable future [43].

One frequently offered solution is to expect increasing amounts of treatment to be provided by primary care professionals – a solution that runs the risk of decreased quality of care.

Another approach that appears to be gathering support is to diversify the workforce with non-professional staff including "health coaches and lay community health workers trained to provide screening and brief interventions for geriatric mental health and substance use disorders" [43]. It is argued that this approach would also make it possible to engage more older adults and diverse groups of lay people as providers, a diversification that probably would contribute to generational and cultural competence. In addition, the use of peers as care co-ordinators, care managers, home visitors, and medical escorts could be of great assistance to professionals who are often office-bound because of the size of their caseloads and because of inadequate reimbursement for off-site services.

In addition, there are technological solutions to the workforce shortage, including telemedicine and Internet-based applications [43].

Public policy implications of the inadequacy of the workforce

Needed public policy changes include:

- Enhanced efforts to recruit, educate, and train a high-quality professional workforce with incentives such as loan forgiveness
- More education regarding older adults and regarding mental and substance use disorders in professional schools
- Development of non-professional alternatives emphasizing the use of older adults and people with a history of schizophrenia or other severe mental or substance use disorders ("peers")
- Modifying regulations regarding funding of telemedicine to make it more widely available
- Encouraging innovation in the use of the internet-based interventions.

Research

Research regarding older adults with schizophrenia or other long-term psychotic disorders is not nearly as abundant as research for younger populations [64]. This probably reflects the facts that: (1) historically, older adults have been a small proportion of the American population and (2) psychiatrists and other mental health professionals have had relatively little interest in geriatric psychiatry, preferring other areas of practice and research.

Now, however, the older adult population is in the process of growing to be 25% of the American population, greater than the population of children under the age of 18 [65]. The number of Americans with serious, long-term mental or substance abuse disorders will grow accordingly. It is past time for there to be as much attention to geriatric behavioral health as to other populations.

What should be the focus of future research?

This is a matter of great controversy. NIMH, which is the primary source of funding for research on mental illness, and NIDA and NIAAA, which are the primary sources of research on substance abuse, are all heavily focused on biomedical research.

Pharmaceutical companies, which are also large funders of research, focus on discovering new and hopefully better patent-protected medications.

It is certainly true that this sort of research has borne some fruit, but not nearly as much as has been promised over the past quarter century when major breakthroughs, or even cures, have appeared to be close at hand. Sadly, there have been no major breakthroughs, and there is very little reason to believe that there will be any time soon.

That suggests that it is time to focus more research on how to increase life expectancy and quality of life for adults with schizophrenia and other serious, long-term behavioral disorders. This would include additional clinical research on the effectiveness and safety of anti-psychotic medications, additional research on the treatment of depression in this population, additional research on the effectiveness of psychotherapy, and more.

But beyond clinical research, it is important to explore psychosocial interventions that promote enhanced survival and quality of life, including housing options, prevention of homelessness, recovery-oriented rehabilitation, case/care management, family support, and more. This should include possible preventive interventions, including suicide prevention, relapse prevention, and wellness promotion.

Evidence-based findings regarding effective interventions unfortunately are not effectively translated into practice. Thus, additional research on how to move from the laboratory to the field is very important.

Evaluation of reorganized systems is also extremely important during the period where there is widespread belief that the integration of physical and behavioral health services will result in better outcomes for patients, as well as overall reduced costs. Will the new initiatives such as health homes and accountable care organizations work? Will they work for older adults as well as younger?

In addition, public education and anti-stigma efforts are high on most agendas. Whether they are effective and how they can be effective is an important topic for future research.

Public policy implications of future research needs

- Develop a federal research plan for older adults with serious behavioral disorders that:
  - Coordinates research in various federal agencies – NIMH, SAMHSA, HRSA, AHRQ, and others
  - Rebalances research priorities by reducing the dominance of biomedical research, and increasing clinical and services research, especially regarding psychosocial interventions
- Protect research funding in the federal budget from cuts that have been proposed by the current administration.

Summary

Promotion of increased life expectancy and quality of life should be the fundamental goals of public policy regarding older adults with schizophrenia and other serious, long-term psychotic conditions. This calls for:

1. Addressing the mortality gap via improved access to improved healthcare, enhanced integration of physical and behavioral health services, increased wellness activities, suicide prevention, reduced homelessness, and more.

2. Securing the future of the Social Security Trust Fund and modifying income support measures to assure stable housing.

3. Expanding community housing programs and non-institutional residential care programs specifically for older adults with co-occurring behavioral and physical health conditions, including those who are homeless, those institutionalized in state hospitals and nursing homes, and those incarcerated in jails and prisons.

4. Expanding the capacity to provide high-quality, integrated behavioral health and medical services to this population, including both treatment services and recovery-oriented psychosocial interventions.

5. Restructuring Medicaid and Medicare to assure that funding is available for psychosocial interventions – especially housing, outreach and engagement, off-site services, rehabilitation, case management, and family support – as well as for traditional treatment interventions.

6. Addressing problems of capacity and quality among service providers including the VA, which has an infamously troubled track record serving veterans who have made great sacrifices in service to the nation.

7. Enhancing public education and anti-stigma campaigns.

8. Addressing workforce inadequacies – both size and clinical and cultural competence – through enhanced training, diversification of the workforce, and pursuing technological alternatives.

9. Increasing and diversifying research to emphasize improving services and translating evidence-based methods into practice.

10. Enhancing coordination of federal and state agencies that oversee the behavioral health and other systems that serve this population and ensuring that each system has leadership specifically regarding geriatric mental health.

References

1. N.H. Liu, G.L. Daumit, T. Dua, et al. Excess mortality in persons with severe mental disorders: a multilevel intervention framework and priorities for clinical practice, policy and research agendas. *World Psychiatry* 2017; **16**(1):30–40.

2. S. Danziger, R. Frank, E. Meara. Mental illness, work, and income support programs. *American Journal of Psychiatry* 2009; **166**(4):398–404.

3. D.P. Folsom, W. Hawthorne, L. Lindamer, et al. Prevalence and risk factors for homelessness and utilization of mental health services among 10,340 patients with serious mental illness in a large public mental health system. *American Journal of Psychiatry* 2005; **162**(2):370–6.

4. G. Browne and M. Courtney. Schizophrenia, housing, and supportive relationships. *International Journal of Mental Health Nursing* 2007; **16**(2):73–80.

5. J.S. Brekke, C. Prindle, S.W. Bae, J.D. Long. Risks for individuals with schizophrenia who are living in the community. *Psychiatric Services* 2001; **52**(10):1358–66.

6. B.A. Palmer, V.S. Pankratz, J.M. Bostwick. The lifetime risk of suicide in schizophrenia: a reexamination. *Archives of General Psychiatry* 2005; **62**(3):247–53.

7. K. Hawton, L. Sutton, C. Haw, J. Sinclair, J.J. Deeks. Schizophrenia and suicide: systematic review of risk factors. *British Journal of Psychiatry* 2005; **187**(1):9–20.

8. D.V. Jeste, J.E. Maglione. Treating older adults with schizophrenia: challenges and opportunities. *Schizophrenia Bulletin* 2013; **39**(5):966–8.

9. C. Crump, M.A. Winkleby, K. Sundquist, J. Sundquist. Comorbidities and mortality in persons with schizophrenia: a Swedish national cohort study. *American Journal of Psychiatry* 2013; **170**(3):324–33.

10. C.I. Cohen, P.D. Meesters, J. Zhao. New perspectives on schizophrenia in later life: implications for treatment, policy, and research. *Lancet Psychiatry* 2015; 2(4):340–50.

11. D.V. Jeste, J.E. Maglione. Atypical antipsychotics for older adults: are they safe and effective as we once thought? *Journal of Comparative Effectiveness Research* 2013; 2(4):355–8.

12. R.G. Frank, S.A. Glied. *Better but not Well: Mental Health Policy in the United States since 1950.* Baltimore, MD: Johns Hopkins University Press, 2006.

13. World Health Organization. Premature death among people with severe mental disorders. 2015. www.who.int/mental_health/management/info_sheet.pdf (accessed October 2018).

14. J. de Leon. Smoking and vulnerability for schizophrenia. *Schizophrenia Bulletin* 1996; **22**(3):405–9.

15. M. Šagud, A. Mihaljević-Peleš, D. Mück-Šeler, et al. Smoking and schizophrenia. *Psychiatria Danubina* 2009; **21**(3):371–5.

16. D.A. Wirshing. Schizophrenia and obesity: impact of antipsychotic medications. *Journal of Clinical Psychiatry* 2003; **65**:13–26.

17. B.A. Cullen, E.E. McGinty, Y. Zhang, et al. Guideline-concordant antipsychotic use and mortality in schizophrenia. *Schizophrenia Bulletin* 2013; **39**(5):1159–68.

18. J.J. O'Connell. Premature mortality in homeless populations: A review of the literature. Nashville, TN: National Health Care for the Homeless Council; 2005. http://santabarbarastreetmedicine.org/wp-content/uploads/2011/04/PrematureMortalityFinal.pdf (accessed October 2018).

19. National Health Care for The Homeless Council. Homelessness and health: what's the connection? 2011. www.nhchc.org/wp-content/uploads/2011/09/Hln_health_factsheet_Jan10.pdf (accessed October 2018).

20. L. Roy, A.G. Crocker, T.L. Nicholls, E.A. Latimer, A.R. Ayllon. Criminal behavior and victimization among homeless individuals with severe mental illness: a systematic review. *Psychiatric Services* 2014; **65**(6):739–50.

21. S. Williams, K. L. Bryant. Sexually transmitted infections among homeless persons: a literature review. In *2012 National STD Prevention Conference.* Atlanta, GA: Centers for Disease Control; 2012. https://cdc.confex.com/cdc/std2012/webprogram/Paper30143.html (accessed October 2018).

22. V. Hausswolff-Juhlin, M. Bjartveit, E. Lindström, P. Jones. Schizophrenia and physical health problems. *Acta Psychiatrica Scandinavica* 2009; **119**(s438):15–21.

23. Substance Abuse and Mental Health Services Administration and Health Resources and Services Administration. *Growing Older: Providing Integrated Care for an Aging Population.* HHS Publication No.: (SMA) 16-4982. Rockville, MD: Department of Health and Human Services; 2016. https://store.samhsa.gov/shin/content//SMA16-4982/SMA16-4982.pdf (accessed October 2018).

24. NYS Center of Excellence for Cultural Competence. Improving the physical health of people with serious mental illness: a systematic review of lifestyle interventions. A report from the NYS Center of Excellence for Cultural Competence at the New York State Psychiatric Institute. New York: NYS Psychiatric Institute; 2010. http://nyculturalcompetence.org/wp-content/uploads/2014/04/ImprovingthePhysicalHealthofPeoplewithSMI-ASystematicReviewofLifestyleInterventions.pdf (accessed October 2018).

25. C.I. Cohen, C.G. Abdallah, S. Diwan. Suicide attempts and associated factors in older adults with schizophrenia. *Schizophrenia Research* 2010; **119**(1):253–7.

26. K. Hawton, L. Sutton, C. Haw, J. Sinclair, J.J. Deeks. Schizophrenia and suicide: systematic review of risk factors. *British Journal of Psychiatry* 2005; **187**(1):9–20.

27. R.K. Heinssen, A.B. Goldstein, S.T. Azrin. *Evidence-based treatments for first episode psychosis: components of coordinated specialty care.* Bethesda, MD: National Institute of Mental Health. 2014. www.nimh.nih.gov/health/topics/schizophrenia/raise/nimh-white-paper-csc-for-fep_147096.pdf (accessed October 2018).

28. M.L. LeFevre. Screening for suicide risk in adolescents, adults, and older adults in primary care: US Preventive Services Task Force recommendation statement. *Annals of Internal Medicine* 2014; **160**(10):719–26.

29. B. Stanley, G.K. Brown. *Safety Plan Treatment Manual to Reduce Suicide Risk: Veteran Version.* Washington, D.C.: United States Department of Veterans Affairs; 2008. www.mentalhealth.va.gov/docs/va_safety_planning_manual.pdf (accessed October 2018).

30. M. Taylor, K. Hor. Suicide and schizophrenia: a systematic review of rates and risk factors. *Journal of Psychopharmacology* 2010; **24**(s4): 81–90.

31. Drexler M.(ed.) Guns and suicide: the hidden toll. *Harvard Public Health Magazine.* 2013:25-31. www.hsph.harvard.edu/magazine/magazine_article/guns-suicide/ (accessed October 2018).

32. S.B. Vyrostek, J.L. Annest, G.W. Ryan. Surveillance for fatal and nonfatal injuries: United States, 2001. *Morbidity and Mortality Weekly Report: Surveillance Summaries.* 2004; **53**(s7):1–57

33. E. Cooper, L. Knott, G. Schaak, L. Sloane, A. Zovistoski. *Priced Out in 2014: The Housing Crisis for People with Disabilities.* Boston, MA: Technical Assistance Collaborative, Inc.; 2015. www.tacinc.org/media/52012/Priced%20Out%20in%20 2014.pdf (accessed October 2018).

34. Social Security Administration. *A Summary of the 2016 Annual Reports: Social Security and Medicare Board of Trustees.* Washington, D.C.: Social Security Administration; 2016. www.ssa.gov/oact/TR/2016/tr2016.pdf (accessed October 2018).

35. U.S. Department of Housing and Urban Development. Housing Choice Vouchers Fact Sheet. https://portal.hud.gov/hudportal/HUD?src=/topics/housing_choice_voucher_program_section_8 (accessed October 2018).

36. R. Schulz, P.R. Sherwood. Physical and mental health effects of family caregiving. *Journal of Social Work Education.* 2008; **44**(s3):105–13.

37. M.B. Friedman. Housing for older adults with psychiatric disabilities: a continuing critical need. *Behavioral Health News.* 2014. http://michaelbfriedman.com/mbf/images/HOUSING_FOR_OLDER_ADULTS_WITH_PSYCHIATRIC_DISABILITIES_Print_Friendly.pdf (accessed January 2019).

38. J. Fellner, P. Vinck. Old behind bars: the aging prison population in the United States. *Human Rights Watch*; 2012. www.hrw.org/sites/default/files/reports/usprisons0112webwcover_0.pdf (accessed October 2018).

39. S.J. Prins. Prevalence of mental illnesses in US state prisons: a systematic review. *Psychiatric Services* 2014; **65**(7):862–72.

40. S.K. Roberts, ed. *Aging in Prison: Reducing Elder Incarceration and Promoting Public Safety.* New York: The Center for Justice at Columbia University. 2015. http://centerforjustice.columbia.edu/files/2015/10/AgingInPrison_FINAL_web.pdf (accessed October 2018).

41. D.A. Sisti, A.G. Segal, E.J. Emanuel. Improving long-term psychiatric care: bring back the asylum. *JAMA.* 2015; **313**(3):243–4.

42. L. Sederer. No Asylum for Asylums: 19th-century measures for treating the mentally ill have no place in today's health care system. 2015. www.usnews.com/opinion/blogs/policy-dose/2015/05/20/bringing-back-asylums-will-not-help-mentally-ill-people (accessed October 2018).

43. S.J. Bartels, J.A Naslund. The underside of the silver tsunami: older adults and mental health care. *New England Journal of Medicine* 2013; **368**(6):493–6.

44. J. Kreyenbuhl, R.W. Buchanan, F.B. Dickerson, L.B. Dixon. The schizophrenia patient outcomes research team (PORT): updated treatment recommendations 2009. *Schizophrenia Bulletin* 2010; **36**(1):94–103.

45. M. Steinberg, C.G. Lyketsos. Atypical antipsychotic use in patients with dementia: managing safety concerns. *American Journal of Psychiatry* 2012; **169**(9):900–6.

46. M. Nardone, S. Snyder, J. Paradise. Integrating physical and behavioral health care: promising Medicaid models. *Kaiser Commission on Medicaid and the Uninsured.* 2014. https://kaiserfamilyfoundation.files.wordpress.com/2014/02/8553-integrating-physical-and-behavioral-health-care-promising-medicaid-models.pdf (accessed October 2018).

47. K.M. Griffiths, B. Carron-Arthur, A. Parsons, R. Reid. Effectiveness of programs for reducing the stigma associated with mental disorders: a meta-analysis of randomized controlled trials. *World Psychiatry* 2014; **13**(2):161–75.

48. Substance Abuse and Mental Health Services Administration and the Administration for Community Living. Older Americans behavioral health. Issue brief 9: financing and sustaining older adult behavioral health and supportive services. 2013. www.acl.gov/sites/default/files/programs/2016-11/Issue%20Brief%209%20Financing%20Sustaining.pdf (accessed October 2018).

49. E. Khaykin, W.W. Eaton, D.E. Ford, C.B. Anthony, G.L. Daumit. Health insurance coverage among persons with schizophrenia in the United States. *Psychiatric Services* 2010; **61**(8):830–4.

50. R. Golden, M. Vail. The implications of the Affordable Care Act for mental health care. *Generations Journal of the American Society on Aging* 2014; **38**(3):96–103.

51. W.A. Anthony. Recovery from mental illness: the guiding vision of the mental health service system in the 1990s. *Psychosocial Rehabilitation Journal* 1993; **16**(4):11.

52. G.R. Bond, R.E Drake. The critical ingredients of assertive community treatment. *World Psychiatry* 2015; **14**(2):240–2.

53. C.I. Cohen, C. Jimenez, S. Mittal. The role of religion in the well-being of older adults with schizophrenia. *Psychiatric Services* 2010; **61**(9):917–22.

54. C. McKay, K.L. Nugent, M. Johnsen, W.W. Eaton, C.W. Lidz. A systematic review of evidence for the clubhouse model of psychosocial rehabilitation. *Administration and Policy in Mental Health and Mental Health Services Research* 2016; **45**:1–20.

55. S.J. Bartels, G.S. Moak, A.R. Dums. Mental health services in nursing homes: models of mental health services in nursing homes: a review of the literature. *Psychiatric Services* 2002; **53**(11):1390–6.

56. D.C. Grabowski, K.A. Aschbrenner, V.F. Rome, S.J. Bartels. Quality of mental health care for nursing home residents: a literature review. *Medical Care Research and Review* 2010; **67**(6):627–56.

57. U.S. Centers for Medicare and Medicaid Services. Physical and mental health integration. [No Date Available] www.medicaid.gov/state-resource-center/innovation-accelerator-program/physical-and-mental-health-integration/physical-and-mental-health-integration.html (accessed October 2018).

58. U.S. Centers for Medicare and Medicaid Services. Health homes. 2017. www.medicaid.gov/medicaid/ltss/health-homes/index.html (accessed October 2018).

59. U.S. Centers for Medicare and Medicaid Services. Accountable care organizations. 2017. www.cms.gov/medicare/medicare-fee-for-service-payment/aco/ (accessed October 2018).

60. Committee on the Mental Health Workforce for Geriatric Populations; Board on Health Care Services; Institute of Medicine. Workforce implications of models of care for older adults with mental health and substance use conditions. In *The Mental Health and*

Substance Use Workforce for Older Adults: In Whose Hands? ed. J. Eden, K. Maslow, M. Le, et al. Washington, D.C., National Academies Press; 2012.

61. M.S. Mittelman. Translating an evidence-based intervention for spouse-caregivers into community settings [PowerPoint Presentation]. Center of Excellence for Brain Aging and Dementia, NYU Langone Medical Center. [No Date Available] www.rosalynncarter.org/UserFiles/MITTELMAN(1).pdf (accessed October 2018).

62. L.T. Kohn. HHS Leadership Needed to Coordinate Federal Efforts Related to Serious Mental Illness: Testimony Before the Subcommittee on Oversight and Investigations, Committee on Energy and Commerce, House of Representatives. United States Government Accountability Office, GAO-15-375T. 2015. www.gao.gov/assets/670/668429.pdf (accessed October 2018).

63. Substance Abuse and Mental Health Services Administration. *Office of the Assistant Secretary for Mental Health and Substance Abuse.* 2017. www.samhsa.gov/about-us/who-we-are/offices-centers/oas (accessed January 2019).

64. National Institutes of Health. Estimates of funding for various research, condition, and disease categories (RCDC). 2017. https://report.nih.gov/categorical_spending.aspx (accessed October 2018).

65. S.L. Colby, J.M. Ortman. *Projections of the size and composition of the US population: 2014 to 2060, Current Population Reports.* Washington, D.C.: U.S. Census Bureau; 2015. www.census.gov/content/dam/Census/library/publications/2015/demo/p25-1143.pdf (accessed October 2018).

Chapter 19

Epilogue: Controversies, Conjectures, and Future Directions

Carl I. Cohen, M.D. and Paul D. Meesters, M.D.

The chapters in this book have captured the appreciable research content that has amassed over the past decade since the last compendium on schizophrenia in older age was published. Moreover, we have added chapters on epidemiology and the assessment and diagnosis of psychotic symptoms in later life, a topic that has not been well covered in the literature. The authors have identified numerous methodological problems and limitations in the literature that demand attention. Moreover, they have posited a variety of conjectures and hypotheses that should be assayed. Below, we highlight some of the findings and concerns posed by the writers of the volume.

1. One of the critical issues involves diagnosis. Older adults may be more prone to develop subthreshold psychiatric disorders that have clinical relevance, but do not meet official diagnostic cut-offs (Chapter 1). Adding a dimensional component, as proposed in DSM5, provides an opportunity to include some symptoms that might easily be overlooked. Diagnosis is also made more complex by the co-occurrence of physical disorders. For example, to what extent do comorbid physical conditions alter the pathogenesis, presentation, and course of depression and cognitive deficits that are found disproportionately in older adults with schizophrenia (OAS)? Many of the writers signaled the lack of uniformity that made generalization across samples more difficult (Chapters 1, 6, and 8). Outcome criteria varied; age ranges varied with many "older samples" including persons in their forties; some included both early- and late-onset disorders, whereas others restricted analysis to older adults with early-onset disorders. Some included inpatients, whereas others focused on community-dwelling residents living at various levels of independence. Clearly, such differences can affect findings. Eliciting of symptoms differed widely with many using self-reported symptoms and only a handful of studies obtained collateral information from informants or prior records. Last, few investigations of OAS have used longitudinal data. Cross-sectional data under-estimate the prevalence of symptoms and disorders that individuals may experience. This is because many patients have symptoms that vary over time and may experience periods of remission of some symptoms (Chapter 8).
2. There is little research addressing the diagnostic challenges of new-onset psychotic disease in later life (Chapters 3 and 4). Especially challenging is being able to distinguish between very-late-onset schizophrenia-like psychosis (VLOS) and early dementia with psychotic features. Although there are subtle differences in

the patterns of cognitive deficits and of psychotic symptoms, it is often clinically challenging to discriminate between the two disorders at an early stage. It is also theoretically plausible that part of the VLOS subtype is a predisposition to develop dementia. Longitudinal studies of VLOS, use of biomarkers, and more sophisticated neuroimaging techniques (e.g. PET scans, fMRIs) might provide some additional insight into possible factors that may help to distinguish schizophrenia from dementia at their onset.

3. A related diagnostic conundrum concerns how we classify older persons with early-onset disorder who have shown gradual cognitive decline, but now meet cognitive and functional criteria for mild neurocognitive disorder or early dementia (Chapters 6 and 8). Does the person with schizophrenia now have two disorders? Have they transitioned into a neurocognitive disorder? Or do they have a new hybrid condition? It should be noted that the dimensional approach in DSM5, currently relegated to a special section, allows for various levels of cognitive impairment as a feature of schizophrenia. Using the latter schema, schizophrenia with cognitive deficits does not necessarily evolve into a neurocognitive disorder. However, how should we classify the subset of patients with schizophrenia, usually with long institutional histories, who show more accelerated cognitive decline after age 65, as well as retaining some features of schizophrenia?

4. It is evident that there are various trajectories that schizophrenia can take into later life. Clinical (e.g., remission, cognitive impairment, depression) and social (e.g., community integration, quality of life) aspects show variability – with somewhat more than half showing stability (either favorable or unfavorable), but with a substantial minority showing fluctuations between these states (Chapters 8 and 10). Since outcomes are mostly independent of each other, hundreds of combinations of outcomes are possible. Is there any way to predict various trajectories? Some potential clinical and social predictor variables have been identified, but longitudinal analyses show that they are surprisingly few (Chapter 8). This may reflect the absence of such predictors or, more likely, our inability to properly identify or measure them. Consequently, larger, and more granular analyses may identify other variables. These differences in clinical and social outcomes are also mirrored at the biological level in samples of younger persons with schizophrenia. Morphological changes in the brain, especially white matter changes that occur with aging, as well as increases in certain inflammatory biomarkers, are consistent with the possibility of an "accelerated aging" process in schizophrenia (Chapter 5). However, these are group trends and there is considerable individual variation. While genetic factors may play a part, lifestyle, medication exposure, or the illness itself may have explanatory roles. Lastly, some of the changes in brain morphology seem to occur early in the disorder, and then decelerate to a pace that resembles their age peers (Chapter 5). Likewise, there is some evidence that positive psychosocial factors are associated with lower levels of biomarkers of inflammation and insulin resistance, especially among individuals with schizophrenia (Chapters 5 and 9). Thus, positive psychosocial factors, generally lower in schizophrenia, may be viable treatment targets and have the potential to improve these individuals' well-being and even their physical/biological health.

5. As alluded to above, an intriguing question raised in this volume is whether OAS show accelerated aging. That is, is there evidence of earlier appearance in

OAS of physical diseases, cognitive deficits, or biomarkers that are found among non-schizophrenic persons that are appreciably older? (Chapter 5). Surprisingly, existing data suggest that the prevalence of many physical disorders in OAS is not higher than in their age peers, although mortality rates in schizophrenia at a more advanced age remain substantially higher than in their age peers, possibly suggesting more severe levels of these physical disorders or inadequate care (Chapter 7). Likewise, whereas OAS have more cognitive deficits than their age peers, there is little evidence of a more rapid decline in later life, except for those individuals with the worst prognosis, often residing in institutions (Chapter 6). Although several biomarkers associated with more rapid aging have been identified in younger samples, few studies have been conducted in OAS and there are limited longitudinal data in later life (Chapter 5). Further research is needed, but what little is known suggests no increase in biomarkers in later life, e.g., a study of hsCRF indicated that higher levels were not associated with age in persons with schizophrenia. An important research question is whether these findings reflect a "survivor effect." In other words, since persons with schizophrenia have higher mortality rates throughout their life span, do those who reach old age have better health habits, more social and financial supports, or better genes? (Chapters 5 and 7). The optimal approach to addressing these questions would be to develop long-term longitudinal studies following individuals across the life span, but especially from middle age into later life. As an interim strategy, cross-sectional comparisons between these age groups might provide some provisionally valuable data. Finally, since we know there is heterogeneity in trajectories among various outcome categories in later life, it is critical to understand why some persons show patterns of accelerated aging and others do not. This is especially striking with respect to cognitive decline.

6. There have been remarkably few randomized controlled trials (RCT) of anti-psychotic medications in OAS (Chapter 13). There seems to be little difference between medications – first or second generation – with respect to efficacy. Moreover, there is now evidence that second-generation medications may cause tardive dyskinesia almost as frequently as first-generation medications, albeit in a milder form (Chapter 5). Although there is anecdotal evidence that persons with late-onset disorder may respond better to anti-psychotic medications than those with an early onset, this has not been demonstrated in any RCTs (Chapter 4). Anti-psychotic medications seem to have minimal or no positive impact on cognitive functioning or depressive symptoms, both common problems in OAS that are known to impact on daily functioning. It is not known which patients might benefit from diminishing or stopping their medications. Persons who have been in persistent clinical remission (roughly one-quarter) might benefit; however, those who continue to have symptoms with no benefit from medications might also be candidates for medication discontinuation. Novel medications include pimavanserin, which is an inverse antagonist at serotonin 5-HT2A receptors and has been approved for use with psychotic symptoms associated with Parkinson's disease. There are RCTs examining its utility with the neurobehavioral symptoms found in Alzheimer's disease and in schizophrenia, and it behooves us to assess whether it is both efficacious and safe in OAS.

7. Likewise, there are only a handful of RCTs of non-pharmacological interventions for OAS (Chapter 14). Most of the first-generation studies have focused on improving adaptive functioning such as communication, and social and daily living skills. An unanswered question is to what extent these training programs help in the real world. Cognitive remediation programs that have been developed so far seem to primarily benefit younger, but not older, persons with schizophrenia (Chapter 6). Although there is evidence that OAS can develop effective coping strategies with respect to psychotic symptoms, there have been no RCTs using cognitive behavior therapy (CBT) to diminish the impact of psychotic symptoms in OAS. A second generation of psychosocial programs have focused on cost-effective illness and self-management approaches that have utilized peer specialists as part of the service delivery (Chapter 14). These promising strategies need to be replicated on a wider scale with a variety of older populations. In addition, shortages in professionals in aging care have spurred the development of novel workforce solutions (e.g., peers and community health workers) and technology, including web-based and smartphone delivery and use of wearable sensors (Chapter 15). All of these approaches will need extensive testing in the real world.

8. Subjective responses by OAS to their illness and current life quality has been a neglected area of research. Like many of the items discussed above, there is considerable heterogeneity in self-appraisal ratings (Chapters 12 and 16). Some persons perceived their life as one of adversity, lost opportunities, and persistent suffering. Others, in later life saw new opportunities for growth and enhanced life quality (Chapter 16). They may regard themselves like other older adults who are taking medications and no longer working, and there is a sense of normalcy and pride in having overcome adversities. Whether these are universal perceptions across national or cultural groups is unknown. Also, to what extent are those persons with negative appraisals amenable to therapy?

9. A related issue for clinical care and public policy is whether subjective appraisals should be the gold standard for assessing needs. While a key component of the recovery model is to rely on patient self-appraisals and goals, it begs the question of whether such evaluations also reflect more objective needs that they may be experiencing. Data indicate that the correlations between objective factors and perceived quality of life may be attenuated by the lower expectations of persons with schizophrenia, in part based on comparisons with how they were doing when they were younger [1]. Moreover, only about three-fifths of OAS consistently acknowledge having a mental illness, and this lack of insight about their disorder may also be reflected in their appraisals about their life circumstances [2]. Thus, future investigations should objectively assess the needs of OAS, and this can complement subjective assessments, both of which can be useful for helping individuals implement changes in their lives.

10. Although there has been much written about the impact of Alzheimer's disease on caregivers, there is a dearth of information and evidence-based practices for addressing the needs of family caregivers of OAS (Chapter 15). These caregivers may be aging parents or older siblings. Many worry about who will assist the patient if they should die or become incapacitated. Until recently, in developing countries, most persons with schizophrenia lived with family (Chapters 15 and 17). However,

with increasing urbanization and industrialization, older adults in general find fewer available social supports in rural areas and some face potential abandonment, and those elders in urban areas likewise may encounter isolation and impoverishment.

11. A perplexing issue is to what extent geographic differences influenced by national health systems and culture affect outcome and treatment strategies (Chapter 17). While somewhat controversial, most evidence supports the view that the outcome of schizophrenia in developing countries is often better than in the developed world. Whether this obtains in later life is not clear. How much do cultural and cross-national differences impact on treatment strategies for OAS? Will local treatment remedies coexist or will they be obliterated over time? Globalization is creating more uniformity in psychiatric treatment, whereas there are no data to assess if this is a good or bad thing for OAS in developing countries.

12. In the past, when most OAS were in mental institutions, the facility provided virtually all their needs. Thus, psychiatric, medical, and dental care, nutrition, socialization, housing, and social and vocational activities were offered on-site. While this was not typically done well, it did not require the array of providers that must be summoned to care for people living in the community.

Table 19.1 provides an illustrative grid of the possible needs of a community-dwelling OAS using an individualized care approach. As described previously, OAS are a heterogeneous group, not only with respect to broad global outcome measures, but within the various subcategories listed in the table (Chapter 12). Thus, for example, a person may have a mild level of positive symptoms, a moderate level of negative symptoms, a moderate level of medical problems, severe housing problems, and so forth. Thus, each of these elements needs to be targeted and most of them are largely independent of each other. Consequently, in this individualized care model, there may be hundreds of potential treatment packages.

As the authors in this volume have repeatedly underscored, there are few RCTs of various interventions for clinical symptoms and little is known about optimal housing settings, day care facilities or other social programs for older people with schizophrenia. In addition, there is a dearth of specific facilities within residential and nursing homes that adequately target the specific needs of older persons with severe mental illnesses. Inspired by the recovery movement, in recent years there has begun to be a shift in the orientation of mental health services, giving more priority to the specific needs and desires of consumers. Psychological and social unmet needs have emerged as prominent concerns. While mental health services clearly have a role in meeting these needs, they are unable on their own to meet them. This will require broader efforts at the political and societal level.

There is a severe shortage of health professionals with skills in caring for older adults and this will grow exponentially as the number of elderly increases over the next few decades (Chapters 17 and 18). Worldwide, there will be as many as 10 million persons aged 60 with schizophrenia by 2050. The surge in the number of older people with schizophrenia is occurring in tandem with the increase of older persons in general that will place enormous strain on the economies and care systems of all nations. An unknown question is to what extent the emerging generation of older adults with schizophrenia will differ from the current generation. This generation will have been exposed to very little time in mental institutions, but may have had greater exposure to drug use, prisons, and homeless shelters. They may have greater access to health care and more education. Various lower-cost alternative treatment strategies have been proposed, such as using

Table 19.1 Clinical and social needs

	Positive symptoms	Negative symptoms	Depression/ suicidality	Cognitive symptoms	Entitlements /finances	Housing	Physical health	Social contacts	Social skills	Daily function- ing	Access to medical/ dental care	Access to psychiatric care
0												
1												
2												
3												

0 = none/not a problem; 1 = mild; 2 = moderate; 3 = severe

"health coaches" or lay community workers to assist with screenings and to do brief interventions, telehealth to reach more geographically isolated and homebound individuals, and IT, especially using mobile phones, which are omnipresent, even in the developing world (Chapters 15, 17 and 18). All these strategies may be useful, but have not been systematically evaluated in OAS.

In summary, despite the substantial expansion of clinical research findings concerning psychotic disorders in later life, especially schizophrenia, only 1% of the schizophrenia literature has been devoted to older adults. As the proportion of persons with schizophrenia aged 55 and over approaches one-quarter of the schizophrenia population in many Western countries and the absolute numbers of older adults with schizophrenia increase dramatically around the globe, more basic scientific research and evidence-based treatment studies are sorely needed. This volume has provided a state-of-the art update on the field that can serve as the foundation for future studies.

References

1. Cohen CI, Vengassery A, Garcia Aracena EF. A longitudinal analysis of quality of life and associated factors in older adults with schizophrenia spectrum disorder. *Am J Geriatr Psychiatry* 2017;25(7):755–65.

2. Mani A, Cohen C. Clinical correlates of insight in older adults in schizophrenia. *Am J Geriatr Psychiatry* 2017; 25(3): S147–S148.

Index